Preventive, Diagnostic and Therapeutic Strategies for Abdominal Surgery Complications

Preventive, Diagnostic and Therapeutic Strategies for Abdominal Surgery Complications

Editor

Orestis Ioannidis

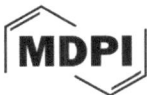

Basel • Beijing • Wuhan • Barcelona • Belgrade • Novi Sad • Cluj • Manchester

Editor
Orestis Ioannidis
Aristotle University of Thessaloniki
Thessaloniki
Greece

Editorial Office
MDPI AG
Grosspeteranlage 5
4052 Basel, Switzerland

This is a reprint of articles from the Special Issue published online in the open access journal *Journal of Clinical Medicine* (ISSN 2077-0383) (available at: https://www.mdpi.com/journal/jcm/special_issues/H71J35SJP2).

For citation purposes, cite each article independently as indicated on the article page online and as indicated below:

Lastname, A.A.; Lastname, B.B. Article Title. *Journal Name* **Year**, *Volume Number*, Page Range.

ISBN 978-3-7258-2383-3 (Hbk)
ISBN 978-3-7258-2384-0 (PDF)
doi.org/10.3390/books978-3-7258-2384-0

© 2024 by the authors. Articles in this book are Open Access and distributed under the Creative Commons Attribution (CC BY) license. The book as a whole is distributed by MDPI under the terms and conditions of the Creative Commons Attribution-NonCommercial-NoDerivs (CC BY-NC-ND) license.

Contents

About the Editor . . . . **vii**

Bo Shi, Qingliang Tai, Junjie Chen, Xinyu Shi, Guoliang Chen, Huihui Yao, et al.
Laparoscopic-Assisted Colorectal Resection Can Reduce the Inhibition of Immune Function Compared with Conventional Open Surgery: A Retrospective Clinical Study
Reprinted from: *J. Clin. Med.* **2023**, *12*, 2320, doi:10.3390/jcm12062320 . . . . **1**

Larsa Gawria, Ahmed Jaber, Richard Peter Gerardus Ten Broek, Gianmaria Bernasconi, Rachel Rosenthal, Harry Van Goor and Salome Dell-Kuster
Appraisal of Intraoperative Adverse Events to Improve Postoperative Care
Reprinted from: *J. Clin. Med.* **2023**, *12*, 2546, doi:10.3390/jcm12072546 . . . . **13**

Luigi Marano, Luigi Verre, Ludovico Carbone, Gianmario Edoardo Poto, Daniele Fusario, Dario Francesco Venezia, et al.
Current Trends in Volume and Surgical Outcomes in Gastric Cancer
Reprinted from: *J. Clin. Med.* **2023**, *12*, 2708, doi:10.3390/jcm12072708 . . . . **27**

Varvara Vasalou, Efstathios Kotidis, Dimitris Tatsis, Kassiani Boulogeorgou, Ioannis Grivas, Georgios Koliakos, et al.
The Effects of Tissue Healing Factors in Wound Repair Involving Absorbable Meshes: A Narrative Review
Reprinted from: *J. Clin. Med.* **2023**, *12*, 5683, doi:10.3390/jcm12175683 . . . . **43**

Antje K. Peters, Mazen A. Juratli, Dhruvajyoti Roy, Jennifer Merten, Lukas Fortmann, Andreas Pascher and Jens Peter Hoelzen
Factors Influencing Postoperative Complications Following Minimally Invasive Ivor Lewis Esophagectomy: A Retrospective Cohort Study
Reprinted from: *J. Clin. Med.* **2023**, *12*, 5688, doi:10.3390/jcm12175688 . . . . **64**

Jasmina Kuvendjiska, Robert Jasinski, Julian Hipp, Mira Fink, Stefan Fichtner-Feigl, Markus K. Diener and Jens Hoeppner
Postoperative Hiatal Hernia after Ivor Lewis Esophagectomy—A Growing Problem in the Age of Minimally Invasive Surgery
Reprinted from: *J. Clin. Med.* **2023**, *12*, 5724, doi:10.3390/jcm12175724 . . . . **76**

Georgios Ntampakis, Manousos-Georgios Pramateftakis, Orestis Ioannidis, Stefanos Bitsianis, Panagiotis Christidis, Savvas Symeonidis, et al.
The Role of Adipose Tissue Mesenchymal Stem Cells in Colonic Anastomosis Healing in Inflammatory Bowel Disease: Experimental Study in Rats
Reprinted from: *J. Clin. Med.* **2023**, *12*, 6336, doi:10.3390/jcm12196336 . . . . **87**

Dragos Serban, Paul Lorin Stoica, Ana Maria Dascalu, Dan Georgian Bratu, Bogdan Mihai Cristea, Catalin Alius, et al.
The Significance of Preoperative Neutrophil-to-Lymphocyte Ratio (NLR), Platelet-to-Lymphocyte Ratio (PLR), and Systemic Inflammatory Index (SII) in Predicting Severity and Adverse Outcomes in Acute Calculous Cholecystitis
Reprinted from: *J. Clin. Med.* **2023**, *12*, 6946, doi:10.3390/jcm12216946 . . . . **103**

Elke Van Daele, Hanne Vanommeslaeghe, Flo Decostere, Louise Beckers Perletti, Esther Beel, Yves Van Nieuwenhove, et al.
Systemic Inflammatory Response and the Noble and Underwood (NUn) Score as Early Predictors of Anastomotic Leakage after Esophageal Reconstructive Surgery
Reprinted from: *J. Clin. Med.* **2024**, *13*, 826, doi:10.3390/jcm13030826 . . . . **118**

Andrew W. Kirkpatrick, Federico Coccolini, Matti Tolonen, Samual Minor, Fausto Catena, Andrea Celotti, et al.
Are Surgeons Going to Be Left Holding the Bag? Incisional Hernia Repair and Intra-Peritoneal Non-Absorbable Mesh Implant Complications
Reprinted from: *J. Clin. Med.* **2024**, *13*, 1005, doi:10.3390/jcm13041005 . . . . **130**

Georgios Koimtzis, Leandros Stefanopoulos, Georgios Geropoulos, Christopher G. Chalklin, Ioannis Karniadakis, Awad A. Alawad, et al.
Mesh Rectopexy or Resection Rectopexy for Rectal Prolapse; Is There a Gold Standard Method: A Systematic Review, Meta-Analysis and Trial Sequential Analysis
Reprinted from: *J. Clin. Med.* **2024**, *13*, 1363, doi:10.3390/jcm13051363 . . . . **146**

Roni Rosen, Felipe F. Quezada-Diaz, Mithat Gönen, Georgios Karagkounis, Maria Widmar, Iris H. Wei, et al.
Oncologic Outcomes of Salvage Abdominoperineal Resection for Anal Squamous Cell Carcinoma Initially Managed with Chemoradiation
Reprinted from: *J. Clin. Med.* **2024**, *13*, 2156, doi:10.3390/jcm13082156 . . . . **160**

Ioannis Baloyiannis, Konstantinos Perivoliotis, Chamaidi Sarakatsianou, Charito Chatzinikolaou and George Tzovaras
The Reduction of Anastomosis-Related Morbidity Using the Kono-S Anastomosis in Patients with Crohn's Disease: A Meta-Analysis
Reprinted from: *J. Clin. Med.* **2024**, *13*, 2461, doi:10.3390/jcm13092461 . . . . **170**

Alexandros Giakoustidis, Menelaos Papakonstantinou, Paraskevi Chatzikomnitsa, Areti Danai Gkaitatzi, Petros Bangeas, Panagiotis Dimitrios Loufopoulos, et al.
The Effects of Sarcopenia on Overall Survival and Postoperative Complications of Patients Undergoing Hepatic Resection for Primary or Metastatic Liver Cancer: A Systematic Review and Meta-Analysis
Reprinted from: *J. Clin. Med.* **2024**, *13*, 3869, doi:10.3390/jcm13133869 . . . . **181**

About the Editor

Orestis Ioannidis

Dr. Ioannidis is currently an Assistant Professor of Surgery at the Medical School of Aristotle University of Thessaloniki, Greece. He studied medicine at the same institution and graduated in 2005. He received his MSC in Medical Research Methodology in 2008 from the Aristotle University of Thessaloniki and his MSC in Surgery of Liver, Biliary Tree and Pancreas from the Democritus University of Thrace in 2016. He received his PhD in 2014 from the Aristotle University of Thessaloniki as valedictorian for his thesis entitled "The effect of combined administration of omega-3 and omega-6 fatty acids in ulcerative colitis. Experimental study in rats." He is a general surgeon with a special interest in laparoscopic surgery and surgical oncology and also surgical infections, acute care surgery, nutrition and ERAS and vascular access. He has received fellowships from the EAES, ESSO, EPC, ESCP and ACS and has published more than 220 articles with more than 9000 citations and has an H-index of 42.

Article

Laparoscopic-Assisted Colorectal Resection Can Reduce the Inhibition of Immune Function Compared with Conventional Open Surgery: A Retrospective Clinical Study

Bo Shi [1,†], Qingliang Tai [1,†], Junjie Chen [2], Xinyu Shi [1], Guoliang Chen [1], Huihui Yao [1], Xiuwei Mi [1], Jinbing Sun [3], Guoqiang Zhou [4], Wen Gu [1] and Songbing He [1,*]

1. Department of General Surgery, The First Affiliated Hospital of Soochow University, Suzhou 215005, China
2. Department of General Surgery, Suzhou Ninth Hospital Affiliated to Soochow University, Suzhou 215000, China
3. Department of General Surgery, Changshu Hospital Affiliated to Soochow University, First People's Hospital of Changshu City, Changshu 215501, China
4. Department of Gastrointestinal Surgery, Changshu No. 2 Hospital, Changshu 215123, China
* Correspondence: hesongbing1979@suda.edu.cn
† These authors contributed equally to this work.

Abstract: Background: Immune function is an important indicator for assessing postoperative recovery and long-term survival in patients with malignancy, and laparoscopic surgery is thought to have a less suppressive effect on the immune response than open surgery. This study aimed to investigate this effect in a retrospective clinical study. Methods: In this retrospective clinical study, we enrolled 63 patients with colorectal cancer in the Department of General Surgery of the First Affiliated Hospital of Soochow University and assessed the changes in their postoperative immune function by measuring $CD3^+T$, $CD4^+T$, $CD8^+T$ lymphocytes, and $CD4^+/CD8^+$ ratio. Results: Compared with open surgery, laparoscopic colorectal surgery was effective in improving the postoperative decline in immune function. We determined that the number of $CD4^+$, $CD8^+T$ lymphocytes, and the $CD4^+/CD8^+$ ratio was not significantly reduced in the laparoscopic group. Conclusion: Laparoscopic-assisted colorectal resection can reduce the inhibition of immune functions compared with conventional open surgery.

Keywords: laparoscopic operation; colorectal cancer; immune function; surgical trauma; T-lymphocyte subsets

1. Introduction

Colorectal cancer is one of the most common malignancies worldwide and the leading cause of cancer-related mortality [1]. In recent years, it has been determined that the occurrence of malignant tumors is related to the tumor microenvironment [2,3]. T cell infiltration, activation, and effector functions are inhibited by tumors when immune evasion occurs, which causes the body to increase immune tolerance, leading to ineffective immune response and tumor progression [4,5]. T cells can be divided into two subpopulations, $CD3^+CD4^+$ and $CD3^+CD8^+$ T cells, according to different surface antigens, and the balance between them is an important insurance for maintaining normal immune system work, and the ratio of the two is an important indicator to assess immune function [6,7]. In a recent study, $CD3^+$ T lymphocytes and $CD4^+/CD8^+$ ratio levels on the second postoperative day were determined to be higher in patients who underwent laparoscopic-assisted natural orifice specimen extraction than in the conventional laparoscopic-assisted radical resection group, thus confirming the early safety after laparoscopic-assisted natural orifice specimen extraction [8]; Gang Wang et al. showed that fast-track surgery had better protection of patients' immune function postoperatively compared to laparoscopic surgery, with less impact on $CD3^+$, $CD4^+T$ lymphocytes, $CD4^+/CD8^+$ ratio and fewer perioperative complications [9]. Hence, detecting changes in T-lymphocyte subsets in peripheral blood and using them to assess immune response have aroused the people's interests.

With the continuous development of minimally invasive surgery, more surgeons prefer laparoscopic surgery. It has been proven that laparoscopic surgery has the advantages of less trauma potential, faster postoperative recovery, and fewer complications [10]. Patients with poor basal immune status have more postoperative complications and more extended hospital stays [11]. Maintaining and improving patients' immune status is important in perioperative management, yet relatively few reports have been published on the relationship between surgical approach and changes in patient immune status. Therefore, we considered 63 cases of patients with colorectal cancer admitted to the First Affiliated Hospital of Soochow University as the study subjects and analyzed the effect of different surgical procedures on the patients' postoperative immune function.

2. Materials and Methods

2.1. Patient Data

We conducted this study by the Declaration of Helsinki and obtained informed consent from all patients. This study was approved by the Ethics Committee of the First Affiliated Hospital of Soochow University (No. 421). The study population included 63 patients who were 18 years or older, had a body mass index (BMI) of 30 or less, had histologically proven colorectal adenocarcinoma with clinical stage II and III at the First Affiliated Hospital of Soochow University between 1 October 2021 and 31 December 2022 (Figure 1). These patients were prospectively included and had their peripheral blood levels of cellular immunity checked during treatment, and all patients had their disease diagnosed by colonoscopy and postoperative pathological biopsy. We excluded patients with a history of other malignant tumors such as cervical, uterine, or bladder; a medical history of Familial Adenomatosis Polyposis Coli, active Crohn's disease, active ulcerative colitis, recent chemotherapy, radiotherapy, or endocrine therapy; the combination of distant metastases such as liver, lung, and bone; the complication of severe heart, lung, and kidney, or due to hematologic disorders thus making them intolerant to surgery; psychiatric or addictive disorders that affected compliance to the protocol; conditions that would limit the success of laparoscopic resection such as multiple previous laparotomies or severe adhesions. After discussing the advantages and disadvantages of various surgical options with the surgeon, the patient chose laparoscopic surgery or open surgery. The patient was admitted to the hospital, the relevant tests were completed, and the patient was prepared for surgery. General anesthesia with tracheal intubation and routine urinary catheterization was used. Postoperative antibacterial drugs were routinely administered to prevent infection.

2.2. Immunological Index Acquisition

The general surgery nurse drew 5 mL of venous blood (15% Ethylene diamine tetraacetic acid tripotassium salt dihydrate anticoagulation) from a fasted, admitted patient at 7 am. Ethylene diamine tetraacetic acid anticoagulated blood was collected in 2 mL tubes. A total of 100 µL of anticoagulated whole blood was collected, 20 µL of $CD45^+/CD3^+/CD4^+/CD8^+$ cells was added, vortexed and mixed, incubated at room temperature and protected from light for 15 min. Then, 500 µL of cell lysate was added to each tube, vortexed and mixed, protected from light at room temperature for 10 min. Afterward, 2 mL of phosphate buffered saline was added to each tube, mixed, and detected by direct immunofluorescence labeling technique using flow cytometry for $CD4^+$ T lymphocytes and $CD8^+$ T lymphocytes to be detected by direct immunofluorescence labeling technique using flow cytometry; the percentages of $CD4^+$ T cells and $CD8^+$ T cells were recorded and the $CD4^+/CD8^+$ ratio was calculated.

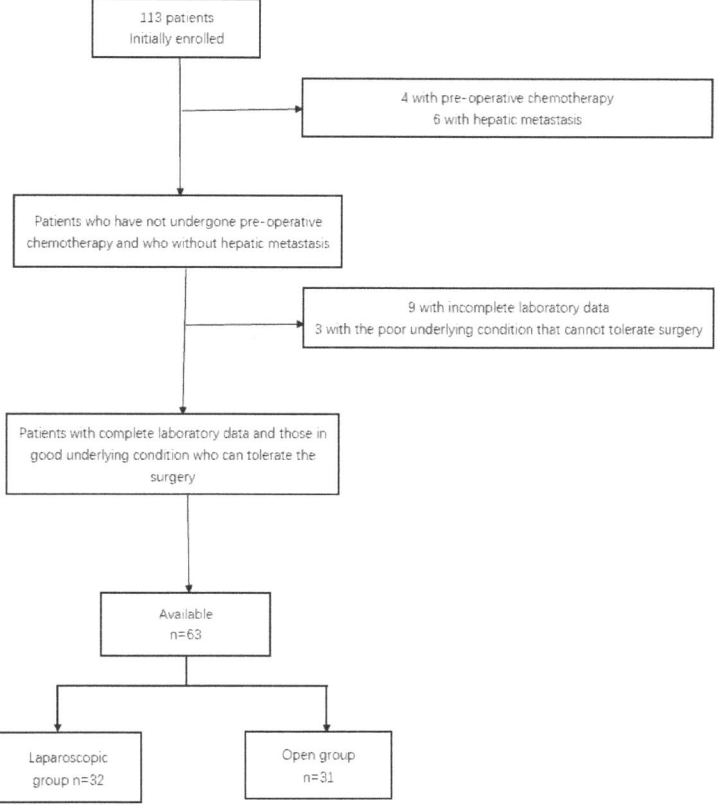

Figure 1. Filtering process of patient data from the initial inclusion of patients.

2.3. Statistical Analysis

All statistical analyses were performed by SPSS software (version 26.0). Measurement data are expressed as $\bar{X} \pm S$. Comparisons between groups were made using independent samples t-test, within-group comparisons before and after treatment were made using paired t-test and Pearson's chi-square test, and p values less than 0.05 were considered significant. Logistic regression was used to eliminate the cofounders. R custom scripts (version 3.5.3) were used to generate all the figures and conducted the power analysis.

3. Results

3.1. Clinical Characteristics

In the Department of General Surgery of the First Affiliated Hospital of Soochow University, we enrolled 63 patients who underwent radical colorectal tumor surgery. All patients were treated according to the standard perioperative care protocol (a total of 31 patients underwent open surgery and 32 patients underwent laparoscopic surgery). Compared with the open group, patients in the laparoscopic group had significantly longer operative time ($p < 0.05$). There was no statistically significant difference in gender, age, BMI, blood type, hospitalization days, degree of tumor differentiation, tumor diameter, N stage, and tumor stage between the laparoscopic group and the open group ($p > 0.05$) (Table 1).

Table 1. General material comparison in perioperative period of the open and laparoscopic groups (x ± s).

Items	Open Group (n = 31)	Laparoscopic Group (n = 32)	p
Gender			0.677+
Male	20	19	
Female	11	13	
Age (years)	68.58 ± 9.135	64.97 ± 8.102	0.102
BMI (kg/m^2)	22.17 ± 2.43	22.49 ± 5.14	0.746
Operation times (min)	156.32 ± 48.10	188.78 ± 65.10	*0.028*
Postoperative hospital stay (days)	12.46 ± 2.41	12.50 ± 3.99	0.753
Tumor differentiation			0.892+
Well or Moderate	14	15	
Poorly	17	17	
Maximal tumor diameter (cm)			0.246+
≤5 cm	19	24	
>5 cm	12	8	
N stage			0.267+
0	18	14	
1	6	12	
2	7	6	
Tumor stage			0.378+
II	18	15	
III	13	17	
Blood Type			0.742+
A	10	10	
B	9	12	
O	7	6	
AB	5	4	
Tumor Location			0.367+
Right colon cancer	7	11	
Left colon cancer	10	9	
Rectal cancer	14	12	

p-values were estimated by t-test; + p-values were estimated by Pearson's chi-square test; $p < 0.05$ are highlighted in bold italic.

3.2. Difference of Immunological Indexes

Compared with the preoperative level, the postoperative number of CD3$^+$ cells in the open group was not significantly different from that of the preoperative level, whereas the number of CD4$^+$, CD8$^+$, and CD4$^+$/CD8$^+$ ratio was significantly lower compared with the preoperative level; the postoperative number of CD3$^+$ cells in the laparoscopic group was significantly higher compared with the preoperative level, whereas the number of CD4$^+$ and CD8$^+$ and the CD4$^+$/CD8$^+$ ratio were not significantly different compared with that of the preoperative level (Table 2).

Table 2. Changes in number of immune cells in open and laparoscopic groups at different time point in pre- and post-surgery (x ± s).

Group	CD3$^+$T (%)	CD4$^+$T (%)	CD8$^+$T (%)	CD4$^+$T/CD8$^+$T
Open group				
The day before operation	66.59 ± 11.05	42.35 ± 9.21	23.08 ± 8.40	2.04 ± 0.78
The third day after operation	63.56 ± 9.72 *	32.86 ± 9.02 *#	20.21 ± 5.80 *#	1.73 ± 0.71 *#
Laparoscopic group				
The day before operation	69.10 ± 10.70	43.76 ± 9.64	24.52 ± 8.13	2.06 ± 1.17
The third day after operation	71.87 ± 10.89 #	42.75 ± 8.70	25.08 ± 7.20	2.01 ± 0.85

* The comparison in laparoscopic group at the same time point, $p < 0.05$. # The comparison in the same group on the day before operation, $p < 0.05$.

The number of CD3$^+$, CD4$^+$, CD8$^+$ cells and the CD4$^+$/CD8$^+$ ratio in the laparoscopic group were not significantly different preoperatively compared to the open group, while they were significantly higher postoperatively compared to the open group (Table 2 and Figure 2).

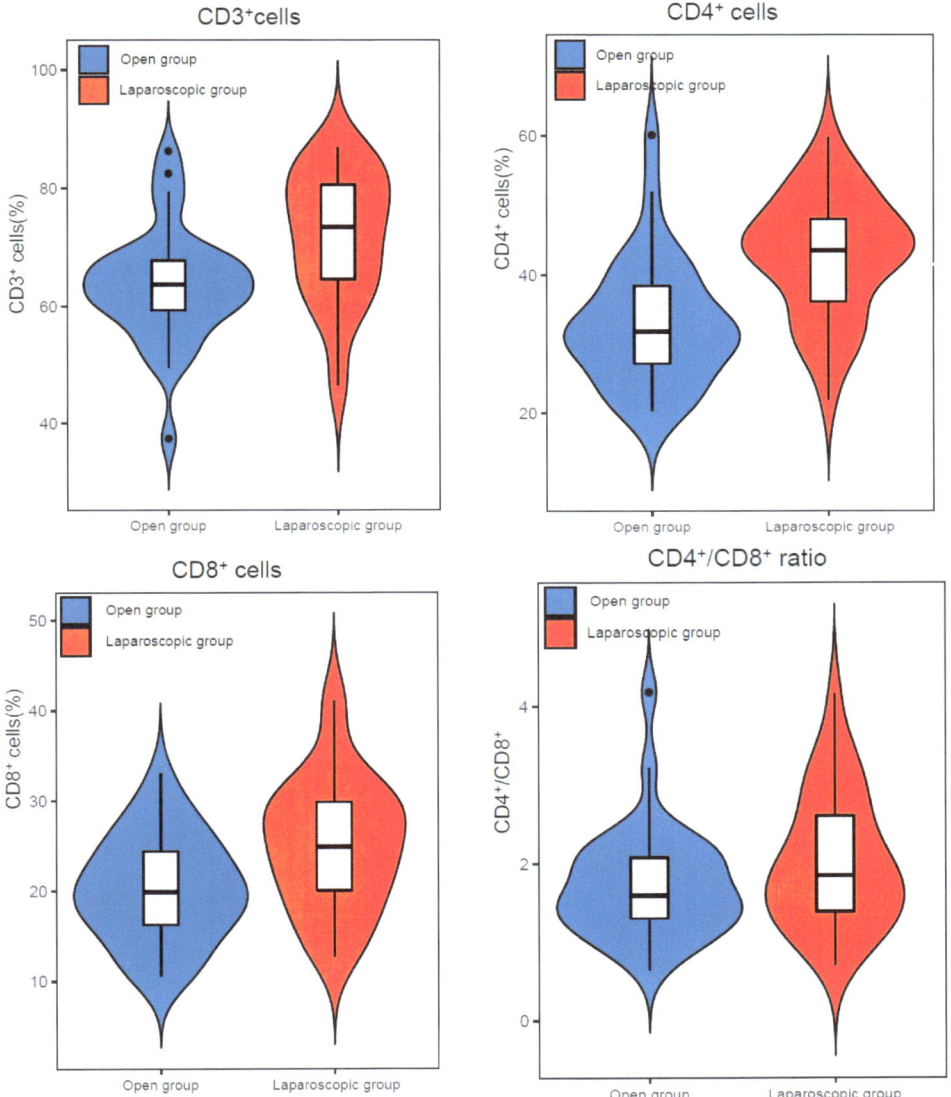

Figure 2. Changes in number of immune cells in open and laparoscopic groups at time point in post-surgery.

The number of CD3$^+$, CD4$^+$, CD8$^+$ cells and the CD4$^+$/CD8$^+$ ratio in the laparoscopic group were not significantly different from those in the open group before operation. In order to confirm that this is not the false negative caused by the low power, we conducted a power analysis, and calculated that the post hoc power of the number of CD3$^+$, CD4$^+$, CD8$^+$ cells and the CD4$^+$/CD8$^+$ ratio were 80.46%, 80.12%, 87.89%, and 81.12%, respectively, which were greater than 80%. Based on this, we could confirm that the number of $CD3^+$, $CD4^+$, $CD8^+$ cells and the $CD4^+/CD8^+$ ratio in the laparoscopic group did not differ from those of the open group before operation.

We also calculated that the post hoc power of the number of $CD3^+$, $CD4^+$, $CD8^+$ cells and the $CD4^+/CD8^+$ ratio in the two groups of patients after surgery were 83.74%, 89.70%, 87.59%, and 40.82%, respectively. Although the post hoc power of the $CD4^+/CD8^+$ ratio was lower than 80%, our independent sample t-test still detected that there was a significant difference in the $CD4^+/CD8^+$ ratio between the two groups of patients after operation.

3.3. Analysis of Influencing Factors

The results of univariate logistic regression analysis showed that the effects of age, tumor location, and types of surgery on patients' postoperative $CD3^+$ T cells were statistically significant. Then, the effect of age and tumor location was excluded by multivariate logistic regression analysis, and it was determined that the effect of types of surgery on patients' postoperative $CD3^+$ T cells remained statistically significant (Table 3). Laparoscopic-assisted surgery can reduce the inhibition of immune functions compared with open surgery.

Table 3. Logistic regression analysis of the patient's postoperative $CD3^+T$.

Items	Postoperative $CD3^+T$			
	Univariate Analysis		Multivariate Analysis	
	OR (95%CI)	p	OR (95%CI)	p
Gender (male/female)	1.379 (0.497~3.825)	0.537		
Age (years, ≤65/>65)	0.930 (0.873~0.991)	0.025	0.933 (0.870~1.001)	0.052
BMI (kg/m², ≤18.5/>18.5)	1.027 (0.906~1.165)	0.676		
Operation times (min, ≤150/>150)	1.003 (0.994~1.011)	0.544		
Tumor differentiation (Well or Moderate/Poor)	1.071 (0.398~2.887)	0.891		
Maximal tumor diameter (≤5 cm/>5 cm)	1.406 (0.484~4.079)	0.531		
Tumor stage (II/III)	0.941 (0.350~2.531)	0.904		
Blood type				
AB	1			
A	2.321 (0.467~11.545)	0.303		
B	0.769 (0.158~3.744)	0.745		
O	1.458 (0.264~8.048)	0.665		
Tumor location				
Rectal cancer	1			
Right colon cancer	4.911 (1.325~18.205)	0.017	5.349 (1.250~22.898)	0.024
Left colon cancer	2.099 (0.626~7.037)	0.230		
Types of surgery (open/laparoscopic)	4.620 (1.599~13.349)	0.005	3.908 (1.225~12.468)	0.021

Similarly, after excluding the effect of operation time, tumor stage as well as tumor location by multivariate logistic regression analysis, the effect of types of surgery on patients' postoperative $CD4^+T$ and $CD8^+T$ remained statistically significant (Tables 4 and 5). These findings suggested that laparoscopic-assisted surgery can reduce the inhibition of immune functions compared with open surgery. However, the results of both univariate logistic regression and multivariate logistic regression analysis showed that the surgical approach of patients had no statistically significant influence on the $CD4^+T/CD8^+T$ ratio of patients after surgery (Table 6).

Table 4. Logistic regression analysis of the patient's postoperative CD4$^+$T.

Items	Postoperative CD4$^+$T			
	Univariate Analysis		Multivariate Analysis	
	OR (95%CI)	p	OR (95%CI)	p
Gender (male/female)	0.612 (0.219~1.710)	0.349		
Age (years, ≤65/>65)	0.959 (0.903~1.017)	0.161		
BMI (kg/m^2, ≤18.5/>18.5)	0.897 (0.771~1.042)	0.155		
Operation times (min, ≤150/>150)	1.012 (1.002~1.023)	0.021	1.012 (0.999~1.024)	0.064
Tumor differentiation (Well or Moderate/Poor)	0.830 (0.308~2.237)	0.712		
Maximal tumor diameter (≤5 cm/>5 cm)	1.895 (0.645~5.569)	0.245		
Tumor stage (II/III)	0.376 (0.136~1.043)	0.060		
Blood type				
AB	1			
A	0.533 (0.109~2.616)	0.438		
B	1.067 (0.221~5.145)	0.936		
O	0.933 (0.169~5.151)	0.937		
Tumor location				
Rectal cancer	1			
Right colon cancer	7.875 (1.964~31.574)	0.004	10.384 (2.076~51.936)	0.004
Left colon cancer	2.5 (0.733~8.524)	0.143		
Types of surgery (open/laparoscopic)	6.247 (2.093~18.641)	0.001	5.656 (1.602~19.982)	0.007

Table 5. Logistic regression analysis of the patient's postoperative CD8$^+$T.

Items	Postoperative CD8$^+$T			
	Univariate Analysis		Multivariate Analysis	
	OR (95%CI)	p	OR (95%CI)	p
Gender (male/female)	1.379 (0.497~3.825)	0.537		
Age (years, ≤65/>65)	0.998 (0.942~1.056)	0.934		
BMI (kg/m^2, ≤18.5/>18.5)	1.012 (0.894~1.146)	0.848		
Operation times (min, ≤150/>150)	0.997 (0.988~1.005)	0.423		
Tumor differentiation (Well or Moderate/Poor)	2.338 (0.848~6.447)	0.101		
Maximal tumor diameter (≤5 cm/>5 cm)	0.711 (0.245~2.065)	0.531		
Tumor stage (II/III)	1.775 (0.654~4.819)	0.260		
Blood type				
AB	1			
A	1.250 (0.257~6.070)	0.782		
B	2.031 (0.417~9.886)	0.380		
O	0.781 (0.139~4.387)	0.779		
Tumor location				
Rectal cancer	1			
Right colon cancer	0.500 (0.144~1.737)	0.275	0.353 (0.090~1.389)	0.136
Left colon cancer	2.167 (0.630~7.454)	0.220		
Types of surgery (open/laparoscopic)	3.471 (1.232~9.782)	0.019	4.780 (1.495~15.280)	0.008

Table 6. Logistic regression analysis of the patient's postoperative CD4$^+$T/CD8$^+$T.

Items	Postoperative CD4$^+$T/CD8$^+$T			
	Univariate Analysis		Multivariate Analysis	
	OR (95%CI)	p	OR (95%CI)	p
Gender (male/female)	1.379 (0.497~3.825)	0.537		
Age (years, ≤65/>65)	0.968 (0.913~1.026)	0.275		
BMI (kg/m^2, ≤18.5/>18.5)	1.006 (0.889~1.139)	0.921		
Operation times (time, ≤150/>150)	1.017 (1.005~1.028)	0.005	1.016 (1.004~1.028)	0.009
Tumor differentiation (Well or Moderate/Poorly)	1.071 (0.398~2.887)	0.891		
Maximal tumor diameter (≤5 cm/>5 cm)	0.711 (0.245~2.065)	0.531		
Tumor stage (II/III)	1.214 (0.451~3.269)	0.701		
Blood type				
AB	1			
A	0.269 (0.051~1.420)	0.122		
B	0.813 (0.157~4.197)	0.804		
O	0.429 (0.073~2.500)	0.346		
Tumor location				
Rectal cancer	1			
Right colon cancer	3.545 (0.974~12.905)	0.055		
Left colon cancer	0.992 (0.299~3.285)	0.989		
Types of surgery (open/laparoscopic)	2.024 (0.742~5.519)	0.168	1.360 (0.451~4.102)	0.586

4. Discussion

It is well known that the stress response induced by surgical trauma affects the immune system and postoperative immunosuppression; it can also make CD3$^+$ and CD4$^+$ cell counts and CD4$^+$/CD8$^+$ ratios decrease [9]. The main immune mechanism against tumors is cellular immunity, which directly reflects anti-tumor activity. Therefore, avoiding suppression of cellular immunity plays an important role in prognosis of colon cancer surgery [12]. Surgery, whether laparoscopic or open, is a controlled trauma that can trigger changes in inflammation, neuroendocrine and immune function. With the advent of laparoscopic surgery, the ability to enter the patient's abdominal cavity through small openings, carefully segment and repair tissue and reduce the risk of bleeding has been greatly enhanced. Laparoscopic radical colorectal cancer surgery is a safe and effective surgical method, and its advantages include the following: (1) the surgical field of view is wide and has a magnifying effect, which can determine the intra-abdominal tissues and lesions; (2) the operation is delicate and gentle, and the interference with the internal organs of the abdominal cavity is small; (3) the operation is less invasive, causes less bleeding, pain, implies less adhesive intestinal obstruction, and fewer postoperative complications and faster recovery [10]; (4) less stress on the patient's organism and less impact on cell mediated immunity [13].

Konstantinos E. and colleagues reportedly studied the acute phase response after open and laparoscopic surgery. Their seminal report compared interleukin-6 (IL-6), tumor necrosis factor-α, c-reactive protein (CRP), Toll-like receptors-2 and Toll-like receptors-4 levels. They concluded that the inflammatory response and resulting stress response after laparoscopic surgery were significantly lower than in patients undergoing open surgery, which has a clear short-term clinical benefit for patients [14]. Mauro P. reviewed the early postoperative and oncological outcomes after laparoscopic colectomy for T4 cancer compared with open surgery, determining that laparoscopic colectomy for T4 colonic cancer is safe and is associated with better clinical outcomes than open surgery and similar oncological outcomes. Mauro's research demonstrates that in regard to long-term clinical benefits, laparoscopic surgery is better for patients than open surgery [15].

The development of malignant tumors is closely related to the immune function affected by the factors such as surgery, trauma, and infection. The immune system mainly includes cell-mediated immunity and humoral immunity. It is believed that cell-mediated immunity is the mainstay of anti-tumor immunity, while humoral immunity only plays a synergistic role in some cases, and some cytokines are also involved in the body's immune response [16]. T-lymphocyte-mediated cell-mediated immunity is involved in the postoperative immune response. $CD3^+$ T-cells are the main marker of mature T-lymphocytes in peripheral blood, representing the overall level of cell-mediated immunity. Human mature T-lymphocytes are divided into $CD4^+$ and $CD8^+$ T-cells depending on their phenotypes. $CD4^+$ T-cells are helper T-cells, which have helper functions and are co-receptors for T cell receptor signaling, and upon activation can release a large number of cytokines, enhancing the antitumor effect. Apart from producing cytokines, different subsets of $CD4^+$ T cell has been identified, including cytotoxic $CD4^+$ T cells, which possess cytotoxic programs and can directly kill cancer cells [17].$CD8^+$ T cells are cytotoxic and suppressive T cells that are involved in the maturation and positive selection of restrictive cytotoxic T lymphocyte for major histocompatibility complex-I [18]. In recent studies, multiple subsets of $CD8^+$ T cells have been detected in tumor microenvironments, called Tc subsets, each with distinct effector functions and cytotoxic potential, possibly influencing the antitumor response and patient outcomes [19]. The $CD4^+/CD8^+$ ratio is approximately 1.2–2.0, which is an important indicator of the body's immune homeostasis. Decrease in this ratio often indicates immune dysfunction, and a significant reduction or inversion is often used as an indicator of severe disease and poor prognosis [20].

Previously, studies on the effects of laparoscopic and open surgery on the immune system have focused on IL-6 and CRP [21]. The IL-6 promotes tumor angiogenesis and reduces inter-tumor cell adherence; it inhibits the body's anti-tumor immunity; it also has anti-apoptotic effects, thus promoting tumorigenesis. IL-6 plays an important role in the metastasis and progression of colorectal cancer [9]. CRP is a more sensitive inflammatory response protein produced by hepatocytes induced by IL-6, and its expression level increases when the body is exposed to trauma or infection [22]. Surgery remains the mainstay of treatment for colorectal cancer; however, it also leads to transient immunosuppression and diminished tumor resistance. Experimental animal studies have shown that immunity is better preserved after laparoscopic colorectal surgery, and open surgery is associated with accelerated tumor growth compared to laparoscopic surgery [23].

The application of pneumoperitoneum requires the introduction of large amounts of CO_2 gas into the abdominal cavity, and studies have shown that CO_2 pneumoperitoneum may produce hypercapnia and have immunological effects on the body [24]. Kim I. and his colleague reported that low intra-abdominal pressure during laparoscopic colorectal surgery, which means less CO_2, preserved innate immune homeostasis and formed a valuable addition to future enhanced recovery [25]. This issue has been controversial; however, from the present study, even though pneumoperitoneum affects the immune function of the organism, its effect is less compared to an open abdominal injury. In general, laparoscopic surgery causes less loss of immune function of the organism compared to open surgery, for better short-term postoperative benefit.

To conclude, we conducted studies on immune function parameters and the results showed that the number of $CD3^+$ cells in the open group, compared with the preoperative level, was not significantly different from that before surgery, while the number of $CD4^+$ and $CD8^+$ cells and the $CD4^+/CD8^+$ ratio was significantly lower. The number of $CD3^+$ cells in the laparoscopic group was significantly higher than that before surgery, while the number of $CD4^+$, $CD8^+$ cells and $CD4^+/CD8^+$ ratio was not significantly different from those before surgery. Compared with the open group, there was no significant difference in the number of $CD3^+$, $CD4^+$, $CD8^+$ cells and the ratio of $CD4^+/CD8^+$ in the laparoscopic group before surgery, but the number was significantly higher than in the open group after surgery. In Gang Wang's study, it was suggested that laparoscopic colon surgery effectively protected postoperative cellular immunity, and the decrease in the number of $CD3^+$ and $CD4^+$ cells and the $CD4^+/CD8^+$ ratio was significantly attenuated compared with open surgery patients. This is consistent with our findings [9]. However, Wichmann and Tang reported no difference in the number of $CD3^+$ and $CD4^+$ cells after laparoscopic surgery compared with open surgery, and only a small difference in the number of compliments, but the difference may exist due to the significantly longer surgery time in the laparoscopic group compared with the open group, thus weakening the function of laparoscopic surgery in reducing immunosuppression because of the excessive surgery time [21,26]. In the surgical treatment of lung cancer, Lian-Bin Zhang et al. determined that the postoperative T-lymphocyte subpopulation cell count was significantly higher in patients in the video-assisted thoracic surgery group compared to the traditional open surgery group, suggesting that the video-assisted thoracic surgery lowers the postoperative acute phase response and reduces immune suppression [27]. Li-Wen Zhou et al. detected higher postoperative $CD4^+$ and $CD8^+$ cell counts in patients on tramadol compared to those operated on without tramadol, which may be due to the perioperative patient's pain-mediated immunosuppression and consequent decrease in immune cell counts, which is also consistent with our findings [28]. Laparoscopic surgery has been shown to have a lower incidence of postoperative pain than open surgery [29], and thus patients undergoing laparoscopic surgery may benefit in terms of immune function.

This study is one of the few reports in which $CD4^+$ and $CD8^+$ cell counts were detected in peripheral blood after many recent studies investigating the relationship between T lymphocyte subsets in tumor microenvironment and tumor development as well as prognosis [30]. However, there are several drawbacks, and although we detected significantly higher numbers of $CD4^+$ and $CD8^+$ cells in the laparoscopic group than in the open group, the reasons for this occurrence cannot be well explained because laparoscopic surgery requires filling the peritoneal cavity with a large amount of CO_2 gas, and West studied cytokine production in peritoneal macrophages incubated in CO_2. Macrophage tumor necrosis factor and interleukin-1 responses to bacterial endotoxin were lower in macrophages incubated in CO_2 than in macrophages incubated in air or helium. West hypothesized that impairment of peritoneal macrophage cytokine production may contribute to the apparent lack of inflammatory systemic response during laparoscopic surgery [31]. We speculate that this may also apply to explain the changes in $CD4^+$ and $CD8^+$ cell numbers during laparoscopic surgery.

Our study has a few limitations. Firstly, we had a relatively small number of patients previously tested for T lymphocytes and the numerous exclusion criteria, and we have now made the detection of T lymphocyte counts in colorectal cancer patients a routine test. We will collect more patient data in the near future to draw more convincing conclusions. Secondly, the blood biomarkers analyzed in this study were nonspecific and may be influenced by various physiological or pathological factors. In addition, there are many blood indicators that can reflect the changes in immune status of patients. IL-6, CRP, reactive oxygen species, superoxide dismutase, etc., have been reported in the literature and are also closely related to the immune function of patients [32–34]. Thus, we subsequently plan to increase the tests in collaboration with clinical laboratory and also to verify them at the tissue level to support our conclusions. In addition, we employed the statistical technique of power analysis, but this power is no longer important because the results have been obtained. Post hoc power calculations were based on the observed effect entirely, but the lack of statistical power may substantially affect the size and even the direction of the observed effect. Finally, because of the lack of long-term prognostic data, we cannot yet determine the impact of the reduction in immunosuppression by laparoscopy on the long-term prognosis of patients, but studies have shown that this advantage of laparoscopy is valuable for the long-term survival of patients [35], and we will continue to follow up this cohort of patients to study the long-term impact of this surgical approach.

There is no doubt that the clinical efficacy of laparoscopic surgery has been established [36] and that the systemic immune impact of laparoscopic surgery may be ever lesser [37]. With increased research at the cellular and molecular levels, the systemic, metabolic, and immune effects of laparoscopic surgery will be better understood and patients will hopefully benefit from it.

In conclusion, this study determined that laparoscopic-assisted surgery can reduce the inhibition of immune functions compared with open surgery. It is clear that laparoscopic surgery is known to provide an immunological advantage, but whether it provides a survival advantage needs further study.

Author Contributions: Conceptualization, B.S., Q.T., J.C. and S.H.; Data curation, B.S., Q.T., J.C., X.M., J.S., G.Z. and W.G.; Formal analysis, B.S. and S.H.; Investigation, B.S., Q.T., J.C., X.S. and G.C.; Methodology, B.S. and S.H.; Supervision, S.H.; Writing—original draft, B.S., Q.T., J.C. and H.Y.; Writing—review and editing, B.S., Q.T., J.C. and S.H. All authors have read and agreed to the published version of the manuscript.

Funding: This work was supported by the Key Laboratory Project of the Clinical Pharmacy of Jiangsu Province of China XZSYSKF2020027 (G. Z.), the Gusu Medical Key Talent Project of Suzhou City of China GSWS2020005 (S. H.), the New Pharmaceutics and Medical Apparatuses Project of Suzhou City of China SLJ2021007 (S. H.), the Science and Technology Development Plan Project of Suzhou City of China SYS2019007 (G. Z.), and the Clinical Medical Expert Team Project of Suzhou City of China CSYJTD202101 (J. S.).

Institutional Review Board Statement: The study was conducted in accordance with the Declaration of Helsinki, and approved by the Ethics Committee of the First Affiliated Hospital of Soochow University (protocol code No. 421 and date of approval 27 October 2022).

Informed Consent Statement: Written informed consent was obtained from all patients.

Data Availability Statement: The data supporting the findings of this study are available from the corresponding author upon reasonable request.

Conflicts of Interest: The authors declare no conflict of interest.

References

1. Siegel, R.L.; Miller, K.D.; Goding Sauer, A.; Fedewa, S.A.; Butterly, L.F.; Anderson, J.C.; Cercek, A.; Smith, R.A.; Jemal, A. Colorectal cancer statistics, 2020. *CA Cancer J. Clin.* **2020**, *70*, 145–164. [CrossRef]
2. Buhrmann, C.; Kraehe, P.; Lueders, C.; Shayan, P.; Goel, A.; Shakibaei, M. Curcumin suppresses crosstalk between colon cancer stem cells and stromal fibroblasts in the tumor microenvironment: Potential role of EMT. *PLoS ONE* **2014**, *9*, e107514. [CrossRef]
3. Maiorino, L.; Daßler-Plenker, J.; Sun, L.; Egeblad, M. Innate Immunity and Cancer Pathophysiology. *Annu. Rev. Pathol.* **2022**, *17*, 425–457. [CrossRef]
4. Scharping, N.E.; Menk, A.V.; Moreci, R.S.; Whetstone, R.D.; Dadey, R.E.; Watkins, S.C.; Ferris, R.L.; Delgoffe, G.M. The Tumor Microenvironment Represses T Cell Mitochondrial Biogenesis to Drive Intratumoral T Cell Metabolic Insufficiency and Dysfunction. *Immunity* **2016**, *45*, 374–388. [CrossRef]
5. Saleh, R.; Elkord, E. Acquired resistance to cancer immunotherapy: Role of tumor-mediated immunosuppression. *Semin. Cancer Biol.* **2020**, *65*, 13–27. [CrossRef]
6. Mkrtichyan, M.; Najjar, Y.G.; Raulfs, E.C.; Liu, L.; Langerman, S.; Guittard, G.; Ozbun, L.; Khleif, S.N. B7-DC-Ig enhances vaccine effect by a novel mechanism dependent on PD-1 expression level on T cell subsets. *J. Immunol.* **2012**, *189*, 2338–2347. [CrossRef] [PubMed]
7. Varanasi, S.K.; Kumar, S.V.; Rouse, B.T. Determinants of Tissue-Specific Metabolic Adaptation of T Cells. *Cell Metab.* **2020**, *32*, 908–919. [CrossRef]
8. Liu, G.; Shi, L.; Wu, Z. Is Natural Orifice Specimen Extraction Surgery Really Safe in Radical Surgery for Colorectal Cancer? *Front. Endocrinol.* **2022**, *13*, 837902. [CrossRef] [PubMed]
9. Wang, G.; Jiang, Z.; Zhao, K.; Li, G.; Liu, F.; Pan, H.; Li, J. Immunologic response after laparoscopic colon cancer operation within an enhanced recovery program. *J. Gastrointest. Surg. Off. J. Soc. Surg. Aliment. Tract* **2012**, *16*, 1379–1388. [CrossRef] [PubMed]
10. Michelucci, A.; Cordes, T.; Ghelfi, J.; Pailot, A.; Reiling, N.; Goldmann, O.; Binz, T.; Wegner, A.; Tallam, A.; Rausell, A.; et al. Immune-responsive gene 1 protein links metabolism to immunity by catalyzing itaconic acid production. *Proc. Natl. Acad. Sci. USA* **2013**, *110*, 7820–7825. [CrossRef]
11. Kobashi, Y.; Shimizu, H.; Ohue, Y.; Mouri, K.; Obase, Y.; Miyashita, N.; Oka, M. Comparison of T-cell interferon-gamma release assays for Mycobacterium tuberculosis-specific antigens in patients with active and latent tuberculosis. *Lung* **2010**, *188*, 283–287. [CrossRef] [PubMed]
12. Ma, R.; Yuan, D.; Guo, Y.; Yan, R.; Li, K. Immune Effects of γδ T Cells in Colorectal Cancer: A Review. *Front. Immunol.* **2020**, *11*, 1600. [CrossRef] [PubMed]
13. Degrandi, D.; Hoffmann, R.; Beuter-Gunia, C.; Pfeffer, K. The proinflammatory cytokine-induced IRG1 protein associates with mitochondria. *J. Interferon Cytokine Res. Off. J. Int. Soc. Interferon Cytokine Res.* **2009**, *29*, 55–67. [CrossRef] [PubMed]

14. Tsimogiannis, K.E.; Tellis, C.C.; Tselepis, A.D.; Pappas-Gogos, G.K.; Tsimoyiannis, E.C.; Basdanis, G. Toll-like receptors in the inflammatory response during open and laparoscopic colectomy for colorectal cancer. *Surg. Endosc.* **2012**, *26*, 330–336. [CrossRef]
15. Podda, M.; Pisanu, A.; Morello, A.; Segalini, E.; Jayant, K.; Gallo, G.; Sartelli, M.; Coccolini, F.; Catena, F.; Di Saverio, S. Laparoscopic versus open colectomy for locally advanced T4 colonic cancer: Meta-analysis of clinical and oncological outcomes. *Br. J. Surg.* **2022**, *109*, 319–331. [CrossRef] [PubMed]
16. Milasiene, V.; Stratilatovas, E.; Norkiene, V. The importance of T-lymphocyte subsets on overall survival of colorectal and gastric cancer patients. *Medicina* **2007**, *43*, 548–554. [CrossRef]
17. Oh, D.Y.; Fong, L. Cytotoxic CD4+ T cells in cancer: Expanding the immune effector toolbox. *Immunity* **2021**, *54*, 2701–2711. [CrossRef]
18. Wu, Z.; Zheng, Y.; Sheng, J.; Han, Y.; Yang, Y.; Pan, H.; Yao, J. CD3(+)CD4(-)CD8(-) (Double-Negative) T Cells in Inflammation Immune Disorders and Cancer. *Front. Immunol.* **2022**, *13*, 816005. [CrossRef]
19. St Paul, M.; Ohashi, P.S. The Roles of CD8+ T Cell Subsets in Antitumor Immunity. *Trends Cell Biol.* **2020**, *30*, 695–704. [CrossRef]
20. Xia, X.J.; Liu, B.C.; Su, J.S.; Pei, H.; Chen, H.; Li, L.; Liu, Y.F. Preoperative CD4 count or CD4/CD8 ratio as a useful indicator for postoperative sepsis in HIV-infected patients undergoing abdominal operations. *J. Surg. Res.* **2012**, *174*, e25–e30. [CrossRef]
21. Wichmann, M.W.; Hüttl, T.P.; Winter, H.; Spelsberg, F.; Angele, M.K.; Heiss, M.M.; Jauch, K.W. Immunological effects of laparoscopic vs open colorectal surgery: A prospective clinical study. *Arch. Surg.* **2005**, *140*, 692–697. [CrossRef]
22. Mölkänen, T.; Rostila, A.; Ruotsalainen, E.; Alanne, M.; Perola, M.; Järvinen, A. Genetic polymorphism of the C-reactive protein (CRP) gene and a deep infection focus determine maximal serum CRP level in Staphylococcus aureus bacteremia. *Eur. J. Clin. Microbiol. Infect. Dis. Off. Publ. Eur. Soc. Clin. Microbiol.* **2010**, *29*, 1131–1137. [CrossRef]
23. Vittimberga, F.J., Jr.; Foley, D.P.; Meyers, W.C.; Callery, M.P. Laparoscopic surgery and the systemic immune response. *Ann. Surg.* **1998**, *227*, 326–334. [CrossRef]
24. Strowitzki, M.J.; Nelson, R.; Garcia, M.P.; Tuffs, C.; Bleul, M.B.; Fitzsimons, S.; Navas, J.; Uzieliene, I.; Ritter, A.S.; Phelan, D. et al. Carbon Dioxide Sensing by Immune Cells Occurs through Carbonic Anhydrase 2-Dependent Changes in Intracellular pH. *J. Immunol.* **2022**, *208*, 2363–2375. [CrossRef] [PubMed]
25. Albers, K.I.; Polat, F.; Helder, L.; Panhuizen, I.F.; Snoeck, M.M.J.; Polle, S.B.W.; de Vries, H.; Dias, E.M.; Slooter, G.D.; de Boer, H.D. et al. Quality of Recovery and Innate Immune Homeostasis in Patients Undergoing Low-pressure Versus Standard-pressure Pneumoperitoneum During Laparoscopic Colorectal Surgery (RECOVER): A Randomized Controlled Trial. *Ann. Surg.* **2022**, *276*, e664–e673. [CrossRef] [PubMed]
26. Tang, C.L.; Eu, K.W.; Tai, B.C.; Soh, J.G.; MacHin, D.; Seow-Choen, F. Randomized clinical trial of the effect of open versus laparoscopically assisted colectomy on systemic immunity in patients with colorectal cancer. *Br. J. Surg.* **2001**, *88*, 801–807. [CrossRef] [PubMed]
27. Zhang, L.B.; Wang, B.; Wang, X.Y.; Zhang, L. Influence of video-assisted thoracoscopic lobectomy on immunological functions in non-small cell lung cancer patients. *Med. Oncol.* **2015**, *32*, 201. [CrossRef]
28. Zhou, L.W.; Ding, H.L.; Li, M.Q.; Jin, S.; Wang, X.S.; Ji, L.J. Effect of tramadol on perioperative immune function in patients undergoing gastric cancer surgeries. *Anesth. Essays Res.* **2013**, *7*, 54–57.
29. Préfontaine, H.; Hélie, P.; Vachon, P. Postoperative pain in Sprague Dawley rats after liver biopsy by laparotomy versus laparoscopy. *Lab Anim.* **2015**, *44*, 174–178. [CrossRef] [PubMed]
30. Toor, S.M.; Murshed, K.; Al-Dhaheri, M.; Khawar, M.; Abu Nada, M.; Elkord, E. Immune Checkpoints in Circulating and Tumor-Infiltrating CD4(+) T Cell Subsets in Colorectal Cancer Patients. *Front. Immunol.* **2019**, *10*, 2936. [CrossRef]
31. West, M.A.; Baker, J.; Bellingham, J. Kinetics of decreased LPS-stimulated cytokine release by macrophages exposed to CO_2. *J. Surg. Res.* **1996**, *63*, 269–274. [CrossRef]
32. Zawadzki, M.; Krzystek-Korpacka, M.; Gamian, A.; Witkiewicz, W. Comparison of inflammatory responses following robotic and open colorectal surgery: A prospective study. *Int. J. Colorectal Dis.* **2017**, *32*, 399–407. [CrossRef] [PubMed]
33. Chen, Y.; Zhou, Z.; Min, W. Mitochondria, Oxidative Stress and Innate Immunity. *Front. Physiol.* **2018**, *9*, 1487. [CrossRef] [PubMed]
34. Al-Kuraishy, H.M.; Al-Gareeb, A.I. Eustress and Malondialdehyde (MDA): Role of Panax Ginseng: Randomized Placebo Controlled Study. *Iran. J. Psychiatry* **2017**, *12*, 194–200. [PubMed]
35. Galon, J.; Fridman, W.H.; Pagès, F. The adaptive immunologic microenvironment in colorectal cancer: A novel perspective. *Cancer Res.* **2007**, *67*, 1883–1886. [CrossRef]
36. Braga, M.; Pecorelli, N.; Frasson, M.; Vignali, A.; Zuliani, W.; Carlo, V.D. Long-term outcomes after laparoscopic colectomy. *World J. Gastrointest. Oncol.* **2011**, *3*, 43–48. [CrossRef] [PubMed]
37. Karanika, S.; Karantanos, T.; Theodoropoulos, G.E. Immune response after laparoscopic colectomy for cancer: A review. *Gastroenterol. Rep.* **2013**, *1*, 85–94. [CrossRef]

Disclaimer/Publisher's Note: The statements, opinions and data contained in all publications are solely those of the individual author(s) and contributor(s) and not of MDPI and/or the editor(s). MDPI and/or the editor(s) disclaim responsibility for any injury to people or property resulting from any ideas, methods, instructions or products referred to in the content.

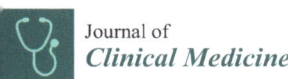

Article

Appraisal of Intraoperative Adverse Events to Improve Postoperative Care

Larsa Gawria [1,2,*], Ahmed Jaber [1,3], Richard Peter Gerardus Ten Broek [1], Gianmaria Bernasconi [4], Rachel Rosenthal [5], Harry Van Goor [1] and Salome Dell-Kuster [3,6,7]

1. Department of Surgery, Radboud University Medical Centre, 6525 GA Nijmegen, The Netherlands
2. Basel Institute for Clinical Epidemiology and Biostatistics, University Hospital Basel, University of Basel, 4051 Basel, Switzerland
3. Department of Surgery, Yitzhak Shamir Medical Centre, Tel Aviv 7030083, Israel
4. Clinic for Anesthesiology and Pain Therapy, Hospital of Fribourg, 1752 Fribourg, Switzerland
5. Faculty of Medicine, University of Basel, 4001 Basel, Switzerland
6. Clinic for Anesthesiology, Intermediate Care, Prehospital Emergency Medicine and Pain Therapy, University Hospital Basel, 4031 Basel, Switzerland
7. Department of Clinical Research, University of Basel, 4031 Basel, Switzerland
* Correspondence: larsa.gawria@radboudumc.nl or larsa.gawria@gmail.com

Abstract: Background: Intraoperative adverse events (iAEs) are associated with adverse postoperative outcomes and cause a significant healthcare burden. However, a critical appraisal of iAEs is lacking. Considering the details of iAEs could benefit postoperative care. We comprehensively analyzed iAEs in a large series including all types of operations and their relation to postoperative complications. Methods: All patients enrolled in the multicenter ClassIntra® validation study (NCT03009929) were included in this analysis. The surgical and anesthesia team prospectively recorded all iAEs. Two researchers, blinded to each other's ratings, appraised all recorded iAEs according to their origin into four categories: surgery, anesthesia, organization, or other, including subcategories such as organ injury, arrhythmia, or instrument failure. They further descriptively analyzed subcategories of all iAEs. Postoperative complications were assessed using the Comprehensive Complication Index (CCI®), a weighted sum of all postoperative complications according to the Clavien–Dindo classification. The association of iAE origins in addition to the severity grade of ClassIntra® on CCI® was assessed with a multivariable mixed-effects generalized linear regression analysis. Results: Of 2520 included patients, 778 iAEs were recorded in 610 patients. The origin was surgical in 420 (54%), anesthesia in 283 (36%), organizational in 34 (4%), and other in 41 (5%) events. Bleeding ($n = 217$, 28%), hypotension ($n = 118$, 15%), and organ injury ($n = 98$, 13%) were the three most frequent subcategories in surgery and anesthesia, respectively. In the multivariable mixed-effect analysis, no significant association between the origin and CCI® was observed. Conclusion: Analyzing the type and origin of an iAE offers individualized and contextualized information. This detailed descriptive information can be used for targeted surveillance of intra- and postoperative care, even though the overall predictive value for postoperative events was not improved by adding the origin in addition to the severity grade.

Keywords: intraoperative adverse events; intraoperative complications; origin of Intraoperative adverse events; classification of intraoperative adverse events

1. Introduction

Intraoperative adverse events (iAEs) are relevant to postoperative care and quality improvement. One-half to two-thirds of all perioperative events are attributed to surgical care, with the majority occurring during surgery and more than one-half of these appearing to be preventable [1–3]. Awareness for safe intraoperative care is raised with the emergence of minimally invasive surgery, the increased complexity of operations, and the higher number of elderly and multimorbid surgical patients [4–6]. Standardized reporting of iAEs is key for identification of repeated occurrence of events and for improving perioperative care [7]. Compared to the reporting of postoperative complications, for which the Clavien–Dindo classification is dominantly applied, iAEs lag behind in uniform and standardized reporting in clinical practice and the available literature [7,8]. This is reflected by the 270-times more cited Clavien–Dindo classification compared to all available classifications of iAEs together [9].

Generally, the operative and anesthesia report is used to report and describe iAEs. However, operative reports have been found to be subjective; events are underreported, and reports rarely include organizational causes such as equipment failure [10,11]. In addition, operative reports may be delayed, resulting in incomplete handovers at transfers to higher-level care or surgical wards [11,12]. Several grading systems for iAEs have been developed. These systems usually have several important drawbacks that hinder their uniform implementation (e.g., not including all sources of iAEs, focusing on specific operations (laparoscopic) or specific iAEs (adhesiolysis), and being complex or not properly validated) [13–16]. Our group recently developed and validated ClassIntra®, an easy-to-use grading system for all types of iAEs, and found a strong association between the severity of intraoperative and postoperative complications in a range of surgical disciplines [17]. This association was further established for visceral surgery [18]. Similar to other grading systems, ClassIntra® does not describe the origin of the iAE. Such a description might add context to the severity grading and possibly strengthen the association with the postoperative outcome. The context can also improve postoperative handovers and early diagnosis of postoperative complications, and may serve as a tool for training and quality improvement [19,20].

The large prospective database of the ClassIntra® study offers the possibility to describe the attributes of iAEs including origins and subcategories as a means for improved postoperative handovers and the development of strategies to prevent postoperative complications. We hypothesized that the addition of the origin to the severity grade of an iAE according to ClassIntra® could strengthen the association between the severity grade of the iAE and the postoperative complication. Therefore, we evaluated the prognostic value of the origin of iAEs on postoperative complications when added to the ClassIntra® grading system.

2. Materials and Methods

Operative data of an international study aimed at validating the ClassIntra® classification for iAEs was used in this analysis [17]. Eighteen centers from 12 countries prospectively enrolled 2520 consecutive in-hospital patients undergoing any type of surgery in whom iAEs were reported and graded according to ClassIntra® (Supplementary Materials Table S1).

This classification defines an iAE as any deviation from the ideal intraoperative course that occurs between skin incision and skin closure, and consists of five severity grades depending on the required intervention and patient symptoms. The attending surgical and anesthesia teams reported the severity grade and a free-text description of the iAE(s) directly after surgery. Patients were assessed daily for postoperative complications until hospital discharge and had one post-discharge follow-up to assess 30-day mortality. Postoperative complications were assessed and graded according to the Clavien–Dindo classification by the physician on the ward [8,21]. A weighted sum of all postoperative complications in a single patient was calculated using the Comprehensive Complication Index (CCI®) [22,23]. The CCI® forms a continuous scale from 0 (no complications) to 100 (postoperative death, based on grades according to Clavien–Dindo [23]. All participating centers in the validation study provided consent to use their data for this study. No approval was required from the local ethical committees of the study centers in addition to the existing approval for the ClassIntra® study (EKNZ Req-2016-00469; ClinicalTrials.gov, NCT03009929).

2.1. Categorization

Free-text descriptions of the iAEs were evaluated to identify the origin of the iAEs. The origin was categorized into four categories: surgical, anesthesia, organizational, and other. Surgical iAEs were defined as events initially arising in the operative field, such as bleeding or an iatrogenic bowel injury. Anesthesia-related iAEs included all medical events not arising in the operative field (e.g., arrhythmia or hypoxemia). iAEs that involved more than one origin were categorized according to the origin causing the sequela. For example, hypotension caused by bleeding was categorized as surgical, while hypotension resulting from anaphylaxis was categorized as anesthesia.

Organizational iAEs were due to errors in logistic or technical failure (e.g., instrument failure). iAEs were categorized as 'other' in cases where the origin was not clear from the description, or if they occurred before skin incision or after skin closure and did not match any set definition [17].

The list of subcategories was designed as an open list with subcategories added to further describe the parent category (e.g., the type of bleeding or hypotension) when appropriate, as outlined below.

As bleeding and hypotension were common heterogeneous subcategories with a range of treatments, the respective iAEs were further specified. For bleeding, a differentiation was made between diffuse and major. If the description stated "minor", "small"-vessel or "diffuse", bleeding was classified as 'diffuse'. When a large caliber vessel was indicated, either by naming the vessel or with the terms "large" or "major", bleeding was classified as 'major'. In case of hypotension, a differentiation was made between mild, profound, or unknown severity, based on the required treatment as mentioned in the description of the iAEs. If the description noted ephedrine or phenylephrine, or "mild" or "transient", hypotension was classified as 'mild'. If the description noted noradrenaline or "strong", hypotension was classified as 'profound'. A description that did not distinguish the type of bleeding or hypotension was left unspecified. The attending team reported conversion from minimally invasive to open surgery when they judged it as an iAE. We categorized this based on the provided context in the free text.

Categorization and subcategories were recorded by two researchers (LG and AJ) who were blinded for each other's assessments. Thirty iAEs were used for training. An intraclass correlation coefficient was used as a reliability measure for categorization of the origin. In case of differences in origins or subcategories, two senior physicians (RtB and SDK) were consulted for surgical and anesthesia iAEs, respectively, to reach consensus. Categorization was recorded in a Microsoft Access database for Office 365, which included the iAEs and relevant patient-related information.

2.2. Outcomes and Statistical Analysis

We used descriptive statistics and frequency tables of all iAEs and their distribution across origins and subcategories.

In an explorative way, we investigated the effects of the origin of an iAE on the CCI® in addition to the severity grade, using multivariable linear mixed-effect regression analyses [23]. The multivariable models with and without the origin of iAEs were compared using a likelihood ratio test. We tested the interaction between the origin and ClassIntra® grade, which was not significant and therefore not included in the model. No extensive testing of the model's predictive ability was conducted due to the exploratory nature.

As more than one iAE of different origins could occur in one patient, we categorized the origin variable for statistical analyses into the following 5 levels: 1 = no iAE, 2 = surgical origin of a single iAE, 3 = anesthesia origin of a single iAE, 4 = organizational origin of a single iAE, 5 = in case more than one iAE of any origin occurred. iAEs in the other origin category were not taken into account as these were insufficiently described or were not considered iAEs according to pre-set definitions [17].

The model was adjusted for predefined potential confounders: patient age, American Society of Anesthesiologists (ASA) physical status [24], complexity graded as one of five categories (minor, intermediate, major, major plus, and complex major operation) according to the British United Provident Association (BUPA) [25], the duration and urgency of the surgical procedure, the wound category [26], and the experience of the surgery and anesthesia teams. The variables for anesthesia and surgical experience were handled as in the validation study of ClassIntra® [17]. In short, anesthesia experience was summed up with anesthesia nurse in training, his/her graduation, and a resident present in the operating room each contributing one point; a consultant added another 2 and a senior consultant added 3 points. Surgical experience was defined by the most senior surgeon present in the operating room, to which the consultant and the resident (in training) were compared.

Complexity grades were not available for 4% of the procedures, for which an alternative grade corresponding to a comparable procedure was used. There were no other missing data. All analyses were performed using Stata/SE 15.1 for Windows (StataCorp College Station, TX, USA). We followed the STROBE guidelines for reporting the results.

3. Results

Out of 2520 patients, 610 (24%) experienced 778 iAEs according to ClassIntra®, of which 198 (25%) were of grade I, 417 (54%) grade II, 142 (18%) grade III, and 21 (2.7%) grade IV. No intraoperative deaths of grade V occurred. Baseline characteristics and postoperative outcomes are described in Tables 1 and 2.

Table 1. Baseline characteristics for the total study population (n = 2520) and for subgroups without intraoperative adverse events (iAEs) (n = 1910) and with at least one iAE (n = 610).

	All Patients (n = 2520)	Patients without iAEs (n = 1910, 76)	Patients with iAE (n = 610, 24)
American Society of Anesthesiologists (ASA) physical status			
ASA I	503 (20)	431 (23)	72 (12)
ASA II	1118 (44)	852 (45)	266 (44)
ASA III	805 (32)	565 (30)	240 (39)
ASA IV	92 (4)	62 (3)	30 (5)
ASA V	2 (0.1)	-	2 (0.3)
Age in adults, median (IQR, range) (n = 2340)	61 (46–72; 18–97)	60 (45–71; 18–97)	64 (49–74; 18–93)
Sex			
Male	1382 (55)	1038 (54)	344 (56)
Female	1138 (45)	872 (46)	266 (44)
Body Mass Index in adults (kg/m^2), median (IQR) (n = 2340)	26 (23–30)	26 (23–30)	26 (23–30)
Surgical discipline			
Gastrointestinal surgery	1437 (57)	1085 (57)	352 (58)
Orthopedic surgery and traumatology	297 (12)	260 (14)	37 (6)
Vascular surgery	169 (7)	121 (6)	48 (8)
Urology	134 (5)	109 (6)	25 (4)
ENT and maxillofacial surgery	122 (5)	99 (5)	23 (4)
Neuro- and spine surgery	96 (4)	53 (3)	43 (7)
Cardiac surgery	73 (3)	41 (2)	32 (5)
Pediatric surgery	54 (2)	48 (3)	6 (1)
Gynecology	46 (2)	29 (2)	17 (3)
Obstetrics	44 (2)	31 (2)	13 (2)
Reconstructive and hand surgery	26 (1)	21 (1)	5 (1)
Thoracic surgery	22 (1)	13 (1)	9 (2)

Table 1. Cont.

	All Patients (n = 2520)	Patients without iAEs (n = 1910, 76)	Patients with iAE (n = 610, 24)
Complexity of surgical procedure			
Minor	105 (4)	94 (5)	11 (2)
Intermediate	437 (17)	383 (20)	54 (9)
Major	790 (31)	613 (32)	177 (29)
Major plus	442 (18)	323 (17)	119 (20)
Complex major operation	648 (26)	431 (23)	217 (36)
Urgency of procedure			
Planned	2153 (85)	1627 (85)	526 (86)
Unplanned	367 (15)	283 (15)	84 (14)
Operating surgeon			
Senior consultant	1662 (66)	1239 (65)	423 (69)
Junior consultant	544 (22)	427 (22)	117 (19)
Resident	314 (12)	244 (13)	70 (11)
Anesthesia consultant present	2311 (92)	1746 (91)	565 (93)
Senior consultant	1481/2311 (64)	1112/1746 (64)	369/565 (65)
Junior consultant	830/2311 (36)	634/1746 (36)	196/565 (35)

All values are frequencies and percentage (n, %) unless stated otherwise. ENT = ear, nose, throat surgery.

Table 2. Origin of intraoperative adverse events (iAEs) according to surgical discipline. Multiple iAEs are possible in one patient. All values are frequencies and row percentages. (n, %).

Disciplines	Total iAEs (n = 778, 24)	Origin			
		Surgery (n = 420, 54)	Anesthesia (n = 283, 36)	Organization (n = 34, 4.4)	Other (n = 41, 5.3)
Gastrointestinal surgery (n = 1437)	442 (24)	289 (65)	117 (26)	17 (4)	19 (4)
Orthopedic surgery (n = 297)	40 (11)	18 (45)	19 (48)	1 (3)	2 (5)
Vascular surgery (n = 169)	64 (28)	35 (55)	24 (38)	2 (3)	3 (5)
Urology (n = 134)	29 (18)	3 (10)	17 (59)	2 (7)	7 (24)
Ear, nose, throat and maxillofacial surgery (n = 122)	25 (19)	9 (36)	12 (48)	2 (8)	2 (8)
Neuro- and spine surgery (n = 96)	58 (45)	15 (26)	38 (66)	2 (2)	3 (5)
Cardiac surgery (n = 73)	62 (44)	26 (42)	36 (58)	-	-
Pediatric surgery (n = 54)	6 (11)	5 (82)	1 (17)	-	-
Gynecology (n = 46)	22 (37)	7 (32)	8 (36)	7 (32)	-
Obstetrics (n = 44)	16 (30)	5 (32)	9 (56)	-	2 (13)
Reconstructive and hand surgery (n = 26)	5 (19)	2 (40)	2 (40)	1 (20)	-
Thoracic surgery (n = 22)	9 (41)	6 (67)	2 (22)	-	1 (11)

3.1. Origin of iAEs

Of all 778 iAEs, the researchers classified a total of 420 (54%) iAEs of surgical origin, 283 (36%) of anesthesia origin, 34 (4.4%) of organizational origin, and 41 (5.0%) of other origin (Figure 1).

Frequency of iAE by severity grade according to ClassIntra® are depicted in Figure 1.

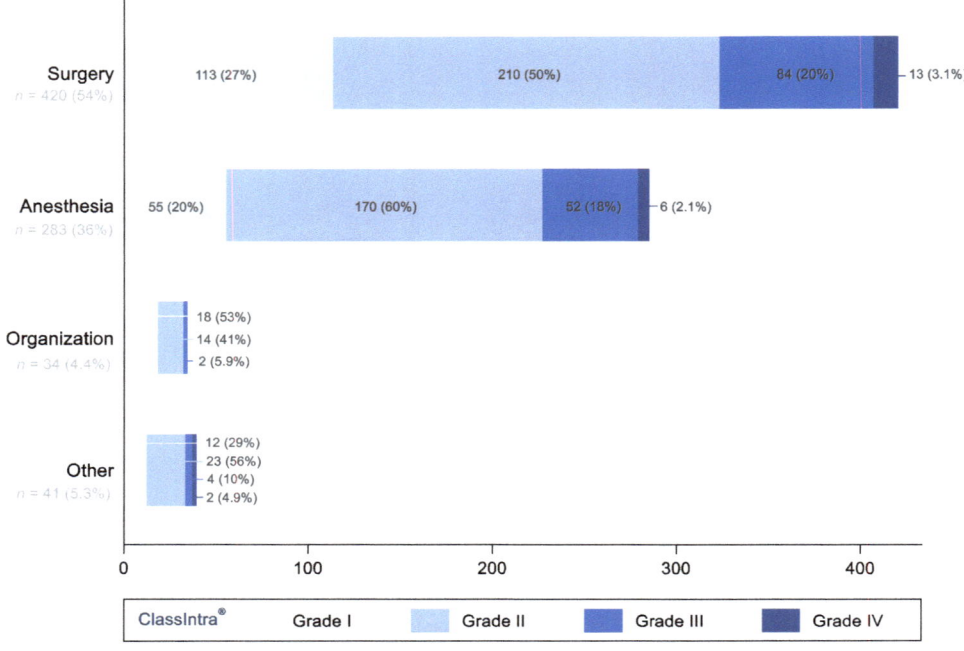

Figure 1. Origin of intraoperative adverse events versus severity grade of intraoperative adverse events according to ClassIntra®. Frequencies and percentages are displayed according to grade.

All grades, except for grade II, were more frequently reported with surgery as the origin as opposed to anesthesia, with grade I at 113 (27%) vs. 55 (19%), grade III at 84 (20%) vs. 52 (18%), and grade IV at 12 (3.1%) vs. 5 (1.8%), respectively. Grade II was less frequently observed to have a surgical origin as compared to anesthesia, with 210 (50%) vs. 172 (60%). Although iAEs with an organizational origin were predominantly of grade I and II, at 18 (53%) and 14 (41%), respectively, we note that 2 (5.8%) grade III iAEs occurred, meaning patients with severe symptoms that were potentially life-threatening. iAEs in the other category occurred before incision or after skin closure and were outside the definitions of ClassIntra® (34, 87%); referred to open-close procedures due to unresectable tumors (3, 7.7%); or were insufficiently described (2, 5.1%). Out of the iAEs that were outside the window, 5/34 (15%) were severe, i.e., grade III or IV.

In the case of unplanned procedures, e.g., emergency or urgent, iAEs of surgical origin occurred twice as often compared to anesthesia, in 65 (15%) and 19 (6.7%) cases, respectively.

Gastrointestinal surgery was the largest discipline and included most iAEs compared to the other surgical disciplines in Table 2.

However, the distribution of the iAE origins varied per discipline.

Regarding the distribution of origin according to the case-mix of patients, surgery related iAEs occurred more than anesthesia-related iAEs in ASA I patients, in 63/430 (15%) and 13/283 (4.2%) cases, respectively (see Table 1). However, for ASA IV patients the incidence rate was reversed. There were fewer surgical and more anesthesia iAEs with 21/420 (5.0%) and 32/283 (11%) cases, respectively. Likewise, fewer unplanned ICU postoperative admissions were reported after surgical iAEs compared with anesthesia, with 170/420 (40%) and 172/283 (60%) cases, respectively, per Table 3.

Table 3. Postoperative outcomes for the total study population ($n = 2520$) and for subgroups without iAEs ($n = 1910$) and with at least one iAE ($n = 610$).

	All Patients ($n = 2520$)	Patients without iAEs ($n = 1910, 76$)	Patients with iAE ($n = 610, 24$)
Origin of procedure (several iAEs per patient possible)			
No iAE	1910 (71)	1910 (100)	-
Surgery	420 (16)	-	420 (54)
Anesthesia	283 (11)	-	283 (3)
Organization	34 (1.3)	-	34 (4.4)
Other	41 (1.6)	-	41 (5.3)
Most severe iAE according to ClassIntra®			
0	1910 (76)	1910 (100)	-
Grade I	161 (6.4)	-	161 (6.4)
Grade II	309 (12)	-	309 (12)
Grade III	122 (4.8)	-	122 (4.8)
Grade IV	19 (0.8)	-	19 (0.8)
Grade V	-	-	-
Most severe postoperative complication			
0	1682 (67)	1367 (72)	315 (52)
Grade I	349 (14)	257 (13)	92 (15)
Grade II	277 (11)	162 (8.5)	115 (19)
Grade IIIa	72 (2.9)	45 (2.4)	27 (4.4)
Grade IIIb	55 (2.2)	40 (2.1)	15 (2.5)
Grade IVa	53 (2.1)	23 (1.2)	30 (4.9)
Grade IVb	7 (0.3)	3 (0.2)	4 (0.7)
Grade V	25 (1.0)	13 (0.7)	12 (2.0)
Duration of surgery, median (IQR, range)	100 (60–170, 4–760)	90 (55–147, 4–760)	151 (93–230, 12–673)
Postoperative length of hospital stay, median (IQR, range)	3 (2–6, 0–191)	3 (1–5, 0–106)	6 (3–9, 1–191)
IMC/ICU during postoperative course	68 (2.7)	40 (2.1)	28 (4.6)
Intermediate care unit (IMC)	18 (26)	15 (38)	3 (11)
Intensive care unit (ICU)	50 (74)	25 (63)	25 (89)
30-day mortality	26 (1.1)	13 (0.7)	13 (2.1)

All values are frequencies and percentage (n, %) unless stated otherwise. iAEs = intraoperative adverse events.

The experience of the surgical or anesthesia teams did not differ among the iAE origins.

A total of 68 (8.7%) iAEs involved more than one origin. Of these, 35 (52%) involved hypotension due to bleeding following an inadvertent injury. In these cases, the origin of the discipline that caused the sequela of the iAEs was accounted for.

The intraclass correlation coefficient for the origins of iAEs between both researchers was 0.60 (95% CI 0.55–0.64). Full consensus was reached after expert consultation.

3.2. Subcategories of Origin of iAEs

Bleeding was the most frequent iAE of surgical origin, with 217 (28%) cases as shown in Table 4.

Approximately one-third of the specified bleeding iAEs were of a major caliber vessel, with 33 (28%) cases. Six bleeding iAEs were of grade IV which needed major and urgent treatment because of life-threatening symptoms, of which five were specified as major and one was unspecified. A similar frequency of major caliber bleeding was observed when categorized by emergency and elective operations.

Table 4. Origin and subcategories of origin of intraoperative adverse events according to severity graded by ClassIntra®. All values are frequencies and column percentages (*n*, %). Organiz. = organization, oth. = other. * Extensive adhesiolysis without organ injury.

	Subcategories	ClassIntra®				
		Total (*n* = 778)	Grade I (*n* = 198, 25%)	Grade II (*n* = 417, 54%)	Grade III (*n* = 142, 19%)	Grade IV (*n* = 21, 3%)
Surgery	Bleeding	217 (55)	65 (59)	99 (50)	47 (60)	6 (55)
	Diffuse	87 (40)	47	37	3	-
	Major	33 (15)	2	12	14	5
	Unspecified	97 (45)	16	50	30	1
	Organ injury	98 (25)	25 (23)	57 (29)	13 (17)	3 (27)
	Seromuscular	28 (29)	1	26	1	-
	Enterotomy	14 (14)	1	8	4	1
	Gallbladder	12 (12)	7	4	1	-
	Urinary system	7 (7)	1	3	3	-
	Spleen	6 (6)	1	3	-	2
	Pulmonal	6 (6)	1	4	1	-
	Liver	4 (4)	1	3	-	-
	Appendix	3 (3)	1	1	1	-
	Nerve	3 (3)	2	-	1	-
	Bone	3 (3)	1	1	1	-
	Stomach	2 (2)	1	1	-	-
	Other organ	10 (10)	7	3	-	-
	Adhesiolysis *	20 (5)	4 (4)	15 (8)	-	1 (9)
	Conversion	13 (3)	2 (2)	2 (1)	9 (12)	-
	Failed insertion of prosthesis	11 (3)	5 (5)	5 (3)	1 (1)	-
	Vessel anastomosis leak	6 (2)	-	4 (2)	2 (2)	-
	Bowel anastomosis leak	4 (1)	-	1 (1)	2 (3)	1 (9)
	Other surgical ****	29 (7)	9 (8)	16 (8)	4 (5)	-
Anesthesia	Cardiovascular circulation	210 (67)	42 (71)	122 (68)	41 (68)	5 (63)
	Hypotension	118 (56)	21	76	20	1
	Hypertension	26 (12)	8	14	4	-
	Arrhythmia	31 (15)	10	11	8	2
	Heart insufficiency	19 (9)	-	12	6	1
	Bradycardia	8 (4)	1	6	1	-
	Tachycardia	5 (2)	2	3	-	-
	Other cardiovascular	3 (1)	-	-	2	1
	Airway and respiratory system	28 (9)	4 (7)	13 (8)	9 (15)	1 (13)
	Hypoventilation	11 (39)	2	4	5	-
	Intubation related	7 (25)	-	5	2	-
	Hypoxemia	3 (11)	-	3	-	-
	Other airway related	7 (25)	1	1	2	1
	Laboratory findings	25 (8)	3 (5)	14 (8)	7 (12)	1 (13)
	Insufficient sedation	14 (5)	2 (3)	12 (7)	-	-
	Conversion to general anesthesia	5 (31)	-	5	-	-
	Need for extra sedation	9 (56)	2	7	-	-
	Systemic reactions	9 (3)	3 (5)	6 (3)	-	-
	Hypothermia	4 (44)	1	3	-	-
	Anaphylaxis	3 (33)	1	2	-	-
	Hyperthermia	2 (22)	1	1	-	-
	Renal system	4 (1)	1 (2)	3 (2)	-	-

Table 4. Cont.

	Subcategories	Total (n = 778)	ClassIntra® Grade I (n = 198, 25%)	Grade II (n = 417, 54%)	Grade III (n = 142, 19%)	Grade IV (n = 21, 3%)
	Lesions	2 (1)	1 (2)	1 (1)	-	-
	Pressure marks	1 (50)	-	1	-	-
	Other lesions	1 (50)	1	-	-	-
	Other anesthesia ****	19 (6)	3 (5)	12 (6)	3 (5)	1 (13)
Organiz.	Instrument failure	12 (43)	7 (41)	5 (45)	-	-
Organiz.	Team communication	10 (36)	8 (47)	2 (18)	-	-
Organiz.	Logistics	6 (21)	2 (12)	4 (36)	-	-
Oth.	Other	41 (5)	12 (6)	23 (6)	4 (3)	2 (10)

**** See Supplementary Materials for descriptions of other surgical and anesthesia iAEs (Table S3).

Organ injury was the second most frequent subcategory of iAEs of surgical origin and included a quarter of the surgical iAEs mainly of low severity, with grade I at 25/98 (26%) and grade II at 57/98 (58%) cases. The majority of injuries were serosa lesion, enterotomy, and gallbladder injury. Adhesiolysis was mentioned in 33 events; in 13 of these cases, adhesiolysis coincided with organ injuries such as serosa injury or enterotomy. A total of 13 (3%) conversions were reported, of which 5 were due to limited overview, 1 to bleeding, 1 to instrument failure, and 6 with no provided context.

In anesthesia, cardiovascular iAEs were most often reported with 210 (67%) cases, including 118 (56%) cases of hypotension and 31 (15%) cases of arrhythmia. Based on the required treatment for hypotension, 53 (45%) cases were mild, 36 (31%) were profound, and 29 (25%) were unspecified. A total of 21 cases of hypotension were severe (grade III or IV) of which 20 were profound and 1 was unspecified. Mild hypotension iAEs were recorded with low severity, namely, 9 grade I and 44 grade II cases. In addition, the unspecified cases were mostly low severity with 5 grade I, 23 grade II, and 1 grade III case.

A total of 28 iAEs were organizational: 12 (43%) were due to instrument failure, 10 (36%) were due to team communication, and 6 (21%) were due to logistics, all of which were grade I or II.

3.3. Multivariable Analysis

The log-likelihood ratio test comparing goodness of fit of the multivariable models including severity grades of ClassIntra® with and without origin was not statistically significant ($p = 0.15$; Table S2).

4. Discussion

The descriptive analysis of 778 iAEs in 610 patients, from an international multicenter prospective cohort study across a wide range of surgical disciplines and anesthesia, offered insights in the incidence and origin of iAEs that occurred between skin incision and skin closure. Surgery encompassed half of all iAEs, and anesthesia accounted for one-third. Almost one in ten iAEs involved both disciplines and seemed interdependent. Organizational iAEs were rarely reported, likely due to the lack of awareness of the origin as an iAE, but still viewed as part of the procedure. Bleeding, hypotension, and organ injury were the most frequently reported subcategories of origin. The addition of origin did not alter the previously reported association between severity of iAEs and postoperative complications [17,18].

The detailed analyses and work-up of the origin of iAEs offer important advantages. While surgery accounted for the majority of iAEs, the proportion of the most severe iAEs was comparable with anesthesia-related iAEs. One in five of surgery- and anesthesia-related iAEs was of major severity, defined as ClassIntra® grade III or IV, which potentially leads to permanent disability. The reporting of well-recognized iAEs (e.g., bleeding and hypotension) was close to reality as reflected by the high incidence. However, with the increasing complexity of procedures and the usage of minimally invasive surgical devices more organizational device-related iAEs were expected but not reported. Only 12 out of 778 iAEs (1.5%) were reported as instrument failure, which is a fraction of the 15% incidence that was reported by direct observation using audio and video recorders, also known as medical data recording [27]. Organizational iAEs might be of lower severity but impact the duration of surgery [28]. Medical data recording of laparoscopic cholecystectomies revealed an average delay of 15 min for each procedure due to workflow interruptions, with a subsequent increase in financial health costs [28].

All study centers participating in the ClassIntra® validation study routinely used a perioperative checklist and an enhanced recovery protocol after surgery whenever applicable for the type of surgery. Yet, a standardized system for reporting iAEs was not developed, possibly leading to small differences in the reported incidences of iAEs between centers. Surgeons have indicated that the most common barriers to reporting iAEs are the fear of litigation, the lack of a standardized reporting system, and the absence of clear definitions for iAEs [29]. Longstanding systemic and cultural practices have hampered adequate reporting of iAEs, but this could be overcome with a positive culture and open communication surrounding iAEs [9,30]. A validated grading system offers a tool for uniform and standardized reporting but falls short of addressing the details of the iAE that could be relevant for postoperative care. Grading an iAE including its origin and describing subcategories may offer structured, relevant, and complete information for postoperative debriefing and handover to the recovery room, general ward, or intensive care unit. More complete information may avoid communication failure at the postoperative handover which is the root cause for 70% of sentinel events in the postoperative course [31]. The simplicity of the ClassIntra® classification with origin and subcategories allows for easy integration in the sign-out of the WHO safety checklists directly after surgery [17,32].

There is a rapid increase in the number of publications investigating iAEs but comparisons are impeded by their heterogeneity [9]. More than 20 different definitions for iAEs are applied and methods vary from chart reviews, (prospective) self-reporting, direct observation by human observers, to medical data recording [3,4,7,17].

With the emergence of checklists, crew resource management protocols, and medical data recording in the operating room, non-surgical iAEs of anesthesia- and non-technical origin (e.g., organizational or communication) have also gained interest [17,33–35]. A prospective evaluation of the characteristics of iAEs of any origin in a large cohort of multiple surgical disciplines is new and may overcome shortcomings of previous studies.

For example, Kaafarani et al. conducted a retrospective chart review of surgery-related iAEs in abdominal surgery and developed a classification for iAEs [14]. They identified an iAE incidence of 1.9%, which is much lower than the 17% incidence of surgery-related iAEs in this study. Moreover, the study did not account for anesthesia-related iAEs and, hence, ignored a significant part of the intraoperative course.

A landmark study by Gawande et al. conducted two decades ago investigated 15,000 surgical patients for iAEs of surgical or other medical origins, including anesthesia. Although Gawande accounted for a range of iAEs, e.g., bleeding, dysrhythmia, acute myocardial infarction, and technique-related complications, they did not differentiate between intra- and postoperative events. Overall, they found that more than half of all iAEs were of surgical origin, of which half were deemed preventable [3]. Despite the lack of further details concerning iAEs, the reported incidences were considerably lower than the 24% incidence rate of iAEs reported in our study. This difference is possibly due to the increased awareness of the impact of iAEs on patient outcomes in the surgical and anesthesia community overall, which is also reflected by the broad implementation of perioperative quality improvement programs such as surgical safety checklists and enhanced recovery after surgery [32,36]. A study investigating reporting bias revealed twice as many intra- and postoperative complications by chart review, compared to self-reporting by the treating perioperative team [37]. The main strength of this study is the detailed information of any type of iAEs in a large and broad surgical cohort across countries, improving the generalization of results. The high incidences reported most likely reflect real occurrences due to the prospective nature of this study and the motivation of participating clinicians to record iAEs [38].

However, this study also has limitations. First, surgical and anesthesia teams may have had different behavior towards a certain event type with a higher interest and knowledge of surgical and anesthesia in contrast to organizational iAEs. This may question the accuracy of the reported incidence of the latter event type [37]. Second, categorization of iAEs may have been wrong in some cases due to the limited context provided in the free-text description, despite two blinded clinical researchers and consensus in all cases after consultation with senior physicians. In addition, categorization of hypotension might be flawed as the optimal blood pressure for adequate perfusion is not individually weighted. Third, an iAE may arise due to an interplay of causal factors including organizational, human, and patient-related factors [39]. In this study, 10% of all iAEs involved multiple origins. Our data did not allow for describing the interaction between the different causative factors of iAEs. In particular, discussing interdependent iAEs with all members of the operative team can reveal insights in the pathogenesis of iAEs and trigger concerted postoperative diagnostic and therapeutic measures, which may enable early decision making to prevent postoperative complications and longer hospital stays [12]. Finally, we acknowledge that adverse events could have occurred outside the defined window between skin incision and skin closure. The definition for this timeframe is based on the results of the Delphi process in which ClassIntra® (formerly CLASSIC) was developed [40]. An additional study is planned to reevaluate the timeframe for assessing iAEs and to extend it beyond skin incision until skin closure.

Introducing content-rich, uniform and adequate reporting, and a positive learning culture allows for benchmarking of iAEs in clinical practice and research. It could enhance open communication and efforts for the development and implementation of strategies to mitigate iAEs.

5. Conclusions

Adding origin and subcategories to the severity grade of ClassIntra® may offer individualized and contextualized information of iAEs, directing surveillance in the postoperative care, however, without altering the prognostic strength of this classification. Simple and complete descriptions of iAEs might be most relevant for easing the postoperative debriefing, handovers, and decision making on the ward or in the ICU.

Supplementary Materials: The following supporting information can be downloaded at: https://www.mdpi.com/article/10.3390/jcm12072546/s1, Table S1: ClassIntra version 1.0 classification of intraoperative adverse events. The classification defines intraoperative adverse events as any deviation from the ideal intraoperative course occurring between skin incision and skin closure. Any event related to surgery and anaesthesia during the index surgery must be considered and should be rated directly after surgery. A requirement is that the indication for surgery and the interventions conform to current guidelines. Table S2: Multivariable linear mixed model of CCI—comparison of models with only ClassIntra® and ClassIntra® including origin of intraoperative adverse event. Table S3: Description of iAEs of the 'Subcategory Other' with origins surgery or anesthesia. This is a supplement to Tables of the main manuscript.

Author Contributions: Conceptualization, L.G., R.P.G.T.B. and S.D.-K.; Methodology, L.G., R.P.G.T.B. and S.D.-K.; Formal analysis, L.G. and S.D.-K.; Investigation, L.G. and S.D.-K.; Data curation, L.G., A.J., R.P.G.T.B. and S.D.-K.; Writing—original draft, L.G.; Writing—review & editing, G.B., R.R., H.V.G. and S.D.-K.; Visualization, L.G.; Supervision, H.V.G. and S.D.-K. All authors have read and agreed to the published version of the manuscript.

Funding: This research received no external funding.

Institutional Review Board Statement: The study was conducted in accordance with the Declaration of Helsinki. All participating centers in the validation study of ClassIntra® gave consent to use the data for this study. No approval was required from the local ethical committees of the study centers in addition to the existing approval for the ClassIntra® study (EKNZ Req-2016-00469; ClinicalTrials.gov NCT03009929).

Informed Consent Statement: Informed consent was obtained from all subjects involved in the study

Data Availability Statement: Data is available upon special request. Anonymized patient level data are available for investigators whose proposed use of the data has been approved by a review committee identified for this purpose.

Conflicts of Interest: The authors have no related conflicts of interest to declare. Rachel Rosenthal is an employee of and may own stock or stock options in F. Hoffmann-La Roche Ltd. The present study has no connection to her employment by the company. Rachel Rosenthal continues to be affiliated to the University of Basel.

ClassIntra® Study Group: R. B. ten Broek, richard.tenbroek@radboudumc.nl, The Netherlands; C. Rosman, camiel.rosman@radboudumc.nl, The Netherlands; M. Aduse-Poku, madusepoku@gmail.com, United Kingdom; S. Aghlamandi, soheila.aghlmandi@usb.ch, Switzerland; I. Bissett i.bissett@auckland.ac.nz, New Zealand; C. Blanc, catherine.blanc@chuv.ch, Switzerland; C. Brandt christian.brandt@spital.so.ch, Switzerland; H. R. Bruppacher, heinz.bruppacher@kws.ch, Switzerland H. C. Bucher, heiner.bucher@usb.ch, Switzerland; C. Clancy, clancyci@tcd.ie, Ireland; P.-A. Clavien pierre-alain.clavien@usz.ch, Switzerland; P. Delrio, p.delrio@istitutotumori.na.it, Italy; E. Espin eespin@mac.com, Spain; A. Engel, alexander.engel@sydney.edu.au, Australia; N. V. Gomes nuno.gomes@usb.ch, Switzerland; K. Galanos-Demiris, kogalanos@gmail.com, Greece; E. Gecim gecimethem@gmail.com, Turkey; S. Ghaffari, shahbaz.ghaffari@bbwien.at, Austria; O. Gié olivier.gie@chuv.ch, Switzerland; B. Goebel, babsigoebel@web.de, Switzerland; D. Hahnloser dieter.hahnloser@chuv.ch, Switzerland; F. Herbst, friedrich.herbst@bbwien.at, Austria; O. Ionnadis, telonakos@hotmail.com, Greece; S. Joller, sonja.joller@ukbb.ch, Switzerland; S. Kang soojin.kang@gstt.nhs.uk, United Kingdom; P. Kirchhoff, kirchhoff@zweichirurgen.ch, Switzerland; B. Loveday, b.loveday@auckland.ac.nz, New Zealand; R. Martín, rociomartin3004@gmail.com, Spain; J. Mayr johannes.mayr@ukbb.ch, Switzerland; S. Meier, sonjaimeier@gmail.com, United Kingdom; J. Murugesan, jothi.murugesan@sswahs.nsw.gov.au, Australia; D. Nally, deirdrenally@rcsi.ie, Ireland; G. O'Grady greg.ogrady@auckland.ac.nz, New Zealand; M. Ozcelik, ozcelikmenekse@yahoo.com, Turkey; U. Pace u.pace@istitutotumori.na.it, Italy; M. Passeri, Michael.Passeri@carolinashealthcare.org, USA; S. Rabanser simone.rabanser@ksgr.ch, Switzerland; B. Ranter, barbara.rantner@med.uni-muenchen.de, Austria D. Rega, daniela.rega@gmail.com, Italy; P. F. Ridgway, paul.ridgway@amnch.ie, Ireland; R. Schmid roger.schmid@szb-chb.ch, Switzerland; P. Schumacher, philippe.schumacher@spital.so.ch Switzerland; A. Solis, alejandro_solis85@hotmail.com, Spain; L. A. Steiner, luzius.steiner@usb.ch Switzerland; L. Villarino, lvillarino@vhebron.net, Spain; D. Vrochides, Dionisios Vrochides@carolinashealthcare.org, USA.

References

1. Leape, L.L.; Brennan, T.A.; Laird, N.; Lawthers, A.G.; Localio, A.R.; Barnes, B.A.; Hebert, L.; Newhouse, J.P.; Weiler, P.C.; Hiatt, H. The nature of adverse events in hospitalized patients. Results of the Harvard Medical Practice Study II. *N. Engl. J. Med.* **1991**, *324* 377–384. [CrossRef] [PubMed]
2. Thomas, E.J.; Studdert, D.M.; Burstin, H.R.; Orav, E.J.; Zeena, T.; Williams, E.J.; Howard, K.M.; Weiler, P.C.; Brennan, T.A. Incidence and types of adverse events and negligent care in Utah and Colorado. *Med. Care* **2000**, *38*, 261–271. [CrossRef] [PubMed]
3. Gawande, A.A.; Thomas, E.J.; Zinner, M.J.; Brennan, T.A. The incidence and nature of surgical adverse events in Colorado and Utah in 1992. *Surgery* **1999**, *126*, 66–75. [CrossRef] [PubMed]
4. ten Broek, R.P.; Strik, C.; Issa, Y.; Bleichrodt, R.P.; van Goor, H. Adhesiolysis-related morbidity in abdominal surgery. *Ann. Surg* **2013**, *258*, 98–106. [CrossRef] [PubMed]
5. Christensen, K.; Doblhammer, G.; Rau, R.; Vaupel, J.W. Ageing populations: The challenges ahead. *Lancet* **2009**, *374*, 1196–1208 [CrossRef] [PubMed]
6. Biere, S.S.; van Berge Henegouwen, M.I.; Maas, K.W.; Bonavina, L.; Rosman, C.; Garcia, J.R.; Gisbertz, S.S.; Klinkenbijl, J.H. Hollmann, M.W.; de Lange, E.S.; et al. Minimally invasive versus open oesophagectomy for patients with oesophageal cancer A multicentre, open-label, randomised controlled trial. *Lancet* **2012**, *379*, 1887–1892. [CrossRef]
7. Jung, J.J.; Elfassy, J.; Jüni, P.; Grantcharov, T. Adverse Events in the Operating Room: Definitions, Prevalence, and Characteristics A Systematic Review. *World J. Surg.* **2019**, *43*, 2379–2392. [CrossRef] [PubMed]

8. Dindo, D.; Demartines, N.; Clavien, P.A. Classification of surgical complications: A new proposal with evaluation in a cohort of 6336 patients and results of a survey. *Ann. Surg.* **2004**, *240*, 205–213. [CrossRef]
9. Cacciamani, G.; Sholklapper, Y.T.; Dell-Kuster, S.; Shekhar Biyani, C.; Francis, N.; Kaafarani, H.; Desai, M.; Sotelo, R.; Gill, I.; on behalf of the ICARUS Global Surgical Collaboration. Standardizing The Intraoperative Adverse Events Assessment to Create a Positive Culture of Reporting Errors in Surgery and Anesthesiology. *Ann. Surg.* **2022**, *275*, 1–3. [CrossRef]
10. Wauben, L.S.; van Grevenstein, W.M.; Goossens, R.H.; van der Meulen, F.H.; Lange, J.F. Operative notes do not reflect reality in laparoscopic cholecystectomy. *Br. J. Surg.* **2011**, *98*, 1431–1436. [CrossRef]
11. ten Broek, R.P.; van den Beukel, B.A.; van Goor, H. Comparison of operative notes with real-time observation of adhesiolysis-related complications during surgery. *Br. J. Surg.* **2013**, *100*, 426–432. [CrossRef] [PubMed]
12. Nagpal, K.; Arora, S.; Abboudi, M.; Vats, A.; Wong, H.W.; Manchanda, C.; Vincent, C.; Moorthy, K. Postoperative handover: Problems, pitfalls, and prevention of error. *Ann. Surg.* **2010**, *252*, 171–176. [CrossRef] [PubMed]
13. Gawande, A.A.; Kwaan, M.R.; Regenbogen, S.E.; Lipsitz, S.A.; Zinner, M.J. An Apgar score for surgery. *J. Am. Coll. Surg.* **2007**, *204*, 201–208. [CrossRef]
14. Kaafarani, H.M.; Mavros, M.N.; Hwabejire, J.; Fagenholz, P.; Yeh, D.D.; Demoya, M.; King, D.R.; Alam, H.B.; Chang, Y.; Hutter, M.; et al. Derivation and validation of a novel severity classification for intraoperative adverse events. *J. Am. Coll. Surg.* **2014**, *218*, 1120–1128. [CrossRef]
15. Lier, E.J.; van den Beukel, B.A.W.; Gawria, L.; van der Wees, P.J.; van den Hil, L.; Bouvy, N.D.; Cheong, Y.; de Wilde, R.L.; van Goor, H.; Stommel, M.W.J.; et al. Clinical adhesion score (CLAS): Development of a novel clinical score for adhesion-related complications in abdominal and pelvic surgery. *Surg. Endosc.* **2021**, *35*, 2159–2168. [CrossRef]
16. Francis, N.K.; Curtis, N.J.; Conti, J.A.; Foster, J.D.; Bonjer, H.J.; Hanna, G.B. EAES classification of intraoperative adverse events in laparoscopic surgery. *Surg. Endosc.* **2018**, *32*, 3822–3829. [CrossRef]
17. Dell-Kuster, S.; Gomes, N.V.; Gawria, L.; Aghlmandi, S.; Aduse-Poku, M.; Bissett, I.; Blanc, C.; Brandt, C.; ten Broek, R.B.; Bruppacher, H.R.; et al. Prospective validation of classification of intraoperative adverse events (ClassIntra): International, multicentre cohort study. *BMJ* **2020**, *370*, m2917. [CrossRef] [PubMed]
18. Gawria, L.; Rosenthal, R.; van Goor, H.; Dell-Kuster, S.; ten Broek, R.B.; Rosman, C.; Aduse-Poku, M.; Aghlamandi, S.; Bissett, I.; Blanc, C.; et al. Classification of intraoperative adverse events in visceral surgery. *Surgery* **2022**, *171*, 1570–1579. [CrossRef]
19. Hutchinson, A.; Young, T.A.; Cooper, K.L.; McIntosh, A.; Karnon, J.D.; Scobie, S.; Thomson, R.G. Trends in healthcare incident reporting and relationship to safety and quality data in acute hospitals: Results from the National Reporting and Learning System. *Qual. Saf. Health Care* **2009**, *18*, 5–10. [CrossRef] [PubMed]
20. Weaver, S.J.; Dy, S.M.; Rosen, M.A. Team-training in healthcare: A narrative synthesis of the literature. *BMJ Qual. Saf.* **2014**, *23*, 359. [CrossRef]
21. Clavien, P.A.; Barkun, J.; de Oliveira, M.L.; Vauthey, J.N.; Dindo, D.; Schulick, R.D.; de Santibanes, E.; Pekolj, J.; Slankamenac, K.; Bassi, C.; et al. The Clavien-Dindo classification of surgical complications: Five-year experience. *Ann. Surg.* **2009**, *250*, 187–196. [CrossRef] [PubMed]
22. Slankamenac, K.; Nederlof, N.; Pessaux, P.; de Jonge, J.; Wijnhoven, B.P.; Breitenstein, S.; Oberkofler, C.E.; Graf, R.; Puhan, M.A.; Clavien, P.A. The comprehensive complication index: A novel and more sensitive endpoint for assessing outcome and reducing sample size in randomized controlled trials. *Ann. Surg.* **2014**, *260*, 757–762; discussion 762–753. [CrossRef] [PubMed]
23. Slankamenac, K.; Graf, R.; Barkun, J.; Puhan, M.A.; Clavien, P.A. The comprehensive complication index: A novel continuous scale to measure surgical morbidity. *Ann. Surg.* **2013**, *258*, 1–7. [CrossRef]
24. American Society of Anesthesiologists. ASA Physical Status Classification System [ASA Web Site]. 15 October 2014. Available online: https://www.asahq.org/resources/clinical-information/asa-physical-status-classification-system (accessed on 3 March 2021).
25. BUPA (British United Provident Association): Schedule of Procedures. Available online: https://bupa.secure.force.com/procedures (accessed on 7 July 2021).
26. Mangram, A.J.; Horan, T.C.; Pearson, M.L.; Silver, L.C.; Jarvis, W.R. Guideline for Prevention of Surgical Site Infection, 1999. *Am. J. Infect. Control* **1999**, *27*, 97–132; quiz 133–134; discussion 196. [CrossRef] [PubMed]
27. Jung, J.J.; Kashfi, A.; Sharma, S.; Grantcharov, T. Characterization of device-related interruptions in minimally invasive surgery: Need for intraoperative data and effective mitigation strategies. *Surg. Endosc.* **2019**, *33*, 717–723. [CrossRef] [PubMed]
28. von Strauss Und Torney, M.; Dell-Kuster, S.; Hoffmann, H.; von Holzen, U.; Oertli, D.; Rosenthal, R. Microcomplications in laparoscopic cholecystectomy: Impact on duration of surgery and costs. *Surg. Endosc.* **2016**, *30*, 2512–2522. [CrossRef]
29. Han, K.; Bohnen, J.D.; Peponis, T.; Martinez, M.; Nandan, A.; Yeh, D.D.; Lee, J.; Demoya, M.; Velmahos, G.; Kaafarani, H.M.A. The Surgeon as the Second Victim? Results of the Boston Intraoperative Adverse Events Surgeons' Attitude (BISA) Study. *J. Am. Coll. Surg.* **2017**, *224*, 1048–1056. [CrossRef]
30. Kachalia, A. Improving Patient Safety through Transparency. *N. Engl. J. Med.* **2013**, *369*, 1677–1679. [CrossRef]
31. Sentinel Event Analysis Statistics. 1995–2004. Available online: http://www.jointcomission.org (accessed on 22 January 2023).
32. Haynes, A.B.; Weiser, T.G.; Berry, W.R.; Lipsitz, S.R.; Breizat, A.-H.S.; Dellinger, E.P.; Herbosa, T.; Joseph, S.; Kibatala, P.L.; Lapitan, M.C.M.; et al. A Surgical Safety Checklist to Reduce Morbidity and Mortality in a Global Population. *N. Engl. J. Med.* **2009**, *360*, 491–499. [CrossRef]

33. van Dalen, A.; Strandbygaard, J.; van Herzeele, I.; Boet, S.; Grantcharov, T.P.; Schijven, M.P. Six Sigma in surgery: How to create a safer culture in the operating theatre using innovative technology. *Br. J. Anaesth.* **2021**, *127*, 817–820. [CrossRef]
34. Leonard, L.D.; Shaw, M.; Moyer, A.; Tevis, S.; Schulick, R.; McIntyre, R., Jr.; Ballou, M.; Reiter, K.; Lace, C.; Weitzel, N.; et al. The surgical debrief: Just another checklist or an instrument to drive cultural change? *Am. J. Surg.* **2022**, *223*, 120–125. [CrossRef] [PubMed]
35. Suliburk, J.W.; Buck, Q.M.; Pirko, C.J.; Massarweh, N.N.; Barshes, N.R.; Singh, H.; Rosengart, T.K. Analysis of Human Performance Deficiencies Associated With Surgical Adverse Events. *JAMA Netw. Open* **2019**, *2*, e198067. [CrossRef] [PubMed]
36. Ljungqvist, O.; Scott, M.; Fearon, K.C. Enhanced Recovery After Surgery: A Review. *JAMA Surg.* **2017**, *152*, 292–298. [CrossRef] [PubMed]
37. Gomes, N.V.; Polutak, A.; Schindler, C.; Weber, W.P.; Steiner, L.A.; Rosenthal, R.; Dell-Kuster, S. Discrepancy in Reporting of Perioperative Complications: A Retrospective Observational Study. *Ann. Surg.* **2023**. published ahead of print. [CrossRef] [PubMed]
38. McCambridge, J.; Witton, J.; Elbourne, D.R. Systematic review of the Hawthorne effect: New concepts are needed to study research participation effects. *J. Clin. Epidemiol.* **2014**, *67*, 267–277. [CrossRef] [PubMed]
39. Zegers, M.; de Bruijne, M.C.; de Keizer, B.; Merten, H.; Groenewegen, P.P.; van der Wal, G.; Wagner, C. The incidence, root-causes and outcomes of adverse events in surgical units: Implication for potential prevention strategies. *Patient Saf. Surg.* **2011**, *5*, 13. [CrossRef]
40. Rosenthal, R.; Hoffmann, H.; Clavien, P.A.; Bucher, H.C.; Dell-Kuster, S. Definition and Classification of Intraoperative Complications (CLASSIC): Delphi Study and Pilot Evaluation. *World J. Surg.* **2015**, *39*, 1663–1671. [CrossRef]

Disclaimer/Publisher's Note: The statements, opinions and data contained in all publications are solely those of the individual author(s) and contributor(s) and not of MDPI and/or the editor(s). MDPI and/or the editor(s) disclaim responsibility for any injury to people or property resulting from any ideas, methods, instructions or products referred to in the content.

Review

Current Trends in Volume and Surgical Outcomes in Gastric Cancer

Luigi Marano [1,†], Luigi Verre [1], Ludovico Carbone [1,*,†], Gianmario Edoardo Poto [1], Daniele Fusario [1], Dario Francesco Venezia [1], Natale Calomino [1], Karolina Kaźmierczak-Siedlecka [2], Karol Polom [3], Daniele Marrelli [1], Franco Roviello [1], Johnn Henry Herrera Kok [4] and Yogesh Vashist [5]

1. Department of Medicine, Surgery and Neuroscience, University of Siena, 53100 Siena, Italy
2. Department of Medical Laboratory Diagnostics-Fahrenheit Biobank BBMRI.pl, Medical University of Gdansk, 80-308 Gdańsk, Poland
3. Department of Surgical Oncology, Medical University of Gdansk, 80-308 Gdańsk, Poland
4. Department of General and Digestive Surgery, Complejo Asistencial Universitario de León, 24071 León, Spain
5. Organ Transplant Center of Excellence, King Faisal Specialist Hospital and Research Center, Riyadh 11211, Saudi Arabia
* Correspondence: ludovicocarbone1@gmail.com
† These authors contributed equally to this work.

Abstract: Gastric cancer is ranked as the fifth most frequently diagnosed type of cancer. Complete resection with adequate lymphadenectomy represents the goal of treatment with curative intent. Quality assurance is a crucial factor in the evaluation of oncological surgical care, and centralization of healthcare in referral hospitals has been proposed in several countries. However, an international agreement about the setting of "*high-volume hospitals*" as well as "*minimum volume standards*" has not yet been clearly established. Despite the clear postoperative mortality benefits that have been described for gastric cancer surgery conducted by high-volume surgeons in high-volume hospitals, many authors have highlighted the limitations of a non-composite variable to define the ideal postoperative period. The textbook outcome represents a multidimensional measure assessing the quality of care for cancer patients. Transparent and easily available hospital data will increase patients' awareness, providing suitable elements for a more informed hospital choice.

Keywords: gastric cancer; gastrectomy; hospital volume; surgical volume; centralization; textbook outcome; quality of care; healthcare

1. State of Art

Gastric cancer represents one of the main causes of cancer mortality worldwide [1]. Although significant advances in diagnostic and therapeutic tools have improved survival outcomes, surgery remains the only curative therapy for gastric cancer patients. Surgical resection of the primary tumor with adequate lymphadenectomy is considered the only curative therapeutic approach for resectable gastric cancer, while preoperative and adjuvant chemotherapies may improve the outcomes aiming at the reduction of recurrence rate and the increase in survival [2,3].

However, the extension of lymphadenectomy is still an open issue between European and Japanese surgical schools [4]. At present, based on scientific and technical outcomes, the Western perspective on lymphadenectomy in gastric cancer surgery has been reversed. Consequently, most national and international scientific societies agree on D2 lymphadenectomy as the standard of treatment with curative intent [5]. Overall, the main goal of gastric cancer surgery is to improve patients' postoperative recovery, resulting in a better quality of life, and to maximize long-term oncological outcomes through a proper surgical approach with a tailored lymphadenectomy [6,7].

Many novel gastric cancer classifications aimed at clinical and prognostic applications have been recently suggested [8]. The new classifications are based on tumor location, histopathology, gene expression, gene amplification, DNA methylation, several cancer-relevant aberrations, and oncogenic pathways [9–14]. The Cancer Genome Atlas (TCGA) and Asian Cancer Research Group (ACRG) [9,10] have proposed a molecular based classification of gastric cancers finding new ways to treat the disease with a more personalized approach. Several reports highlighted specific demographic and pathological features (such as age, tumor location, invasion, and stage) shown by distinct molecular subgroups [9,10,15–19]. Similarly, the project High-tech Omics-based Patient Evaluation (HOPE) has established an updated molecular classification that predicts disease-specific and overall survival in patients undergoing radical gastrectomy [20].

Notwithstanding, despite advancements in surgical techniques [21,22], active involvement in clinical, translational, and basic research together with the improvements in perioperative care, short- and long-term outcomes still vary considerably among different providers and countries [23–26]. In an effort to reduce these variations and pursue the provision of high-quality cancer care, volume-based referral has been advocated as an adequate predictor for good quality of care [27]. In 1979, Luft HS et al. [28] introduced the concept of *"surgical volume"* stating that high-volume hospitals have better outcomes than low-volume hospitals for complex surgical procedures.

2. Centralization

"Centralization" is defined as a process of concentration of resources, including staff materials, infrastructures, knowledge, research, and expertise to enhance the quality of care achieving better financial efficiency. The centralization of major cancer surgery in hospitals with a high annual volume of procedures significantly reduces the risk of perioperative morbidity and mortality [29–31]. As a result, a plethora of research papers have investigated the relationship between surgical volume and outcome, and several policy strategies particularly those designed to limit complex surgery to certified high-volume hospital and/or surgeons, have been debated. In 1999, the US National Cancer Policy Board of the Institute of Medicine published a statement to *"ensure that patients undergoing procedures that are technically difficult to perform and have been associated with greater mortality in lower-volume settings receive care at facilities with extensive experience"* [32].

Therefore, between the 1990s and 2000s, there was a shift also in private practice such as the Leapfrog Group, for referrals being based on hospital volume [33]. Given these assumptions, some authors have recommended the creation of minimum volume thresholds to limit the number of centers with low levels of activity [34,35]. In 2008 Bilimoria KY et al. analyzed the distribution of 27,420 gastrectomies collected in the US National Cancer Database, identifying the lowest volume hospitals as those performing less than four and highest volume centers when performing more than seventeen gastric resections per year [36]. It was estimated that 179 perioperative deaths and 493 long term deaths could have been avoided in high-volume centers, showing a higher risk of perioperative death and a worse 5-year survival for patients treated in low-volume hospitals [36,37].

Quality assurance has been increasingly recognized as a critical factor in the oncological surgical care process and, also for gastric cancer surgery, these associations between volume and outcome have been described [23,24,26]. In 2001, the Association of Upper Gastrointestinal Surgeons of Great Britain and Ireland (AUGIS) set the ideal threshold of volume standards for gastric cancer surgery at a minimum of 15–20 resections per year [38]. Subsequently, in 2003, research from Denmark highlighted the strong relationship between volume and outcomes, reporting less anastomotic leakages, a decreased 30-day mortality, and improved lymph node harvesting after the centralization of cases [38,39]. However, the cut-off point for the minimum number of surgical procedures was not exactly defined. On the other hand, several North American studies have reported conflicting results [31,40–43]. Past definition of high-volume center referred to a cut-off between 15 and 35 annual cases [31,40,41,43–45], whereas a recent international panel [46] defined consensus guidelines on the standard of care for gastric cancer surgery, setting the appropriate threshold for high-volume centers at more than 15 gastrectomies per year. In the Netherlands, the Dutch Health Care Inspectorate imposed a minimum of 10 gastrectomies per institution per year in 2012, and 20 per year from 2013. As a result, the total number of institutions performing gastric cancer surgery decreased, and the annual procedural volume per high-volume hospital increased [30,47]. In Italy, a minimum of 20 cases is considered the cut-off for referral centers treating gastric cancer. In 2017, a systematic evaluation of Italian hospital data, covering the years 2012 to 2015, identifies 40 cases per hospital as the cut-off for a relevant decrease in mortality [48]. These data need to be interpreted with caution because, according to this threshold, only 10.7% of total gastrectomies were performed in high-volume centers.

Even though the centralization of complex surgical oncology into high-volume hospitals has been prompted globally [38,49–51], an international agreement about the clear identification of high-volume hospitals as well as minimum volume standards has not yet been established. No study was able to identify specific thresholds on which outcomes change clearly and causally., and volume thresholds are usually set arbitrarily.

Centralization is important for surgeons to gain sufficient experience and proficiency in order to develop their expertise and achieve high-quality surgery [52]. Most studies about trends in volume and surgical outcomes have assessed mortality as the primary indicator, suggesting that this variable has a positive association with the length of hospital stay [53], recovery time [54], cost of the hospitalization [55], related morbidity [56,57] and disease-free survival [58,59]. However, mortality alone, investigated through a simple logistic model, may be insufficient to establish surgical activity thresholds. or to encourage potential modification of organizational structures [60]. A regression that does not control for organizational effectiveness will find a positive relationship between volume–outcome, whereas it is organizational skills and proven internal protocols, not higher hospital volume, that drives improved patient outcomes [61]. The opportunity of having standardized clinical pathways and healthcare professionals perfectly integrated into the tumor board, such as digestive endoscopy, trained anesthetists, and interventional radiology, guarantees the optimization of the perioperative process and a timely and effective management of postoperative complications [62–64].

Another interesting issue is that health planning aimed at the centralization of rare diseases may increase the probability that patients will be treated in hospitals with a comprehensive range of experienced specialists (nursing, radiology, pathology, and geriatrics), services to support the provision of care (physiotherapy, dietetics, and psychosocial support) and free access to new technological advances [65,66]. Over the past decades, minimally invasive gastrectomy has become increasingly utilized, as lower complication rates and shorter hospital stays have been described, despite similar long-term survival [67–69]. Robotic-assisted gastrectomy might overcome some challenges, by offering improved visualization through 3D images and increased magnification, instrument articulation, superior ergonomics, and tremor filtration. Minimally invasive surgery has been demonstrated to be safe and effective, mainly if performed in referral centers, even if further trials are required to establish the superiority of robotic gastrectomy on long-term outcomes [70]. On a population level, the introduction of robotics is expected to have contributed to the centralization of cases in an unintended but potentially beneficial way. To date, Italy boasts more than 100 da Vinci surgical robotic systems, most of them from northern regions with an unequal distribution across the country. On the other hand, its true impact on cancer control, functional outcomes, and access to care is still opaque. Potential risks are longer waiting times from referral to surgery to having the surgical procedure and increased medical tourism [71]. New robotic systems are currently being developed, which will make surgical technologies more widely available, facilitate collaboration among surgeons, who may be separated by distance, in real-time, and decrease patient travel. On a professional level, recent evolutions in care, such as remote surgery, requires continuous training, creation, and revision of specific guidelines and protocols, bringing new challenges to surgical equipment and to their work [72].

Overall, the evidence from clinical data to support the advantages of centralization has not been proven beyond any doubt, showing previous studies on the "*gastrectomy case volume*" conflicting and heterogeneous results [73–77]. It is gradually becoming clear that a mere concentration of the number of cases per hospital or per surgeon is not enough.

3. Predictors for Good Quality of Care

In Europe, the mortality rate after gastric cancer surgery ranges from 2% in specialized centers [78] to 10% in certain nationwide registries [26]. Quality assurance has been regarded as the current main challenge for surgeons [27], in order to pursue the so-called "*rescue phenomenon*", i.e., the ability to prevent minor postoperative events from developing into severe complications and death.

Standardized surgical therapy is supported in surgical oncology, due to the weak evidence of the surgical randomized control trials, especially those focusing on chemotherapy. Many international initiatives, such as the new platform SURGCARE, a collaborative project between the European Society of Surgical Oncology (ESSO) and the Japanese Clinical Oncology Group (JCOG) [79,80], invested their resources and promoted quality assurance In gastric cancer, the pursuit of evidence-based medicine and the shift toward precision surgery [81] have advocated the standardization of gastric cancer treatment and the creation of a standard level of competence. This application includes multimodal aspects of treatment, surgical competence with particular attention to the application of minimally invasive approaches, the establishment of a registry of complications as well as a medical database including follow-up [82].

For this purpose, the risk-adjusted and case mix-adjusted American College of Surgeons National Surgical Quality Improvement Program (ACS-NSQIP) has been established with the aim to collect data that provide an accurate, correct, and thorough analysis, in order to help surgeons and hospitals to better understand the quality of their care than similar hospitals with similar patients [83]. Each hospital assigns a trained Surgical Clinical Reviewer to collect 30-day perioperative data on a web-based platform. Blinded information is shared with participant hospitals, allowing them to nationally benchmark their complication rates and surgical outcomes [84].

Over the past years, several studies have investigated the effect of hospital volume on gastric cancer surgery outcomes, leading to the concept that centralization results in better outcomes, acting as a proxy measure for various processes and providing the advantages of a qualified multidisciplinary team and a comprehensive multidimensional assessment [85,86], easier access to sophisticated cancer imaging equipment, availability of skilled surgeons, and better postoperative care facilities [30,87–90]. In this regard, an experienced radiologist with dedicated skills in gastric cancer metastasis detection (i.e. gastric carcinomatosis) is fundamental to allow for better patient selection [91]. Similarly it has been proven that intensive care units (ICUs) with dedicated board-certified staff are associated with a lower post-gastrectomy mortality rate [92,93]. Additionally, early diagnosis as well as successful and effective management of postoperative complications might be better in high-volume hospitals [94]. Moreover, in an attempt to guarantee high quality oncologic care, the discussion of clinical cases within a regional multidisciplinary expert panel is advocated [95].

In addition, the existing research does not focus on the patients-perceived quality of care [96]. A Swedish analysis emphasized that patient satisfaction arises from well functioning care pathways, individualized care plans, continuity of treatment with local providers, accessibility for contact and information, involvement in the care process, and limited waiting time. A dramatic disadvantage of centralization is an increase in travel demands. A recent experiment conducted in England highlighted that patients were prepared to travel an average of 75 min longer to decrease their risk of complications by 1%, and over 5 h longer to reduce the risk of death by 1%, in line with the centralization trend [97]. Additionally, centralization should address real-life issues, such as postoperative continuity of care, long-term follow-up, and the possible need for urgent readmission [98]. The literature data suggested that most patients were prepared to travel long distances to receive specific care, but information on clinical outcomes of different hospitals is not widely available for the patients.

The present finding raises the possibility to shift from *"output"* (maximizing the number of *"stuff"* produced and of tasks in the guidelines), to *"outcomes"* mindsets (applying to understanding your patients' needs and solving their clinical problems). A clear focus on outcomes helps organizations succeed better by achieving *"patient centricity"* and maximizing the bottom line in terms of efficiency and costs. However, an organization that focuses primarily on solving its own problems (*"impact"*), will lose sight of its patients. Considering such evidence, it is mandatory to detect adequate predictors for good quality of care.

3.1. Hospital Volume

Despite the lack of unanimity [73,99], there is a growing recognition that multidisciplinary care in high hospital volume can improve postoperative mortality for gastrectomy [51,100,101].

Nelen SD et al. [77] reported a study aimed at investigating the outcomes of 250 gastric cancer patients after the centralization of surgery in the Netherlands since the introduction of the centralization policy in 2012. The treatment in high-volume hospitals resulted in an improvement in the percentage of patients treated with appropriate lymphadenectomy (21% vs. 93%, respectively), and a successful introduction of laparoscopic gastrectomies (6% vs. 40%, respectively). However, centralization did not realize an improvement in 30-day mortality as well as complication requiring a reintervention. More recently, the same Dutch study group reported the impact of centralization of gastric cancer surgery in a population-based setting. In this updated study comparing 3777 gastric cancer patients treated between 2009–2011 and 3427 between 2013–2015, the impact of the centralization was more evident in terms of improvement in surgical outcomes (lymph node retrieval and R0 resection rate), lower postoperative mortality and increased overall survival for all gastric cancer patients [102].

On the other hand, Claassen YHM et al. [39] did not report differences in morbidity and mortality rates between the hospital volume categories, ranked as very low (1–10 gastrectomies/year), low (11–20), medium (21–30), and high (31 or more). They postulated that patients referring to medium and high-volume centers had major comorbidities (comorbidity score ≥ 3) or more frequently underwent total gastrectomy surgery. Moreover, a retrospective review of the CRITICS trial reclassified hospitals as low-volume (1–20 gastrectomies/year) and high-volume (21 or more) finding higher overall survival and disease-free survival from high-volume hospitals [103].

Agnes A et al. argued that the high-volume status is referred to surgeons performing a high number of gastric resections and to other measurable and non-measurable variables, such as case mix (complexity of operation, comorbidities), well-organized perioperative process (ICU, trained anesthesiologist, radiologist, and nurses, availability of other specialists around the clock), timely management of postoperative complications (continuous assistance from experienced physicians, interventional radiology, digestive endoscopy) and appropriateness of the indication resulting from multidisciplinary cancer boards [104]. Most of these aspects could directly improve early postoperative outcomes and influence failure to rescue phenomenon [105].

The UK National Esophago-Gastric Cancer Audit registered a 90-day mortality of <5% and an anastomotic leakage rate of 6.3% in gastric cancer surgery. Moreover, after adjustment, lower 30-day mortality and anastomotic leak rate were observed in hospitals with higher volumes, while higher surgeon volume was associated with a lower anastomotic leak rate [106]. A German observational study revealed that treatment in a very high volume is associated with lower in-hospital mortality compared to low-volume hospitals [107]. Similar results arose from the Taiwan National Insurance Research Database [108]. Interestingly, postoperative mortality was low for each hospital volume category in a retrospective French study [109] that reported the impact of institution volume on 90-day postoperative mortality after gastric cancer surgery. Postoperative mortality rate ranged from 4.3 to 10.2% and resulted in 7.9% in very high-volume hospitals (at least 60 resections/year). Those data suggest the role of other factors, such as hospital facilities, or timely recognition of complications, in determining outcomes [30]. It could be argued that death or complication after surgery are imperfect measures of surgical quality.

On the other hand, a Japanese perspective on a total of 145,523 patients who underwent distal gastrectomy for gastric cancer by 11,914 surgeons at 2182 institutions has been recently published [110]. Hospital volumes were divided into 3 tertiles (low, 1–22 cases per year, medium, 23–51 and high, 52–404): An inversely proportional relationship between mortality rate and hospital volume was registered, resulting in the operative mortality of 1.9% in low-volume hospitals, 1.0% in medium and 0.5% in high ($p < 0.001$). Similarly, surgical complications such as anastomotic leakage, pneumonia, and surgical site infection were significantly higher in low-volume hospitals ($p < 0.001$) [110,111]. The same group recently analyzed a cohort of 71,307 patients undergoing total gastrectomy at 2051 institutions. Hospital volumes were divided into three tertiles: low, 0–11 cases per year; medium, 12–26, and high, 27–146. The peri-operative mortality rate passed from 3.1% in low-volume hospitals to 1.7% and 1.2% in medium and high volumes, respectively ($p < 0.001$). Surprisingly, the anastomotic leakage rate was not significantly different between low- and high-volume hospitals, while the rate of septic shock and medical complications of the nervous system were significantly higher in low-volume hospitals ($p < 0.001$) [112].

However, if Persi Diaconis and Frederick Mosteller's *"law of truly large numbers"* was true, with a sufficiently large number of samples, any highly implausible result would be likely to be observed. Since the occurrence of probable events is never surprising, we highlight fewer probable events [113].

A South Korean study, using National Health Insurance Service (NHIS) Sampling Cohort data during 2004–2013, noted that if mortality decreased with increasing hospital volume, the risk of mortality increased again after reaching some level of surgery volume [35].

Another interesting topic is the assessment of procedure volume effect on patient outcomes after the perioperative period. Long-term outcomes could be strongly influenced by the appropriateness of patient selection for peri-operative therapies, the type of surgery, the technical skills of the surgeon, and the availability of a specialized pathologist to appropriate stage the disease. To date, only a limited number of studies investigating the relationship between hospital volume and long-term survival after gastrectomy have been published, with scarce and conflicting results [43,51,73,99,102]. Birkmeyer JD et al. [31] explored the relationship between hospital volume and late survival after different types of cancer resections, using the national Surveillance Epidemiology and End Results (SEER)-Medicare-linked database. They found a statistically significant association between 5-year survival and hospital volume, reporting a lower survival rate in low-volume compared with high-volume centers (25.6% vs. 32.0%, respectively), irrespective of differences in the use of adjuvant radiation and chemotherapy [31]. On the contrary, a prospective population-based study of 3293 consecutive patients with esophageal or gastric cancer endorsed by the Scottish Audit of Gastric and Oesophageal Cancer (SAGOC) failed to demonstrate any correlation between hospital volume and postoperative morbidity or mortality, nor between survival and volume of patients neither for the hospital of diagnosis nor hospital of surgery [73].

There is much debate if positive relationship volume–outcome results from a practice makes-perfect or a selective-referral mechanism. Under the first hypothesis, repeatedly performing procedures yields experience and enhances the organization of the surgical team, improving future outcomes. Under the second hypothesis, better outcomes attract more patients. Of course, practice-makes-perfect supports centralization, whereas selective referral does not.

3.2. Surgeon Volume

The hospital volume and outcome relationship does not maintain its correlation at the individual surgeon level. As for hospital volume, similar attention was paid to the relationship between mortality rate and surgeon volume. Several reports have demonstrated an impact of surgeon activity on postoperative short- as well as long-term outcomes among patients undergoing gastric cancer surgery [110,114,115]. Even though 10-15 gastrectomies per year were suggested as a minimum surgeon volume for gastrectomy, [50,116], further evaluation in a large-scale cohort is needed [110].

Furthermore, it is hard to apply the same caseload threshold to clinical practice in different countries since the differences in epidemiology, biology, and treatment strategy can influence the cut-off value.

In the Western setting, the lower incidence of gastric cancer also resulted in a lower average volume, which ultimately led to poorer opportunities for surgical trainees. In terms of postoperative results, the learning curve is considered optimized once the minimum threshold of 15–25 cases is exceeded [117–119]. In the minimally invasive era, a significant reduction of the conversion rate and an increase in the lymph node yield was reported after the 10th case [120]. Moreover, comparing well-trained laparoscopic surgeons working in high- and low-volume hospitals, perioperative outcomes were not influenced, underlining that hospital volume is not a decisive factor [121].

In Japan, the National Clinical Database (NCD) was established in 2010 with the aim of recording all procedures performed by national surgeons. From this project, data on 11,300,000 Japanese patients with gastric cancer were extracted to discuss how surgical and hospital volume impact mortality following surgery for gastric cancer [110]. Interestingly, Iwatsuki M et al. disclosed a strong impact of hospital and surgeon volume on mortality and morbidity rates [110,112]. Particularly, dividing surgeon volume into four groups, S1 (0–2 cases per year), S2 (3–9 cases), S3 (10–25 cases), and S4 (>26 cases), the operative mortality rate after a total gastrectomy decreased from 2.5% in S1 to 0.6% in S4. By contrast, after proper statistical analysis adjusted by risk model variables (demographic factors, preoperative functional status, pre-existing comorbidities, operative factors, and preoperative laboratory data), only hospital volume showed a crucial role in improving outcomes compared with the surgeon volume. In other words, surgeons with low volumes could obtain lower morbidity and mortality rates compared to surgeons with high volumes and worse results.

Urbach DR et al. assumed that low-volume surgeons may have excellent outcomes because of experience or because they performed a high volume of similar operations requiring similar technical skills [122]. Interestingly, the best postoperative outcomes were obtained by high-volume surgeons in high-volume hospitals, followed by low-volume surgeons in high-volume hospitals [123]. These results may influence surgical training programs and the centralization of advanced surgical procedures.

However, a more precise standardization of surgical training is needed through dedicated fellowships or the establishment of a minimum skill–volume load for performing certain surgical procedures. If no doubt exists that the accreditation of hospitals improves surgical quality and safety, surgeons' accreditation programs are currently lacking. The ESSO Core Curriculum, since its conception in 2013 by ESSO, the European Society for Radiotherapy and Oncology (ESTRO), and the European Society of Medical Oncology (ESMO), has served as a guidance document for surgical oncologists to obtain the level of knowledge needed both for surgical oncology practice but also for the European Board of Surgery Qualification (EBSQ) in surgical oncology. In October 2021, an update on ESSO Core Curriculum was published [124], with the aim to give the candidate an idea of expectations and areas for in-depth study, in addition to the practical requirements to *"permit flexibility to suit the needs of the different regions of the world with their inherently diverse sociocultural, financial and cultural differences"*—Audisio R. In this way, the paradox of having a particular hospital accredited to perform several complex procedures without having qualified accredited surgeons can be avoided. It is time to shift from the pursuit of high-volume to high-quality centers.

On the other hand, the annual surgeon activity can only represent a surrogate marker for medical care quality [125], since it may not cover the complexity of this issue consisting of hospital volume, specialization, and mentorship opportunities [114]. Quality of care, in fact, consists of more than the performance of a single surgeon. Organizational effectiveness, perioperative care, anesthesia, ICU staffing, the experience of the nursery staff, nutritional evaluation, comprehensive geriatric assessment [85], and collaboration between different disciplines all contribute to the outcomes of the performed procedure [25].

3.3. Textbook Outcome

In 2017 the Dutch Upper Gastrointestinal Cancer Audit (DUCA) group designed the Textbook Outcome (TO), a multidimensional scale that provides an ideal route after esophagogastric cancer surgery [126]. It comprises ten perioperative quality-of-care parameters:

(1) Complete, potentially curative, resection as judged by the surgeon at the time of surgery;
(2) No intraoperative complication;
(3) Negative resection margin;
(4) Greater than 15 lymph nodes sampled;
(5) No severe postoperative complications (Clavien–Dindo grade II or higher);
(6) No re-intervention (surgical, endoscopic, or radiological) $\leq$30 days after surgery;
(7) No unplanned ICU or medium-care unit (MCU) admission $\leq$30 days after surgery;
(8) Duration of stay not exceeding 21 days;
(9) No 30-day readmission;
(10) No 30-day mortality following surgery.

They demonstrated that the quality of surgical care for patients with gastric cancer is multidimensional, and it is possible to generate supplementary information when different outcome parameters are combined into a single comprehensive outcome measure. TO was achieved in 48.6% (569/1172 patients) of patients with gastric cancer, resulting in a good match of 30-day postoperative mortality (5.5%) and severe postoperative complications (11.7%) when compared with other contemporary results [25,127].

In van der Kaaij's RT series, TO was associated with long-term overall survival (OS) after surgery for gastric cancer. Patients with a TO had 1-, 2-, and 3-year overall survival rates of 85%, 70%, and 64%, respectively, versus 64%, 49%, and 42% for patients with no TO respectively. Good patient selection, well-performed surgery, and optimal postoperative care can ensure a rapid discharge, optimize long-term outcomes, and reduce costs for the healthcare system. Interestingly, the DUCA group achieved TO in 23% of patients in hospitals performing 0 to 19 gastrectomies per year, 29% in hospitals performing 20 to 39 gastrectomies per year, and 27% in hospitals performing more than 40 gastrectomies per year [128,129].

The next update of the Population Registry of Esophageal and Stomach Tumors of Ontario (PRESTO) group did not include radical resection according to the surgeon and intraoperative complications (previously not unambiguously differentiated from postoperative complications) [130]. Overall, the new TO definition included eight points in total and was achieved in 24.6% of patients with gastric cancer. First, the proportion achieving TO varied significantly by year of surgery and displayed a significant and positive trend (20.3% in 2004 and 29.3% in 2015, $p < 0.001$). Secondly, surgeons and hospitals were ranked into quintiles (Q): surgeon Q1 performing 0 gastrectomies per year to surgeon Q5 performing 3.5–9.5 gastrectomies per year, and hospital Q1 with 0–2 volume per year to hospital Q5 with 12–22 procedures. TO was achieved in a higher percentage of patients treated in the highest volume hospitals compared to the lowest volume ones (Hospital Q5 23.5% vs. Q1 16.2%), while similar TO results were obtained by the highest and lowest volume surgeons (Surgeon Q5 24.0% vs. Q1 20.8%). This discrepancy was due to the adequate lymph node sampling rate, the lower rate of unplanned ICU admissions, and lesser 30-day mortality

However, neither TO nor 30-day postoperative morbidity, readmission, and mortality were associated with surgeon or hospital volumes.

In 2022, the same group concluded that achieving TO is strongly associated with improved long-term survival in 1836 gastric cancer patients, with a 41% reduction in 3-year mortality ($p < 0.001$) [131].

According to Levy J et al., the volume–outcome relationship is analogous to practice-makes-perfect, whereas *"perfect practice makes perfect"* may be more effective [130]. Future policies should be focused more on meeting quality parameters than on absolute volume.

Anyway, new scientific evidence is shedding light on the grey zones of the management of gastric cancer, focusing researchers' efforts on new outcomes. This is the premise for setting a new TO for gastric cancer.

4. European Recommendations

Vonlanthen R, on behalf of members of the European Surgical Association (ESA), presented 12 recommendations for future development strategies in centralization:

(1) The definition should be based on disease (i.e., pancreatic cancer) or on organ systems (i.e., complex HPB diseases) rather than a procedure (i.e., esophagectomy or pancreatectomy);
(2) Planning is based on a minimum number of cases per center and well distributed among the various regions, taking into account the demographic and cultural specificities of a country;
(3) Planning should include at least two centers per country to secure choice and competition (except for small countries and very rare diseases);
(4) Adequate resources must be ensured with an appropriate assessment of the available infrastructure and personnel;
(5) Centers must offer fully functioning multidisciplinary teams (MDTs) of specialists able to deal with all aspects of the diseases throughout the year;
(6) Adequate care and follow-up are ensured by the presence of the centers connected to a network of hospitals;
(7) Centralization specifications must be legally applied for adherence to the specifications applied locally and regionally and for private and non-private hospitals;
(8) The centralization process must be accompanied by mainstream media activities to ensure adequate public awareness;
(9) Centers are required to have an externally verified database, to be actively involved in clinical studies (including RCTs), and should be supported to contribute to laboratory research;
(10) Quality control must be accompanied by international benchmark comparative studies;
(11) Equal accessibility to centralized healthcare should be monitored;
(12) Centers are expected to participate in surgical training and provide specialized training, as well as rotation of general surgeons [132].

Furthermore, an obvious gap between regulations for centralization and implementation was registered, especially in the private sector compared to publicly "subsidized" hospitals. Overall, obstacles to centralization could be recognized at different levels: (a) healthcare provider (insufficient infrastructure, lack of specialized personnel, long waiting time), (b) patient (resistance to longer travel distance, to cultural and language changes, lack of awareness of better outcome), (c) payer, i.e., insurance, government (concerns from increased cost or charges), (d) political level (political decision are not enforced, regional interests outweigh centralization policies, legal divergences, conflict of interest, overwhelming bureaucracy, lack of specialization boards and of board recognition among countries) [132].

There are at least two possible solutions to the fragmentation of the care process and to patient trends and geographical needs consequent to an increase in centralization: on one hand, the implementation of surgical fellowships and training of medical staff in higher volume hospitals and younger surgeons working in lowest volume centers; on the other hand, the creation of hospital and territorial clinical and oncological networks, to ensure standard and multidisciplinary care [133]

5. Italian Perspective

How centralization should be implemented remains a controversy and in many countries, the focus lies on the centralization of complex surgical procedures.

The Italian National Health Care Outcomes Program (*Programma Nazionale Esiti*, PNE, https://pne.agenas.it, accessed on 14 March 2023), a tool developed by the National Agency for Regional Health Services (AGENAS), evaluates the outcome measurements in Italian hospitals. In 2021, PNE recorded a total of 5075 gastrectomies performed in Italian hospitals, with a higher prevalence of cases treated in hospitals in the north of the country. According to the volume of interventions, 274 (54.9%) institutions registered more than 5 gastrectomies per year; of these, only 60 hospitals (21.9%) performed more than 20 gastrectomies per year

Overall postoperative 30-day mortality was 5.62%. Low-volume centers' mortality rate ranged from 10 to 20%, while in high-volume centers a mortality rate of 3–5% was registered. The threshold of low adherence to quality standards was accordingly set at 10%.

Since there are no strict regulations due to the absence of a formal policy of centralization, gastric cancer surgery is still executed anywhere in Italy. Nowadays, a referral pathway for cancer patients has been introduced only in several Italian regions, i.e., Campania, Lazio, Liguria, Lombardia, Toscana, Piemonte, Veneto, Valle d'Aosta, with the vast majority organized according to a hub and spoke model. As a result, differently from other countries, an Italian agreement about the minimum volume standards of gastrectomies has yet to be established and attempts for its definition come from scientific societies, such as the Italian Society of Surgery (SIC) and the Italian Society of Surgical Oncology (SICO).

Lorenzon L et al. reported that 40.4% of the hospitals treating patients with gastric cancer performed less than five procedures/year in 2018. Classifying institutions by volume, the mean mortality was 7.7% in institutions performing 1–3 resections, compared to 4.7% in the highest volume institutions, 17–127 resections/year ($p < 0.001$) [134]. Moreover, the authors noted that the number of gastrectomies in each Italian province does not reflect the actual number of gastric cancers diagnosed in the same zone and that the pattern of health-related travels usually follows a south-to-north trend.

The Italian Research Group on Gastric Cancer (GIRCG) is implementing an Italian centralization policy for gastric cancer surgery, acting on the national healthcare system and with the support of the scientific community. Its recent guidelines can be a useful tool to address physicians in managing gastric cancer patients [3]. Based on the principles set forth in these statements, physicians will adhere to the best, internationally accepted effective standard of care.

6. Conclusions

Interpretations of studies on this topic require caution. Hospital and surgeon volumes act as a proxy measure and a surrogate of technical and non-technical items to be identified and evaluated in both low- and high-volume centers. It is time to drop Birkmeyer's aphorism "*the more I do, the better I do*" [135,136], to share "*perfect practice make perfect*" [130]. Careful selection of outcomes is essential for decision-makers, clinical professionals, and patients to improve clinical practice, guide health policy, and drive healthcare choices. The textbook outcome is a novel quality measure, reflecting the "ideal" surgical outcome.

Although the centralization of complex surgical procedures is totally sensible, since it is potentially associated with a higher quality of care, clear criteria are still lacking on what, where, and whom to centralize. The ESA recommendations may serve as a basis for discussion to improve healthcare in surgical oncology.

Emphasis on multidisciplinary evaluations and clinical decision-making such as prehabilitation, standardized clinical pathways, and perioperative noninvasive management has improved the hospital care of patients with gastric cancer. High-volume centers boast the cooperation of healthcare professionals and services to support the provision of care.

The definition of centers of excellence equally distributed across the country, well-organized multidisciplinary networks, and centralization of high-risk procedures, as well as advanced training for new generations, accreditation of surgeons, and monitoring of surgical performance, should be the priorities.

Author Contributions: Conceptualization, L.M. and L.C.; methodology, L.M.; validation, N.C. and K.K.-S.; investigation, L.V. and L.C.; data curation, G.E.P. and D.M.; writing—original draft preparation, L.M. and L.C.; writing—review and editing, L.V., G.E.P. and D.M.; visualization, D.F. and D.F.V.; supervision, K.P., J.H.H.K. and F.R.; project administration, Y.V. All authors have read and agreed to the published version of the manuscript.

Funding: This research received no external funding.

Institutional Review Board Statement: Not applicable.

Informed Consent Statement: Not applicable.

Data Availability Statement: Not applicable.

Acknowledgments: The authors express their special thanks to Antonia Carbone, a native English speaker, for assistance in language revision.

Conflicts of Interest: The authors declare no conflict of interest.

References

1. Fock, K.M. Review Article: The Epidemiology and Prevention of Gastric Cancer. *Aliment. Pharmacol. Ther.* **2014**, *40*, 250–260. [CrossRef] [PubMed]
2. Japanese Gastric Cancer Association. Japanese Gastric Cancer Treatment Guidelines 2018 (5th Edition). *Gastric Cancer* **2021**, *24*, 1–21. [CrossRef] [PubMed]
3. De Manzoni, G.; Marrelli, D.; Baiocchi, G.L.; Morgagni, P.; Saragoni, L.; Degiuli, M.; Donini, A.; Fumagalli, U.; Mazzei, M.A.; Pacelli, F.; et al. The Italian Research Group for Gastric Cancer (GIRCG) Guidelines for Gastric Cancer Staging and Treatment: 2015. *Gastric Cancer* **2017**, *20*, 20–30. [CrossRef]
4. Degiuli, M.; De Manzoni, G.; Di Leo, A.; D'Ugo, D.; Galasso, E.; Marrelli, D.; Petrioli, R.; Polom, K.; Roviello, F.; Santullo, F.; et al. Gastric Cancer: Current Status of Lymph Node Dissection. *World J. Gastroenterol.* **2016**, *22*, 2875. [CrossRef] [PubMed]
5. Marano, L.; Marrelli, D.; Roviello, F. Focus on Research: Nodal Dissection for Gastric Cancer-A Dilemma Worthy of King Solomon! *Eur. J. Surg. Oncol.* **2016**, *42*, 1623–1624. [CrossRef] [PubMed]
6. Ohdaira, H.; Nimura, H.; Mitsumori, N.; Takahashi, N.; Kashiwagi, H.; Yanaga, K. Validity of Modified Gastrectomy Combined with Sentinel Node Navigation Surgery for Early Gastric Cancer. *Gastric Cancer* **2007**, *10*, 117–122. [CrossRef]
7. D'Antonio, A.; Addesso, M.; Memoli, D.; Liguori, P.; Cuomo, R.; Boscaino, A.; Nappi, O. Lymph Node-Based Disease and HHV-8/KSHV Infection in HIV Seronegative Patients: Report of Three New Cases of a Heterogeneous Group of Diseases. *Int. J. Hematol.* **2011**, *93*, 795–801. [CrossRef]
8. Russi, S.; Marano, L.; Laurino, S.; Calice, G.; Scala, D.; Marino, G.; Sgambato, A.; Mazzone, P.; Carbone, L.; Napolitano, G.; et al. Gene Regulatory Network Characterization of Gastric Cancer's Histological Subtypes: Distinctive Biological and Clinically Relevant Master Regulators. *Cancers* **2022**, *14*, 4961. [CrossRef]
9. Cancer Genome Atlas Research Network; Thorsson, V.; Shmulevich, I.; Reynolds, S.M.; Miller, M.; Bernard, B.; Hinoue, T.; Laird, P.W.; Curtis, C.; Shen, H.; et al. Comprehensive Molecular Characterization of Gastric Adenocarcinoma. *Nature* **2014**, *513*, 202–209. [CrossRef]
10. Cristescu, R.; Lee, J.; Nebozhyn, M.; Kim, K.-M.; Ting, J.C.; Wong, S.S.; Liu, J.; Yue, Y.G.; Wang, J.; Yu, K.; et al. Molecular Analysis of Gastric Cancer Identifies Subtypes Associated with Distinct Clinical Outcomes. *Nat. Med.* **2015**, *21*, 449–456. [CrossRef]
11. Wang, G.; Hu, N.; Yang, H.H.; Wang, L.; Su, H.; Wang, C.; Clifford, R.; Dawsey, E.M.; Li, J.-M.; Ding, T.; et al. Comparison of Global Gene Expression of Gastric Cardia and Noncardia Cancers from a High-Risk Population in China. *PLoS ONE* **2013**, *8*, e63826. [CrossRef]
12. Liu, J.; McCleland, M.; Stawiski, E.W.; Gnad, F.; Mayba, O.; Haverty, P.M.; Durinck, S.; Chen, Y.-J.; Klijn, C.; Jhunjhunwala, S.; et al. Integrated Exome and Transcriptome Sequencing Reveals ZAK Isoform Usage in Gastric Cancer. *Nat. Commun.* **2014**, *5*, 3830. [CrossRef]
13. Roviello, F.; Marano, L.; Ambrosio, M.R.; Resca, L.; D'Ignazio, A.; Petrelli, F.; Petrioli, R.; Costantini, M.; Polom, K.; Macchiarelli, R.; et al. Signet Ring Cell Percentage in Poorly Cohesive Gastric Cancer Patients: A Potential Novel Predictor of Survival. *Eur. J. Surg. Oncol.* **2022**, *48*, 561–569. [CrossRef]
14. Marano, L.; Ambrosio, M.R.; Resca, L.; Carbone, L.; Carpineto Samorani, O.; Petrioli, R.; Savelli, V.; Costantini, M.; Malaspina, L.; Polom, K.; et al. The Percentage of Signet Ring Cells Is Inversely Related to Aggressive Behavior and Poor Prognosis in Mixed-Type Gastric Cancer. *Front. Oncol.* **2022**, *12*, 897218. [CrossRef]

15. Kim, H.-H.; Han, S.-U.; Kim, M.-C.; Hyung, W.J.; Kim, W.; Lee, H.-J.; Ryu, S.W.; Cho, G.S.; Song, K.Y.; Ryu, S.Y. Long-Term Results of Laparoscopic Gastrectomy for Gastric Cancer: A Large-Scale Case-Control and Case-Matched Korean Multicenter Study. *J. Clin. Oncol.* **2014**, *32*, 627–633. [CrossRef]
16. Polom, W.; Markuszewski, M.; Rho, Y.S.; Matuszewski, M. Use of Invisible near Infrared Light Fluorescence with Indocyanine Green and Methylene Blue in Urology. Part 2. *Cent. Eur. J. Urol.* **2014**, *67*, 310–313. [CrossRef]
17. Voyant, C.; Julian, D.; Roustit, R.; Biffi, K.; Lantieri, C. Biological Effects and Equivalent Doses in Radiotherapy: A Software Solution. *Rep. Pract. Oncol. Radiother.* **2014**, *19*, 47–55. [CrossRef]
18. Polom, K.; Marano, L.; Marrelli, D.; De Luca, R.; Roviello, G.; Savelli, V.; Tan, P.; Roviello, F. Meta-Analysis of Microsatellite Instability in Relation to Clinicopathological Characteristics and Overall Survival in Gastric Cancer. *Br. J. Surg.* **2018**, *105*, 159–167 [CrossRef]
19. Polom, K.; Marrelli, D.; Pascale, V.; Ferrara, F.; Voglino, C.; Marini, M.; Roviello, F. The Pattern of Lymph Node Metastases in Microsatellite Unstable Gastric Cancer. *Eur. J. Surg. Oncol.* **2017**, *43*, 2341–2348. [CrossRef]
20. Furukawa, K.; Hatakeyama, K.; Terashima, M.; Nagashima, T.; Urakami, K.; Ohshima, K.; Notsu, A.; Sugino, T.; Yagi, T.; Fujiya, K.; et al. Molecular Classification of Gastric Cancer Predicts Survival in Patients Undergoing Radical Gastrectomy Based on Project HOPE. *Gastric Cancer* **2022**, *25*, 138–148. [CrossRef]
21. Marano, L.; Fusario, D.; Savelli, V.; Marrelli, D.; Roviello, F. Robotic versus Laparoscopic Gastrectomy for Gastric Cancer: An Umbrella Review of Systematic Reviews and Meta-Analyses. *Updat. Surg.* **2021**, *73*, 1673–1689. [CrossRef] [PubMed]
22. Marano, L.; Ricci, A.; Savelli, V.; Verre, L.; Di Renzo, L.; Biccari, E.; Costantini, G.; Marrelli, D.; Roviello, F. From Digital World to Real Life: A Robotic Approach to the Esophagogastric Junction with a 3D Printed Model. *BMC Surg.* **2019**, *19*, 153. [CrossRef] [PubMed]
23. Verlato, G.; Roviello, F.; Marchet, A.; Giacopuzzi, S.; Marrelli, D.; Nitti, D.; de Manzoni, G. Indexes of Surgical Quality in Gastric Cancer Surgery: Experience of an Italian Network. *Ann. Surg. Oncol.* **2009**, *16*, 594–602. [CrossRef] [PubMed]
24. Sant, M.; Allemani, C.; Santaquilani, M.; Knijn, A.; Marchesi, F.; Capocaccia, R.; EUROCARE Working Group EUROCARE-4 Survival of Cancer Patients Diagnosed in 1995–1999. Results and Commentary. *Eur. J. Cancer* **2009**, *45*, 931–991. [CrossRef]
25. Dikken, J.L.; Stiekema, J.; van de Velde, C.J.H.; Verheij, M.; Cats, A.; Wouters, M.W.J.M.; van Sandick, J.W. Quality of Care Indicators for the Surgical Treatment of Gastric Cancer: A Systematic Review. *Ann. Surg. Oncol.* **2013**, *20*, 381–398. [CrossRef]
26. Lepage, C.; Sant, M.; Verdecchia, A.; Forman, D.; Esteve, J.; Faivre, J. Operative Mortality after Gastric Cancer Resection and Long-Term Survival Differences across Europe. *Br. J. Surg.* **2010**, *97*, 235–239. [CrossRef]
27. Peeters, K.C.M.J.; van de Velde, C.J.H. Quality Assurance of Surgery in Gastric and Rectal Cancer. *Crit. Rev. Oncol. Hematol.* **2004** *51*, 105–119. [CrossRef]
28. Luft, H.S.; Bunker, J.P.; Enthoven, A.C. Should Operations Be Regionalized? *N. Engl. J. Med.* **1979**, *301*, 1364–1369. [CrossRef]
29. Chowdhury, M.M.; Dagash, H.; Pierro, A. A Systematic Review of the Impact of Volume of Surgery and Specialization on Patient Outcome. *Br. J. Surg.* **2007**, *94*, 145–161. [CrossRef]
30. Busweiler, L.A.D.; Dikken, J.L.; Henneman, D.; van Berge Henegouwen, M.I.; Ho, V.K.Y.; Tollenaar, R.A.E.M.; Wouters, M.W.J.M. van Sandick, J.W. The Influence of a Composite Hospital Volume on Outcomes for Gastric Cancer Surgery: A Dutch Population based Study. *J. Surg. Oncol.* **2017**, *115*, 738–745. [CrossRef]
31. Birkmeyer, J.D.; Sun, Y.; Wong, S.L.; Stukel, T.A. Hospital Volume and Late Survival after Cancer Surgery. *Ann. Surg.* **2007**, *245* 777–783. [CrossRef]
32. Institute of Medicine (US); National Research Council (US) National Cancer Policy Board. *Ensuring Quality Cancer Care*; National Academies Press: Washington, DC, USA, 1999; ISBN 978-0-309-06480-4.
33. Birkmeyer, J.D.; Dimick, J.B. Potential Benefits of the New Leapfrog Standards: Effect of Process and Outcomes Measures. *Surgery* **2004**, *135*, 569–575. [CrossRef]
34. Dixon, M.; Mahar, A.; Paszat, L.; McLeod, R.; Law, C.; Swallow, C.; Helyer, L.; Seeveratnam, R.; Cardoso, R.; Bekaii-Saab, T. et al. What Provider Volumes and Characteristics Are Appropriate for Gastric Cancer Resection? Results of an International RAND/UCLA Expert Panel. *Surgery* **2013**, *154*, 1100–1109. [CrossRef]
35. Choi, H.; Yang, S.-Y.; Cho, H.-S.; Kim, W.; Park, E.-C.; Han, K.-T. Mortality Differences by Surgical Volume among Patients with Stomach Cancer: A Threshold for a Favorable Volume-Outcome Relationship. *World J. Surg. Oncol.* **2017**, *15*, 134. [CrossRef]
36. Bilimoria, K.Y.; Bentrem, D.J.; Feinglass, J.M.; Stewart, A.K.; Winchester, D.P.; Talamonti, M.S.; Ko, C.Y. Directing Surgical Quality Improvement Initiatives: Comparison of Perioperative Mortality and Long-Term Survival for Cancer Surgery. *J. Clin. Oncol.* **2008** *26*, 4626–4633. [CrossRef]
37. Gabriel, E.; Narayanan, S.; Attwood, K.; Hochwald, S.; Kukar, M.; Nurkin, S. Disparities in Major Surgery for Esophagogastric Cancer among Hospitals by Case Volume. *J. Gastrointest. Oncol.* **2018**, *9*, 503–516. [CrossRef]
38. Jensen, L.S.; Nielsen, H.; Mortensen, P.B.; Pilegaard, H.K.; Johnsen, S.P. Enforcing Centralization for Gastric Cancer in Denmark. *Eur. J. Surg. Oncol. (EJSO)* **2010**, *36*, S50–S54. [CrossRef]
39. Claassen, Y.H.M.; van Sandick, J.W.; Hartgrink, H.H.; Dikken, J.L.; De Steur, W.O.; van Grieken, N.C.T.; Boot, H.; Cats, A.; Trip A.K.; Jansen, E.P.M.; et al. Association between Hospital Volume and Quality of Gastric Cancer Surgery in the CRITICS Trial. *Br J. Surg.* **2018**, *105*, 728–735. [CrossRef]
40. Callahan, M.A.; Christos, P.J.; Gold, H.T.; Mushlin, A.I.; Daly, J.M. Influence of Surgical Subspecialty Training on In-Hospital Mortality for Gastrectomy and Colectomy Patients. *Ann. Surg.* **2003**, *238*, 629–636, discussion 636–639. [CrossRef]

41. Smith, D.L.; Elting, L.S.; Learn, P.A.; Raut, C.P.; Mansfield, P.F. Factors Influencing the Volume-Outcome Relationship in Gastrectomies: A Population-Based Study. *Ann. Surg. Oncol.* **2007**, *14*, 1846–1852. [CrossRef]
42. Ju, M.R.; Blackwell, J.-M.; Zeh, H.J.; Yopp, A.C.; Wang, S.C.; Porembka, M.R. Redefining High-Volume Gastric Cancer Centers: The Impact of Operative Volume on Surgical Outcomes. *Ann. Surg. Oncol.* **2021**, *28*, 4839–4847. [CrossRef] [PubMed]
43. Hannan, E.L.; Radzyner, M.; Rubin, D.; Dougherty, J.; Brennan, M.F. The Influence of Hospital and Surgeon Volume on In-Hospital Mortality for Colectomy, Gastrectomy, and Lung Lobectomy in Patients with Cancer. *Surgery* **2002**, *131*, 6–15. [CrossRef] [PubMed]
44. Ghaferi, A.A.; Birkmeyer, J.D.; Dimick, J.B. Complications, Failure to Rescue, and Mortality with Major Inpatient Surgery in Medicare Patients. *Ann. Surg.* **2009**, *250*, 1029–1034. [CrossRef] [PubMed]
45. Sabesan, A.; Petrelli, N.J.; Bennett, J.J. Outcomes of gastric cancer resections performed in a high volume community cancer center. Surgical oncology. *Surg. Oncol.* **2015**, *24*, 16–20. [CrossRef]
46. Brar, S.S.; Mahar, A.L.; Helyer, L.K.; Swallow, C.; Law, C.; Paszat, L.; Seevaratnam, R.; Cardoso, R.; McLeod, R.; Dixon, M.; et al. Processes of Care in the Multidisciplinary Treatment of Gastric Cancer: Results of a RAND/UCLA Expert Panel. *JAMA Surg.* **2014**, *149*, 18–25. [CrossRef]
47. DICA Jaarrapportage 2014-DUCA. Available online: https://dica.nl/jaarrapportage-2014/duca.html (accessed on 1 December 2019).
48. Amato, L.; Fusco, D.; Acampora, A.; Bontempi, K.; Rosa, A.C.; Colais, P.; Cruciani, F.; D'Ovidio, M.; Mataloni, F.; Minozzi, S.; et al. Volume and Health Outcomes: Evidence from Systematic Reviews and from Evaluation of Italian Hospital Data. *Epidemiol. Prev.* **2013**, *41*, 1–128. [CrossRef]
49. Geraedts, M.; de Cruppé, W.; Blum, K.; Ohmann, C. Implementation and Effects of Germany's Minimum Volume Regulations: Results of the Accompanying Research. *Dtsch. Arztebl. Int.* **2008**, *105*, 890–896. [CrossRef]
50. Mamidanna, R.; Ni, Z.; Anderson, O.; Spiegelhalter, S.D.; Bottle, A.; Aylin, P.; Faiz, O.; Hanna, G.B. Surgeon Volume and Cancer Esophagectomy, Gastrectomy, and Pancreatectomy: A Population-Based Study in England. *Ann. Surg.* **2016**, *263*, 727–732. [CrossRef]
51. Dikken, J.L.; Dassen, A.E.; Lemmens, V.E.P.; Putter, H.; Krijnen, P.; van der Geest, L.; Bosscha, K.; Verheij, M.; van de Velde, C.J.H.; Wouters, M.W.J.M. Effect of Hospital Volume on Postoperative Mortality and Survival after Oesophageal and Gastric Cancer Surgery in the Netherlands between 1989 and 2009. *Eur. J. Cancer* **2012**, *48*, 1004–1013. [CrossRef]
52. Langer, B. Role of Volume Outcome Data in Assuring Quality in HPB Surgery. *HPB* **2007**, *9*, 330–334. [CrossRef]
53. Modrall, J.G.; Minter, R.M.; Minhajuddin, A.; Eslava-Schmalbach, J.; Joshi, G.P.; Patel, S.; Rosero, E.B. The Surgeon Volume-Outcome Relationship. *Ann. Surg.* **2018**, *267*, 863–867. [CrossRef]
54. Balentine, C.J.; Naik, A.D.; Robinson, C.N.; Petersen, N.J.; Chen, G.J.; Berger, D.H.; Anaya, D.A. Association of High-Volume Hospitals with Greater Likelihood of Discharge to Home Following Colorectal Surgery. *JAMA Surg.* **2014**, *149*, 244. [CrossRef]
55. Sutton, J.M.; Hoehn, R.S.; Ertel, A.E.; Wilson, G.C.; Hanseman, D.J.; Wima, K.; Sussman, J.J.; Ahmad, S.A.; Shah, S.A.; Abbott, D.E. Cost-Effectiveness in Hepatic Lobectomy: The Effect of Case Volume on Mortality, Readmission, and Cost of Care. *J. Gastrointest. Surg.* **2016**, *20*, 253–261. [CrossRef]
56. Gourin, C.G.; Stewart, C.M.; Frick, K.D.; Fakhry, C.; Pitman, K.T.; Eisele, D.W.; Austin, J.M. Association of Hospital Volume with Laryngectomy Outcomes in Patients with Larynx Cancer. *JAMA Otolaryngol. Head Neck Surg.* **2019**, *145*, 62. [CrossRef]
57. Odagiri, H.; Yasunaga, H.; Matsui, H.; Matsui, S.; Fushimi, K.; Kaise, M. Hospital Volume and Adverse Events Following Esophageal Endoscopic Submucosal Dissection in Japan. *Endoscopy* **2016**, *49*, 321–326. [CrossRef]
58. Borowski, D.W.; Bradburn, D.M.; Mills, S.J.; Bharathan, B.; Wilson, R.G.; Ratcliffe, A.A.; Kelly, S.B. Volume–Outcome Analysis of Colorectal Cancer-Related Outcomes. *Br. J. Surg.* **2010**, *97*, 1416–1430. [CrossRef]
59. Van der Werf, L.R.; Cords, C.; Arntz, I.; Belt, E.J.T.; Cherepanin, I.M.; Coene, P.-P.L.O.; van der Harst, E.; Heisterkamp, J.; Langenhoff, B.S.; Lamme, B.; et al. Population-Based Study on Risk Factors for Tumor-Positive Resection Margins in Patients with Gastric Cancer. *Ann. Surg. Oncol.* **2019**, *26*, 2222–2233. [CrossRef]
60. Levaillant, M.; Marcilly, R.; Levaillant, L.; Michel, P.; Hamel-Broza, J.-F.; Vallet, B.; Lamer, A. Assessing the Hospital Volume-Outcome Relationship in Surgery: A Scoping Review. *BMC Med. Res. Methodol.* **2021**, *21*, 204. [CrossRef]
61. Kim, W.; Wolff, S.; Ho, V. Measuring the Volume-Outcome Relation for Complex Hospital Surgery. *Appl. Health Econ. Health Policy* **2016**, *14*, 453–464. [CrossRef]
62. Baiocchi, G.L.; Giacopuzzi, S.; Marrelli, D.; Reim, D.; Piessen, G.; Matos da Costa, P.; Reynolds, J.V.; Meyer, H.-J.; Morgagni, P.; Gockel, I.; et al. International Consensus on a Complications List after Gastrectomy for Cancer. *Gastric Cancer* **2019**, *22*, 172–189. [CrossRef]
63. Kim, Y.-I.; Lee, J.Y.; Khalayleh, H.; Kim, C.G.; Yoon, H.M.; Kim, S.J.; Yang, H.; Ryu, K.W.; Choi, I.J.; Kim, Y.-W. Efficacy of Endoscopic Management for Anastomotic Leakage after Gastrectomy in Patients with Gastric Cancer. *Surg. Endosc.* **2022**, *36*, 2896–2905. [CrossRef] [PubMed]
64. Messager, M.; Warlaumont, M.; Renaud, F.; Marin, H.; Branche, J.; Piessen, G.; Mariette, C. Recent Improvements in the Management of Esophageal Anastomotic Leak after Surgery for Cancer. *Eur. J. Surg. Oncol. (EJSO)* **2017**, *43*, 258–269. [CrossRef] [PubMed]
65. Fulop, N.J.; Ramsay, A.I.G.; Vindrola-Padros, C.; Aitchison, M.; Boaden, R.J.; Brinton, V.; Clarke, C.S.; Hines, J.; Hunter, R.M.; Levermore, C.; et al. Reorganising Specialist Cancer Surgery for the Twenty-First Century: A Mixed Methods Evaluation (RESPECT-21). *Implement. Sci.* **2016**, *11*, 155. [CrossRef] [PubMed]
66. Melnychuk, M.; Vindrola-Padros, C.; Aitchison, M.; Clarke, C.S.; Fulop, N.J.; Levermore, C.; Maddineni, S.B.; Moore, C.M.; Mughal, M.M.; Perry, C.; et al. Centralising Specialist Cancer Surgery Services in England: Survey of Factors That Matter to Patients and Carers and Health Professionals. *BMC Cancer* **2018**, *18*, 226. [CrossRef] [PubMed]

67. Hu, H.-T.; Ma, F.-H.; Xiong, J.-P.; Li, Y.; Jin, P.; Liu, H.; Ma, S.; Kang, W.-Z.; Tian, Y.-T. Laparoscopic vs. Open Total Gastrectomy for Advanced Gastric Cancer Following Neoadjuvant Therapy: A Propensity Score Matching Analysis. *World J. Gastrointest. Surg.* **2022**, *14*, 161–173. [CrossRef]
68. Huang, C.; Liu, H.; Hu, Y.; Sun, Y.; Su, X.; Cao, H.; Hu, J.; Wang, K.; Suo, J.; Tao, K.; et al. Laparoscopic vs. Open Distal Gastrectomy for Locally Advanced Gastric Cancer: Five-Year Outcomes From the CLASS-01 Randomized Clinical Trial. *JAMA Surg.* **2022**, *157*, 9. [CrossRef]
69. Son, S.-Y.; Hur, H.; Hyung, W.J.; Park, Y.-K.; Lee, H.-J.; An, J.Y.; Kim, W.; Kim, H.-I.; Kim, H.-H.; Ryu, S.W.; et al. Laparoscopic vs Open Distal Gastrectomy for Locally Advanced Gastric Cancer: 5-Year Outcomes of the KLASS-02 Randomized Clinical Trial. *JAMA Surg.* **2022**, *157*, 879. [CrossRef]
70. Collins, J.W.; Ghazi, A.; Stoyanov, D.; Hung, A.; Coleman, M.; Cecil, T.; Ericsson, A.; Anvari, M.; Wang, Y.; Beaulieu, Y.; et al. Utilising an Accelerated Delphi Process to Develop Guidance and Protocols for Telepresence Applications in Remote Robotic Surgery Training. *Eur. Urol. Open Sci.* **2020**, *22*, 23–33. [CrossRef]
71. Rokni, L.; Yun, J.-Y. Healthcare Mobility between East and West, Two Forthcoming Challenges. *Iran J. Public Health* **2017**, *46*, 1437–1439.
72. Marano, L.; Carbone, L.; Poto, G.E.; Restaino, V.; Piccioni, S.A.; Verre, L.; Roviello, F.; Marrelli, D. Extended Lymphadenectomy for Gastric Cancer in the Neoadjuvant Era: Current Status, Clinical Implications and Contentious Issues. *Curr. Oncol.* **2023**, *30*, 875–896. [CrossRef]
73. Thompson, A.M.; Rapson, T.; Gilbert, F.J.; Park, K.G.M. Hospital Volume Does Not Influence Long-Term Survival of Patients Undergoing Surgery for Oesophageal or Gastric Cancer. *Br. J. Surg.* **2007**, *94*, 578–584. [CrossRef]
74. Chan, D.S.Y.; Reid, T.D.; White, C.; Willicombe, A.; Blackshaw, G.; Clark, G.W.; Havard, T.J.; Escofet, X.; Crosby, T.D.L.; Roberts, S.A.; et al. Influence of a Regional Centralised Upper Gastrointestinal Cancer Service Model on Patient Safety, Quality of Care and Survival. *Clin. Oncol. R Coll. Radiol.* **2013**, *25*, 719–725. [CrossRef]
75. Boddy, A.P.; Williamson, J.M.L.; Vipond, M.N. The Effect of Centralisation on the Outcomes of Oesophagogastric Surgery—A Fifteen Year Audit. *Int. J. Surg.* **2012**, *10*, 360–363. [CrossRef]
76. Coupland, V.H.; Lagergren, J.; Lüchtenborg, M.; Jack, R.H.; Allum, W.; Holmberg, L.; Hanna, G.B.; Pearce, N.; Møller, H. Hospital Volume, Proportion Resected and Mortality from Oesophageal and Gastric Cancer: A Population-Based Study in England 2004–2008. *Gut* **2013**, *62*, 961–966. [CrossRef]
77. Nelen, S.D.; Heuthorst, L.; Verhoeven, R.H.A.; Polat, F.; Kruyt, P.M.; Reijnders, K.; Ferenschild, F.T.J.; Bonenkamp, J.J.; Rutter, J.E.; de Wilt, J.H.W.; et al. Impact of Centralizing Gastric Cancer Surgery on Treatment, Morbidity, and Mortality. *J. Gastrointest. Surg.* **2017**, *21*, 2000–2008. [CrossRef]
78. Degiuli, M.; Sasako, M.; Ponti, A. Italian Gastric Cancer Study Group Morbidity and Mortality in the Italian Gastric Cancer Study Group Randomized Clinical Trial of D1 versus D2 Resection for Gastric Cancer. *Br. J. Surg.* **2010**, *97*, 643–649. [CrossRef]
79. Evrard, S.; Audisio, R.; Poston, G.; Caballero, C.; Kataoka, K.; Fontein, D.; Collette, L.; Nakamura, K.; Fukuda, H.; Lacombe, D. From a Comic Opera to Surcare an Open Letter to Whom Clinical Research in Surgery Is a Concern: Announcing the Launch of SURCARE. *Ann. Surg.* **2016**, *264*, 911–912. [CrossRef]
80. Tanis, E.; Caballero, C.; Collette, L.; Verleye, L.; den Dulk, M.; Lacombe, D.; Schuhmacher, C.; Werutsky, G. The European Organization for Research and Treatment for Cancer (EORTC) Strategy for Quality Assurance in Surgical Clinical Research Assessment of the Past and Moving towards the Future. *Eur. J. Surg. Oncol.* **2016**, *42*, 1115–1122. [CrossRef]
81. Japanese Gastric Cancer Association, J.G.C. Japanese Gastric Cancer Treatment Guidelines 2014 (Ver. 4). *Gastric Cancer* **2017**, *20*, 1–19. [CrossRef]
82. Zhang, K.C.; Chen, L. Emphasis on Standardization of Minimally Invasive Surgery for Gastric Cancer. *Zhonghua Wai Ke Za Zhi* **2018**, *56*, 262–264.
83. Papenfuss, W.A.; Kukar, M.; Oxenberg, J.; Attwood, K.; Nurkin, S.; Malhotra, U.; Wilkinson, N.W. Morbidity and Mortality Associated with Gastrectomy for Gastric Cancer. *Ann. Surg. Oncol.* **2014**, *21*, 3008–3014. [CrossRef] [PubMed]
84. American College of Surgeons National Surgical Quality Improvement Program. Available online: https://www.facs.org/quality-programs/data-and-registries/acs-nsqip/ (accessed on 7 November 2022).
85. Boccardi, V.; Marano, L. The Geriatric Surgery: The Importance of Frailty Identification Beyond Chronological Age. *Geriatrics* **2020**, *5*, 12. [CrossRef] [PubMed]
86. Marano, L.; Carbone, L.; Poto, G.E.; Gambelli, M.; Nguefack Noudem, L.L.; Grassi, G.; Manasci, F.; Curreri, G.; Giuliani, A.; Piagnerelli, R.; et al. Handgrip Strength Predicts Length of Hospital Stay in an Abdominal Surgical Setting: The Role of Frailty beyond Age. *Aging Clin. Exp. Res.* **2022**, *34*, 811–817. [CrossRef] [PubMed]
87. Siriwardena, A.K. Centralisation of Upper Gastrointestinal Cancer Surgery. *Ann. R. Coll. Surg. Engl.* **2007**, *89*, 335–336. [CrossRef] [PubMed]
88. Mesman, R.; Westert, G.P.; Berden, B.J.M.M.; Faber, M.J. Why Do High-Volume Hospitals Achieve Better Outcomes? A Systematic Review about Intermediate Factors in Volume-Outcome Relationships. *Health Policy* **2015**, *119*, 1055–1067. [CrossRef]
89. Halm, E.A.; Lee, C.; Chassin, M.R. Is Volume Related to Outcome in Health Care? A Systematic Review and Methodologic Critique of the Literature. *Ann. Intern. Med.* **2002**, *137*, 511–520. [CrossRef]
90. Finlayson, S.R.G. The Volume-Outcome Debate Revisited. *Am. Surg.* **2006**, *72*, 1038–1042, discussion 1061–1069, 1133–1148. [CrossRef]

91. Van Vliet, E.P.M.; Hermans, J.J.; De Wever, W.; Eijkemans, M.J.C.; Steyerberg, E.W.; Faasse, C.; van Helmond, E.P.M.; de Leeuw, A.M.; Sikkenk, A.C.; de Vries, A.R.; et al. Radiologist Experience and CT Examination Quality Determine Metastasis Detection in Patients with Esophageal or Gastric Cardia Cancer. *Eur. Radiol.* **2008**, *18*, 2475–2484. [CrossRef]
92. Pronovost, P.J.; Angus, D.C.; Dorman, T.; Robinson, K.A.; Dremsizov, T.T.; Young, T.L. Physician Staffing Patterns and Clinical Outcomes in Critically Ill Patients: A Systematic Review. *JAMA* **2002**, *288*, 2151–2162. [CrossRef]
93. Needleman, J.; Buerhaus, P.; Mattke, S.; Stewart, M.; Zelevinsky, K. Nurse-Staffing Levels and the Quality of Care in Hospitals. *N. Engl. J. Med.* **2002**, *346*, 1715–1722. [CrossRef]
94. Ghaferi, A.A.; Birkmeyer, J.D.; Dimick, J.B. Hospital Volume and Failure to Rescue with High-Risk Surgery. *Med. Care* **2011**, *49*, 1076–1081. [CrossRef]
95. Koëter, M.; van Steenbergen, L.N.; Lemmens, V.E.P.P.; Rutten, H.J.T.; Roukema, J.A.; Wijnhoven, B.P.L.; Nieuwenhuijzen, G.A.P. Hospital of Diagnosis and Probability to Receive a Curative Treatment for Oesophageal Cancer. *Eur. J. Surg. Oncol.* **2014**, *40*, 1338–1345. [CrossRef]
96. Svederud, I.; Virhage, M.; Medin, E.; Grundström, J.; Friberg, S.; Ramsberg, J. Patient Perspectives on Centralisation of Low Volume, Highly Specialised Procedures in Sweden. *Health Policy* **2015**, *119*, 1068–1075. [CrossRef]
97. Vallejo-Torres, L.; Melnychuk, M.; Vindrola-Padros, C.; Aitchison, M.; Clarke, C.S.; Fulop, N.J.; Hines, J.; Levermore, C.; Maddineni, S.B.; Perry, C.; et al. Discrete-Choice Experiment to Analyse Preferences for Centralizing Specialist Cancer Surgery Services. *Br. J. Surg.* **2018**, *105*, 587–596. [CrossRef]
98. Choi, Y.Y.; Cheong, J.H. Beyond precision surgery: Molecularly motivated precision care for gastric cancer. *Eur. J. Surg. Oncol.* **2017**, *43*, 856–864. [CrossRef]
99. Finlayson, E.V.A. Hospital Volume and Operative Mortality in Cancer Surgery. *Arch. Surg.* **2003**, *138*, 721. [CrossRef]
100. Learn, P.A.; Bach, P.B. A Decade of Mortality Reductions in Major Oncologic Surgery: The Impact of Centralization and Quality Improvement. *Med. Care* **2010**, *48*, 1041–1049. [CrossRef]
101. Smith, J.K.; McPhee, J.T.; Hill, J.S.; Whalen, G.F.; Sullivan, M.E.; Litwin, D.E.; Anderson, F.A.; Tseng, J.F. National Outcomes after Gastric Resection for Neoplasm. *Arch. Surg.* **2007**, *142*, 387–393. [CrossRef]
102. Van Putten, M.; Nelen, S.D.; Lemmens, V.E.P.P.; Stoot, J.H.M.B.; Hartgrink, H.H.; Gisbertz, S.S.; Spillenaar Bilgen, E.J.; Heisterkamp, J.; Verhoeven, R.H.A.; Nieuwenhuijzen, G.A.P. Overall Survival before and after Centralization of Gastric Cancer Surgery in the Netherlands. *Br. J. Surg.* **2018**, *105*, 1807–1815. [CrossRef]
103. Claassen, Y.H.M.; van Amelsfoort, R.M.; Hartgrink, H.H.; Dikken, J.L.; de Steur, W.O.; van Sandick, J.W.; van Grieken, N.C.T.; Cats, A.; Boot, H.; Trip, A.K.; et al. Effect of Hospital Volume with Respect to Performing Gastric Cancer Resection on Recurrence and Survival. *Ann. Surg.* **2019**, *270*, 1096–1102. [CrossRef]
104. Agnes, A.; Lorenzon, L.; Belia, F.; Biondi, A.; D'Ugo, D. Impact of Hospital and Surgeon Volume on the Outcomes of Gastric Cancer Surgery. In *Gastric Cancer: The 25-Year R-Evolution*; Springer: Berlin/Heidelberg, Germany, 2021; pp. 127–136. ISBN 978-3-030-73157-1.
105. Diers, J.; Baum, P.; Wagner, J.C.; Matthes, H.; Pietryga, S.; Baumann, N.; Uttinger, K.; Germer, C.-T.; Wiegering, A. Hospital Volume Following Major Surgery for Gastric Cancer Determines In-Hospital Mortality Rate and Failure to Rescue: A Nation-Wide Study Based on German Billing Data (2009–2017). *Gastric Cancer* **2021**, *24*, 959–969. [CrossRef] [PubMed]
106. Fischer, C.; Lingsma, H.; Klazinga, N.; Hardwick, R.; Cromwell, D.; Steyerberg, E.; Groene, O. Volume-Outcome Revisited: The Effect of Hospital and Surgeon Volumes on Multiple Outcome Measures in Oesophago-Gastric Cancer Surgery. *PLoS ONE* **2017**, *12*, e0183955. [CrossRef]
107. Nimptsch, U.; Haist, T.; Gockel, I.; Mansky, T.; Lorenz, D. Complex Gastric Surgery in Germany—Is Centralization Beneficial? Observational Study Using National Hospital Discharge Data. *Langenbecks Arch. Surg.* **2019**, *404*, 93–101. [CrossRef] [PubMed]
108. Wu, J.-M.; Ho, T.-W.; Tien, Y.-W. Correlation Between the Increased Hospital Volume and Decreased Overall Perioperative Mortality in One Universal Health Care System. *World J. Surg.* **2019**, *43*, 2194–2202. [CrossRef] [PubMed]
109. Pasquer, A.; Renaud, F.; Hec, F.; Gandon, A.; Vanderbeken, M.; Drubay, V.; Caranhac, G.; Piessen, G.; Mariette, C. FREGAT Working GroupFRENCH Is Centralization Needed for Esophageal and Gastric Cancer Patients with Low Operative Risk? *Ann. Surg.* **2016**, *264*, 823–830. [CrossRef]
110. Iwatsuki, M.; Yamamoto, H.; Miyata, H.; Kakeji, Y.; Yoshida, K.; Konno, H.; Seto, Y.; Baba, H. Effect of Hospital and Surgeon Volume on Postoperative Outcomes after Distal Gastrectomy for Gastric Cancer Based on Data from 145,523 Japanese Patients Collected from a Nationwide Web-Based Data Entry System. *Gastric Cancer* **2019**, *22*, 190–201. [CrossRef]
111. Marano, L.; Carbone, L.; Poto, G.E.; Calomino, N.; Neri, A.; Piagnerelli, R.; Fontani, A.; Verre, L.; Savelli, V.; Roviello, F.; et al. Antimicrobial Prophylaxis Reduces the Rate of Surgical Site Infection in Upper Gastrointestinal Surgery: A Systematic Review. *Antibiotics* **2022**, *11*, 230. [CrossRef]
112. Iwatsuki, M.; Yamamoto, H.; Miyata, H.; Kakeji, Y.; Yoshida, K.; Konno, H.; Seto, Y.; Baba, H. Association of Surgeon and Hospital Volume with Postoperative Mortality after Total Gastrectomy for Gastric Cancer: Data from 71,307 Japanese Patients Collected from a Nationwide Web-Based Data Entry System. *Gastric Cancer* **2021**, *24*, 526–534. [CrossRef]
113. Diaconis, P.; Mosteller, F. *Methods for Studying Coincidences*; Springer: New York, NY, USA, 1989; pp. 853–961. [CrossRef]
114. Mehta, A.; Efron, D.T.; Canner, J.K.; Dultz, L.; Xu, T.; Jones, C.; Haut, E.R.; Higgins, R.S.D.; Sakran, J.V. Effect of Surgeon and Hospital Volume on Emergency General Surgery Outcomes. *J. Am. Coll. Surg.* **2017**, *225*, 666–675.e2. [CrossRef]

115. Liang, Y.; Wu, L.; Wang, X.; Ding, X.; Liang, H. The Positive Impact of Surgeon Specialization on Survival for Gastric Cancer Patients after Surgery with Curative Intent. *Gastric Cancer* **2015**, *18*, 859–867. [CrossRef]
116. Bachmann, M.O.; Alderson, D.; Edwards, D.; Wotton, S.; Bedford, C.; Peters, T.J.; Harvey, I.M. Cohort Study in South and West England of the Influence of Specialization on the Management and Outcome of Patients with Oesophageal and Gastric Cancers *Br. J. Surg.* **2002**, *89*, 914–922. [CrossRef]
117. Parikh, D.; Johnson, M.; Chagla, L.; Lowe, D.; McCulloch, P. D2 Gastrectomy: Lessons from a Prospective Audit of the Learning Curve. *Br. J. Surg.* **2005**, *83*, 1595–1599. [CrossRef]
118. Degiuli, M.; Sasako, M.; Calgaro, M.; Garino, M.; Rebecchi, F.; Mineccia, M.; Scaglione, D.; Andreone, D.; Ponti, A.; Calvo, F. Morbidity and Mortality after D1 and D2 Gastrectomy for Cancer: Interim Analysis of the Italian Gastric Cancer Study Group (IGCSG) Randomised Surgical Trial. *Eur. J. Surg. Oncol. (EJSO)* **2004**, *30*, 303–308. [CrossRef]
119. Luna, A.; Rebasa, P.; Montmany, S.; Navarro, S. Learning Curve for D2 Lymphadenectomy in Gastric Cancer. *ISRN Surg.* **2013**, *2013*, 508719. [CrossRef]
120. Brenkman, H.J.F.; Ruurda, J.P.; Verhoeven, R.H.A.; van Hillegersberg, R. Safety and Feasibility of Minimally Invasive Gastrectomy during the Early Introduction in the Netherlands: Short-Term Oncological Outcomes Comparable to Open Gastrectomy. *Gastric Cancer* **2017**, *20*, 853–860. [CrossRef]
121. Lee, H.H.; Son, S.-Y.; Lee, J.H.; Kim, M.G.; Hur, H.; Park, D.J. Surgeon's Experience Overrides the Effect of Hospital Volume for Postoperative Outcomes of Laparoscopic Surgery in Gastric Cancer: Multi-Institutional Study. *Ann. Surg. Oncol.* **2017**, *24*, 1010–1017. [CrossRef]
122. Urbach, D.R.; Baxter, N.N. Does It Matter What a Hospital Is "High Volume" for? Specificity of Hospital Volume-Outcome Associations for Surgical Procedures: Analysis of Administrative Data. *BMJ* **2004**, *328*, 737–740. [CrossRef]
123. Ji, J.; Shi, L.; Ying, X.; Lu, X.; Shan, F. Associations of Annual Hospital and Surgeon Volume with Patient Outcomes After Gastrectomy: A Systematic Review and Meta-analysis. *Ann. Surg. Oncol.* **2022**, *29*, 8276–8297. [CrossRef]
124. Van der Hage, J.; Sandrucci, S.; Audisio, R.; Wyld, L.; Søreide, K.; Amaral, T.; Audisio, R.; Bahadoer, V.; Beets, G.; Benstead, K.; et al. The ESSO Core Curriculum Committee Update on Surgical Oncology. *Eur. J. Surg. Oncol.* **2021**, *47*, e1–e30. [CrossRef]
125. Jha, A.K. Back to the Future: Volume as a Quality Metric. *JAMA* **2015**, *314*, 214–215. [CrossRef]
126. Busweiler, L.A.D.; Schouwenburg, M.G.; van Berge Henegouwen, M.I.; Kolfschoten, N.E.; de Jong, P.C.; Rozema, T.; Wijnhoven, B.P.L.; van Hillegersberg, R.; Wouters, M.W.J.M.; van Sandick, J.W.; et al. Textbook Outcome as a Composite Measure in Oesophagogastric Cancer Surgery. *Br. J. Surg.* **2017**, *104*, 742–750. [CrossRef] [PubMed]
127. Messager, M.; de Steur, W.O.; van Sandick, J.W.; Reynolds, J.; Pera, M.; Mariette, C.; Hardwick, R.H.; Bastiaannet, E.; Boelens, P.G.; van deVelde, C.J.H.; et al. Variations among 5 European Countries for Curative Treatment of Resectable Oesophageal and Gastric Cancer: A Survey from the EURECCA Upper GI Group (EUropean REgistration of Cancer CAre). *Eur. J. Surg. Oncol.* **2016**, *42*, 116–122. [CrossRef] [PubMed]
128. Van der Kaaij, R.T.; de Rooij, M.V.; van Coevorden, F.; Voncken, F.E.M.; Snaebjornsson, P.; Boot, H.; van Sandick, J.W. Using Textbook Outcome as a Measure of Quality of Care in Oesophagogastric Cancer Surgery. *Br. J. Surg.* **2018**, *105*, 561–569. [CrossRef] [PubMed]
129. Van der Werf, L.R.; Wijnhoven, B.P.L.; Fransen, L.F.C.; van Sandick, J.W.; Nieuwenhuijzen, G.A.P.; Busweiler, L.A.D.; van Hillegersberg, R.; Wouters, M.W.J.M.; Luyer, M.D.P.; van Berge Henegouwen, M.I. A National Cohort Study Evaluating the Association Between Short-Term Outcomes and Long-Term Survival After Esophageal and Gastric Cancer Surgery. *Ann. Surg* **2019**, *270*, 868–876. [CrossRef] [PubMed]
130. Levy, J.; Gupta, V.; Amirazodi, E.; Allen-Ayodabo, C.; Jivraj, N.; Jeong, Y.; Davis, L.E.; Mahar, A.L.; De Mestral, C.; Saarela, O.; et al. Gastrectomy Case Volume and Textbook Outcome: An Analysis of the Population Registry of Esophageal and Stomach Tumours of Ontario (PRESTO). *Gastric Cancer* **2020**, *23*, 391–402. [CrossRef]
131. Levy, J.; Gupta, V.; Amirazodi, E.; Allen-Ayodabo, C.; Jivraj, N.; Jeong, Y.; Davis, L.E.; Mahar, A.L.; De Mestral, C.; Saarela, O.; et al. Textbook Outcome and Survival in Patients with Gastric Cancer. *Ann. Surg.* **2022**, *275*, 140–148. [CrossRef]
132. Vonlanthen, R.; Lodge, P.; Barkun, J.S.; Farges, O.; Rogiers, X.; Soreide, K.; Kehlet, H.; Reynolds, J.V.; Käser, S.A.; Naredi, P.; et al. Toward a Consensus on Centralization in Surgery. *Ann. Surg.* **2018**, *268*, 712–724. [CrossRef]
133. Choi, Y.Y.; Cho, M.; Kwon, I.G.; Son, T.; Kim, H.-I.; Choi, S.H.; Cheong, J.-H.; Hyung, W.J. Ten Thousand Consecutive Gastrectomies for Gastric Cancer: Perspectives of a Master Surgeon. *Yonsei Med. J.* **2019**, *60*, 235. [CrossRef]
134. Lorenzon, L.; Biondi, A.; Agnes, A.; Scrima, O.; Persiani, R.; D'Ugo, D. Quality Over Volume: Modeling Centralization of Gastric Cancer Resections in Italy. *J. Gastric Cancer* **2022**, *22*, 35. [CrossRef]
135. Birkmeyer, J.D.; Siewers, A.E.; Finlayson, E.V.A.; Stukel, T.A.; Lucas, F.L.; Batista, I.; Welch, H.G.; Wennberg, D.E. Hospital Volume and Surgical Mortality in the United States. *N. Engl. J. Med.* **2002**, *346*, 1128–1137. [CrossRef]
136. Birkmeyer, J.D.; Stukel, T.A.; Siewers, A.E.; Goodney, P.P.; Wennberg, D.E.; Lucas, F.L. Surgeon Volume and Operative Mortality in the United States. *N. Engl. J. Med.* **2003**, *349*, 2117–2127. [CrossRef]

Disclaimer/Publisher's Note: The statements, opinions and data contained in all publications are solely those of the individual author(s) and contributor(s) and not of MDPI and/or the editor(s). MDPI and/or the editor(s) disclaim responsibility for any injury to people or property resulting from any ideas, methods, instructions or products referred to in the content.

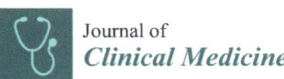

Review

The Effects of Tissue Healing Factors in Wound Repair Involving Absorbable Meshes: A Narrative Review

Varvara Vasalou [1,2], Efstathios Kotidis [1], Dimitris Tatsis [1,3], Kassiani Boulogeorgou [4], Ioannis Grivas [5], Georgios Koliakos [6], Angeliki Cheva [4], Orestis Ioannidis [1,*], Anastasia Tsingotjidou [5] and Stamatis Angelopoulos [1]

1. Fourth Surgical Department, School of Medicine, Aristotle University of Thessaloniki, 57010 Thessaloniki, Greece
2. Andreas Syggros Hospital, 11528 Athens, Greece
3. Oral and Maxillofacial Surgery Department, School of Dentistry, Aristotle University of Thessaloniki, 57010 Thessaloniki, Greece
4. Department of Pathology, School of Medicine, Aristotle University of Thessaloniki, 54124 Thessaloniki, Greece; siliaboulog@gmail.com (K.B.)
5. Laboratory of Anatomy, Histology & Embryology, School of Veterinary Medicine, Aristotle University of Thessaloniki, 54124 Thessaloniki, Greece
6. Department of Biochemistry, School of Medicine, Aristotle University of Thessaloniki, 54124 Thessaloniki, Greece
* Correspondence: telonakos@hotmail.com

Abstract: Wound healing is a complex and meticulously orchestrated process involving multiple phases and cellular interactions. This narrative review explores the intricate mechanisms behind wound healing, emphasizing the significance of cellular processes and molecular factors. The phases of wound healing are discussed, focusing on the roles of immune cells, growth factors, and extracellular matrix components. Cellular shape alterations driven by cytoskeletal modulation and the influence of the 'Formin' protein family are highlighted for their impact on wound healing processes. This review delves into the use of absorbable meshes in wound repair, discussing their categories and applications in different surgical scenarios. Interleukins (IL-2 and IL-6), CD31, CD34, platelet rich plasma (PRP), and adipose tissue-derived mesenchymal stem cells (ADSCs) are discussed in their respective roles in wound healing. The interactions between these factors and their potential synergies with absorbable meshes are explored, shedding light on how these combinations might enhance the healing process. Recent advances and challenges in the field are also presented, including insights into mesh integration, biocompatibility, infection prevention, and postoperative complications. This review underscores the importance of patient-specific factors and surgical techniques in optimizing mesh placement and healing outcomes. As wound healing remains a dynamic field, this narrative review provides a comprehensive overview of the current understanding and potential avenues for future research and clinical applications.

Keywords: IL-2; IL-6; CD31; CD34; absorbable meshes; tissue healing; wound repair

1. Introduction

The intricate process of wound healing involves a meticulous sequence of steps encompassing three fundamental phases: inflammation, proliferation, and remodeling [1,2]. During the inflammatory phase, neutrophils, monocytes, and macrophages are activated to eliminate cellular debris and counteract microbial intrusion, thereby averting infections [1,3,4]. The proliferative phase lasts three to 21 days, during which quiescent cells like fibroblasts, keratinocytes, and endothelial cells (ECs), which are involved in the re-epithelization process, proliferate and migrate to the site of injury [4,5]. Growth factors (GFs) like keratinocyte growth factor (KGF), transforming growth factor-β (TGF-β), and vascular endothelial growth factor (VEGF), along with cytokines like interleukin-1 (IL-1) and tumor necrosis factor-α (TNF-α) are also prominently expressed [3,6,7]. VEGF, for instance, instigates angiogenesis, ensuring nutrient supply to emerging tissue and orchestrating the reconstitution of the extracellular matrix (ECM) through synthesizing proteoglycans, collagen III, elastin, and laminin [4,6]. Finally, in the remodeling phase, spanning months to years, ECM undergoes gradual degradation, with type I collagen replacing type III collagen and a reorganization of dermal collagen fibers, processes under the precise regulation of matrix metalloproteinases (MMPs) and their inhibitors (TIMPs) that modulate apoptosis rates and new cell differentiation [3,4,8].

Throughout these phases, cellular shape and arrangement alterations are mediated by the modulation of cytoskeletal filaments, encompassing actin networks and microtubules, along with their specific binding proteins [9]. It provides mechanical support essential for determining polarity, inducing proliferation, promoting migration, enhancing differentiation, and maintaining proper functioning of the various types of cells synthesized in the wound bed [10–12], potentially orchestrated by the 'Formin' family, a protein group that becomes attached to microtubules and actins impacting on their nucleation, polymerization, and stabilization. As a result, different wound healing processes are regulated through these formin groups of proteins influencing cell polarity, chemotaxis, morphogenesis, proliferation, kinesis, proliferation, migration, and phagocytosis [13].

Wound healing is also involved in forming and remodeling new tissues through inflammation, which reduces the proliferation and migration of fibroblasts, which is vital for forming new tissues [14,15]. Activation and degranulation of platelets occur instantly after an injury, thus releasing chemokines and GFs (e.g., PDGF), which form a localized fibrin clot and suppress blood loss [3,4]. The spatial and temporal coordination of cytokines with various types of cells is crucial for tissue healing [13]. Wounding promotes changes in the function and dynamics of mitochondria, which modulate the downstream signals that participate in the wound healing process by generating reactive oxygen species (ROS), which affect protein function by regulating gene expression or post-transcriptional modifications [14].

Three categories of meshes are currently available for wound repair: non-absorbable synthetic meshes, absorbable synthetic meshes, and absorbable biological meshes [15,16] Absorbable meshes serve as scaffolds for regenerative functions such as the deposition of collagen, the promotion of growth of novel tissues leading to neovascularization, and the formation of a new mesothelial layer [16,17]. Absorbable synthetic meshes have advantages like consistent material characteristics, predictable resorption profiles, rapid tissue integration, and the promotion of rapid host bacterial clearance [18]. The classification of bioabsorbable meshes has been divided into three types based on strength loss versus absorption rates. The three categories include long-term meshes having high strength retaining potential but remaining in situ > 18 months; meshes losing strength in a period of 6–8 weeks; medium-term meshes where strengths are maintained for 3–4 months but the absorption rate is high allowing the mesh to be absorbed within a year [19]. For example the absorbable long-term polylactide mesh (LTS-mesh) demonstrated higher endurance (mechanically stable) and reduced formation of connective tissue than the absorbable short-term polyglactin mesh (PG-mesh) when applied in a standardized rat model of full-thickness abdominal wall defects [20]. Absorbable biological (Strattice, Surgisis, and Tachosil) or absorbable synthetic (Gore® Bio-A® and TIGR®) meshes have been employed for the repair of inguinal hernias (IHs) demonstrating lesser chronic pain and promising results in patients with a high risk of infections [16]. TIGR showed enhanced biocompatibility, lesser local tissue effects, better time-dependent mechanical, and enhanced overall performance when compared to a non-absorbable polypropylene mesh on implantation in a sheep model [21] and when used in Lichtenstein repair of lateral inguinal hernias (LIHs), was found to be safe, without recurrent infections, and with lesser pain and discomfort in patients [22]. Gore Bio-A, TIGR Matrix, and Phasix® meshes, when used to prevent or treat small, non-contaminated abdominal wall defects in experimental animals, were observed to be safe with no serious complications [23]. In treating incisional hernias, GORE BIO-A and Phasix meshes were reported to be safe in a surgical environment contaminated with microbes, both postoperatively and over a year later [24,25]. Treatment of paraesophageal hernias using laparoscopic crural reinforcement with synthetic or biological absorbable meshes resulted in an improved safety profile, with a majority of the patients remaining asymptomatic, with a good quality of life, lesser requirement of follow-up surgeries, and diminished long-term recurrence rates [26]. However, it has been noted that the mass of the meshes could substantially impact the occurrence of extended complications during the treatment of inguinal hernias (IHs), as opposed to the classification of the meshes as non-absorbable, partially absorbable, or completely absorbable [27].

Furthermore, diabetic individuals often face challenges in wound healing due to compromised blood circulation and reduced immune response. Absorbable meshes, serving as scaffolds, introduce a novel dimension to the healing process [28]. These meshes not only provide mechanical support to the wound site but also act as vehicles for the controlled release of growth factors and cytokines, thereby fostering a conducive environment for tissue regeneration. By influencing aspects like angiogenesis, collagen synthesis, and cell migration, these healing factors within the context of absorbable meshes can significantly expedite wound closure and minimize the risk of infection, offering renewed hope for enhanced recovery in diabetic patients grappling with chronic wounds.

The selection of an appropriate mesh type is guided by patient-specific factors, tissue characteristics, and the nature of the surgery. Optimal mesh integration with surrounding tissues is ensured through precise placement techniques, meticulous fixation, and proper sizing. The critical factors governing mesh biocompatibility and weight are the filament type, tensile strength, and porosity level. Notably, the actual tensile strength employed is lower than assumed. Meshes exhibit enhanced flexibility when lightweight, leading to diminished discomfort. Moreover, greater porosity has proven pivotal in reducing infections and shrinkage. Therefore, the most dependable choice is a lightweight mesh with substantial pores and minimal surface area [29].

Despite the advantages, attention needs to be given to postoperative complications of mesh integration, such as infections and seromas. Infections can manifest around the mesh, giving rise to symptoms such as redness, swelling, pain, and fever. Addressing these infections might necessitate antibiotic treatment and, in severe instances, even mesh removal [30]. Additionally, the formation of seromas can impede wound healing and heighten infection susceptibility [31]. Chronic pain at the mesh site, attributed to nerve irritation or entrapment, is observed in certain patients, thereby highlighting the importance of prudent mesh selection, precise placement, and surgical methodology to mitigate this concern [32]. Despite mesh implementation, the occurrence of wound dehiscence remains possible. However, meticulous tension management, adherence to postoperative directives, and comprehensive patient education regarding activity limitations stand as crucial measures in averting this complication [33].

2. Role of Interleukins in Wound Healing

Interleukins (ILs) are a group of signaling molecules that play a crucial role in the immune response, inflammation, and tissue repair processes, including wound healing. The wound-healing process begins with inflammation, during which immune cells are recruited to the wound site. Interleukins, such as IL-1, IL-6, and IL-8, play a significant role in initiating and regulating the inflammatory response. These cytokines promote the migration of immune cells to the wound site and help in removing debris and pathogens. These interleukins might influence the recruitment of immune cells to the mesh site and contribute to the breakdown of the mesh material. The mesh material itself can trigger an immune response, leading to the secretion of various interleukins and other cytokines. The presence of these interleukins can influence the recruitment of immune cells, the proliferation of fibroblasts, and the remodeling of tissue around the mesh. Proper modulation of interleukin activity is essential to ensure that the healing process occurs without excessive inflammation or fibrosis.

a. IL-2 and tissue healing role.

IL-2 in humans is translated as a 153-amino-acid precursor, then processed to a 15.5 kD 133-amino-acid long, four-α-helix bundle glycoprotein [34]. IL-2 is a cytokine involved in the signaling pathways associated with the immune system, plays essential roles in several key functions of the immune system, and interacts with multiple cytokines to modulate the generation and activation of immune cells, which may also impact wound healing. IL-2 is majorly produced by CD8+ and CD4+ T-cells in an active state [35]. IL-2 mediates its action by binding to a specific receptor (IL-2R), a heterotrimeric protein expressed on the surface of certain immune cells, such as lymphocytes [34]. The IL-2 signal can be transduced through three signaling pathways: JAK-STAT, PI3K/Akt/mTOR, and MAPK/ERK [36]. It induces activation-induced cell death (AICD) and prevents autoimmune diseases by promoting the differentiation of immature T-cells into regulatory T-cells [30]. It plays a vital role in the differentiation of naive CD8+ T-cells into effector and memory T-cells, thus improving immunity [37], stimulating the differentiation of naïve CD4+ T-cells into T helper cells (Th-cells), and enhancing the cytotoxic activity of both natural killer cells and cytotoxic T-cells [37,38]. IL-2 production by T-cells is promoted by fibroblast growth factors (FGFs)-1 or -2, which are crucial for wound healing and angiogenesis [39]. IL-2 may be a crucial factor in the growth of fibroblasts via autophagy or through wound components derived from damaged wound organelles being digested and reallocated [40]. IL-2 stimulates the maturation of (Interferon-γ) IFN-γ-producing TH1 cells, thus augmenting the release process of IFN-γ, which leads to the production of IL-1 and helps in the wound-healing process [41].

IL-2 levels correlate positively with the percentage of burn wounds [42], act locally and not systemically, and reduced IL-2 levels are preferable at certain stages of the burn healing process [43]. In accordance with these, lower levels of IL-2 were observed at the sites of bone fractures [44], along with changes in the phosphorylation of certain proteins of the downstream IL-2 signaling pathways [45]. Wounds receiving IL-2 treatment demonstrated increased hydroxyproline, indicating increased collagen fiber cross-linking and enhanced ECM deposition [46]. On the contrary, low IL-2 levels and slow action of IL-2-regulated collagen fibers cross-linking in cell proliferation may enhance the wound closure quality [47,48]. Research has reported IL-2 signaling alterations to impact disease pathology that implicates tissue and skin damage, like systemic lupus erythematosus, diabetes mellitus, sarcoidosis, and myocardial infarction [49].

b. Role of IL-6 in tissue healing.

IL-6 acts as a pro-inflammatory, pleiomorphic cytokine, and anti-inflammatory myokine [50]. It is encoded by the IL6 gene located on chromosome 7 in humans [51]. Though IL-6 usually occurs as a 212-amino acid-long [52], 26-kD glycoprotein, its iso forms purified from various tissues have different molecular weights ranging from 19 to 70-kD due to alternate splicing of the IL-6gene and tissue-specific, post-translational modifications like phosphorylation and glycosylation [53–55]. IL-6 is produced by almost every cell and tissue type in humans in response to a wide variety of stimulating factors; however, several compounds also inhibit its expression [55]. IL-6 expresses its pleiotropic effects by binding to a specific receptor complex (IL-6R) located either on the membrane of the target cell (mIL-6R) through the "classical pathway" or to the soluble IL-6R (sIL-6R) through the "trans-signalling" pathway; this receptor complex consists of two transmembrane domains: CD126, a ligand binding α-chain, and CD130 or gp130, a signal-transducing β-chain [53–55]. The binding of IL-6 to the receptor complex results in either (i) the activation of gp130, which in turn leads to activation of the JAK/STAT/SOCS pathway, or (ii) the activation of the tyrosine phosphatase, SHP2 which in turn activates the RAS/RAF/MEK/MAPK/SOCS pathway [55–57]. IL-6 plays a major role in various cell functions: plasma cell development, B-cell differentiation, T-cell proliferation, maturation of cytotoxic T-cells, Ig class switching, hepatic acute phase response, inducing the synthesis of serum amyloid A and C-reactive protein thrombopoiesis, antimicrobial activity of monocytes and neutrophils, maintenance of bodyweight, and protection against mortality in endotoxin-mediated shock and toxic shock syndrome [56].

IL-6 levels are elevated in the inflammatory and proliferative stages of wound healing, during which it involves multiple functions but returns to normal levels in the remodeling stage [58]. IL-6 plays a pivotal role in inducing acute inflammation and is, therefore, necessary for the timely activation of the process [59,60]. IL-6, on being released very early in response to injury, induces the chemotaxis of leukocytes into the wound and the differentiation of macrophages, B-cells, and T-cells, stimulates the growth of keratinocytes, the release of other pro-inflammatory cytokines from macrophages, keratinocytes, endothelial cells, and stromal cells residing in the wounded tissue, inhibition of proliferation of fibroblasts, induction of acute-phase protein synthesis, simulation of hematopoiesis and angiogenesis, and the release of adrenocorticotropic hormone [61–64].

IL-6 plays an intrinsic role in the acute-phase wound response, may modulate local and systemic post-injury events by being the most persistent cytokine to mediate post-injury complications; and is robustly correlated with adverse clinical events and outcomes after mechanical trauma, burn injury, and elective surgery [55]. On wounding, elevated levels of IL-6 were detected within 24 h of bacterial infection during the initial inflammatory phase, which gradually diminished by the eighth day [65]. IL-6 was the only pro-inflammatory cytokine, the levels of which were persistently elevated post-burn injury; IL-6 levels in the serum peaked during the first few hours after injury and correlated directly with the area of the burn injury, the magnitude of the trauma, the duration of surgery, and the risk of postoperative complications [66]. IL-6 activity in human wound fluids was observed to peak within eight hours of surgery and return to baseline by the third day, a temporal pattern that may suppress the proliferation of fibroblasts in later stages [67]. IL-6 levels in the serum enhanced significantly after either laparoscopic or open IH surgery, more prominently in the latter [53], were highest on day one and fell sharply after the third day [68]. The equilibrium between pro-inflammatory cytokines like IL-6 may induce the transition from the inflammation to the proliferation phase, thus improving the healing process in skin wounds [69]. For instance, in liver transplants for treating chronic liver diseases, IL-6 engages in early graft regeneration and enhances the growth of hepatic tissue by inducing the hepatocyte stem cells to regenerate the liver parenchyma [70,71].

Higher IL-6 levels were observed more in non-healing wounds than in healing wounds [8], during the inflammatory phase in skin wounds in humans [72], and in both the inflammatory and granulating phases in venous leg ulcers [73]. Elevated levels of IL-6 observed in diabetic patients with foot ulcers than those without them indicate that it may play a role in their pathogenesis and development [73]. IL-6 promotes fibrosis due to an improper tissue healing process [58], stimulates the chemo-attraction of neutrophils and mitogenic activity of keratinocytes, which is linked to scar formation [8], and synergistically with hyaluronic acid affects the migration of keratinocytes through the activation of the ERK and NF-kB signalling pathway [74]. Reduced IL-6 synthesis can provide an environment conducive to scarless wound healing, as seen in the lack of inflammation observed in the fetal stages [75].

3. Role of CD31

Cluster of Differentiation 31 (CD31), also known as Platelet Endothelial Cell Adhesion Molecule-1 (PECAM-1), is a protein that is encoded by the PECAM1 gene located on chromosome 17 in humans [76]. CD31 is a highly glycosylated, 130 kD protein [77], consisting of six extracellular immunoglobulin-like domains, a 574 amino acid long N-terminal domain, a 19 amino acid long transmembrane domain, and a 118 amino acid long C-terminal cytoplasmic domain [76]. CD31 engages in cell–cell adhesion by interacting with other CD31 proteins present in other cells via homophilic and heterophilic interactions with CD-31 proteins [78,79]. CD31 is located on the surface of several cell types like platelets, monocytes, neutrophils, leucocytes, and certain T-cells and is constitutively expressed on the vascular endothelium [80]. Cell–cell signaling mediated through CD31 activates neutrophils, leukocytes, and monocytes [81]. CD31 also facilitates the migration of monocytes and neutrophils [82], natural killer cells [82], and T lymphocytes [83] through homophilic interactions mediated through endothelial cells. CD31 impacts cellular adhesion in the endothelium, cell transmigration, and diapedesis, resulting in angiogenesis and maintenance of vascular stability in the early stages [84–86]. Circulating CD31+ endothelial cells participate in blood vessel formation during wound healing, mediating through inflammation [87].

4. Role of CD34

CD34 is a transmembrane phospho-glycoprotein encoded by the CD34 gene located on chromosome 1 in humans [88]. CD34 is a member of the single-pass, transmembrane, sialomucin family of proteins; it was first identified in hematopoietic stem cells (HSCs) and is involved in cell–cell adhesion by participating in the attachment of HSCs to bone marrow ECM or directly to stromal cells; expression of CD34 is commonly associated with early hematopoietic and late-hematopoietic stem cells, and other non-hematopoietic, tissue-specific stem cells like muscle satellite cells, epidermal precursors, vascular-associated progenitor cells, endothelial progenitor cells, endothelial cells of blood vessels, masT-cells, dendritic cells, corneal keratocytes, and adipose cells which can be used to identify both newly formed and pre-existing blood vessels; CD34 facilitates the migration of various cell types, especially the chemokine-dependent migration of eosinophils and dendritic cell precursors [89–96]. Human aging can negatively impact adipose tissue-derived CD45−/CD34+/CD133+ progenitor cells availability as their number reduces with age and significantly reduces their angiogenic functional capacity [97].

CD34+ mesenchymal cells in the intestinal epithelium are genetically programmed to maintain an inductive environment for intestinal epithelial stem cells (IESCs) at homeostasis and facilitate repair post-injury and inflammation in intestines [98]. CD34+ structures with a vessel-like appearance in the mucosal epithelia and striated muscles were identified in human fetuses [99]. Fibrocytes are innovative blood-endured cells that demonstrate a unique cell surface phenotype (collagen+/CD13+/CD34+/CD45+), differentiate, and rapidly accelerate wound repair and scar formation through rapid migration [100,101]. Identifying CD34+ oral mucosa stem or progenitor cells suggests increased angiogenesis after corrective surgery for cleft lip and palate [96]. CD34+ EPCs were initially observed in human skin wounds after two days. Their numbers enhanced in lesions with increasing wound age, and more than 20 EPCs can indicate a wound age of 7–12 days [102].

5. Role of Platelet Rich Plasma (PRP)

Platelets or thrombocytes, originating from the bone marrow, contain several secretory granules, GFs, and cytokines that, in addition to their main function of homeostasis, can affect inflammation, angiogenesis, migration of stem cells, and cell proliferation [103] Platelet-rich plasma (PRP) (also known as platelet-rich fibrin matrix, platelet-rich growth factors, platelet concentrate, and autologous conditioned plasma) is the supernatant obtained after centrifugation of whole blood samples to remove red blood cells and consists of a PRP protein concentrate [103]. Activation of the platelets in PRP by thrombin or calcium causes the platelet granules to degranulate and release GFs and cytokines, which influence the microenvironment [104]. Some of the most important GFs released by platelets in PRP include VEGF, epidermal GF (EGF), hepatocyte GF (HGF), fibroblast GF (FGF) -a and b, platelet-derived GF (PGDF) -a and b, transforming GF (TGF)-α and β, insulin-like GF (IGF)-1 and 2, MMP-2 and 9, SDF-1α/CXCL12, andIL-8 [103,104].

PRP, a rich source of signaling molecules like GFs, cytokines, chemokines, and other plasma proteins, demonstrates significant mitogenic, angiogenic, and chemotactic properties that can stimulate the healing of wounds in both soft tissues and joints [104]. These GFs play a crucial role in all three phases, thus ensuring complete wound healing [105] PRP was initially used to treat thrombocytopenia, then in sports injuries, and nowadays is also employed in cardiac, pediatric, plastic surgery, gynecology, urology, ophthalmology, and dermatology [106–108]. Since various protocols are available for preparing PRPs, they could result in PRPs with different levels of bioactive compounds, which may modulate the final extent of wound healing [109,110]. The residual plasma and platelet-bound fibronectin may act as bioactive proteins, which may directly influence the remodeling of the ECM, thus exerting a synergistic effect on the repair of chronic wounds [111]. Hence, all components of blood, like the plasma, platelets, RBCs, and WBCs, have important individual roles in tissue repair, and PRP cannot function alone [112]. Further research on various techniques of PRP preparation, the exact mechanisms of action of GFs, their application in combination therapy, and related clinical trials is required [113]. Since PRP variations regarding the platelet content and the donor are observed, and due to the lack of standardized preparation methods, PRP use has been specific [114].

Autologous PRP demonstrates a great similarity to the natural healing process, is safe, and can be produced as and when required from the patient's blood [115]. Platelet-derived preparations such as PRP or platelet lysate (PL) may help stimulate regeneration in engineered tissue constructs, and activated PRP has been reported as a potential autologous cell carrier [115]. Due to its potential to stimulate and accelerate the process, PRP is gaining interest in skin wound regenerative therapy [116]. In a clinical setting, PRP and platelet-rich fibrin accelerate healing, thus not only reducing the discomfort of patients but also the probability of adverse outcomes such as infections, poor wound closure, and delay in the formation of sufficiently strong bone for subsequent procedures (such as implants); they may improve long-term outcomes in patients with impaired healing due to diseases (e.g., diabetes, osteoporosis, and atherosclerosis), medications (e.g., steroids), lifestyle choices (e.g., smoking), and aging by supplementing the wound environment to restore proper healing [117]. A systematic review of in vitro, in vivo, and clinical studies highlighted the additive effects of PRF on soft tissue regeneration, augmentation, and wound healing for regenerative therapy in medicine and dentistry [118].

PRP-derived molecules and activated PRP can release various antimicrobial proteins for resolving necrotic tissues and promoting wound healing [119], but in vivo and in vitro studies are required to provide sufficient data for the accurate designing and conducting of RCTs in humans regarding specific pathogens and wound types [120]. For instance, in AIDS patients, PRP may be used to sanitize wounds to induce neovascularization and re-epithelialization and prepare the base and edges of unhealed ulcers for consequent skin grafting procedures and tissue expansion [121]. Activated PRP leads to the production of extracellular micro vesicles, which can fully replicate the pro-healing effects of PRP, suggesting their applicability as an alternative to PRP [122]. The risk factors and contraindications associated with the use of PRP have also been reviewed [123].

Co-culture of human skin fibroblasts with PRP in vivo enhanced the accumulation of type I collagen, MMPs-1, and -2. The G1 cell-cycle regulators-cyclin E and CDK4 may improve wound healing in vitro [124]. Since wounds have a pro-inflammatory environment characterized by high protease activities, which decrease GF levels, PRP, a good source of GFs, is a promising alternative for treating recalcitrant wounds [122], especially in patients with Necrobiosis lipoidica diabeticorum [123]. For treating recalcitrant diabetic foot ulcers and venous foot ulcers, the use of PRP was successful [124], was safe as it does not significantly alter the blood hematology or blood chemistry [125], injections of autologous PRP along with the topical application of PRP gel enhanced wound healing and a reduction in wound size [126] PRP with vacuum-assisted closure dressings were more efficient than conventional dressings [127], homologous platelet-gel (PG) enhanced vascularization and re-epithelialization [128], and resulted in better healing outcomes and lower amputation rates [129]. In the healing of chronic ulcers, the local application of PRP improved the quality of life in patients through effective pain relief [130], combined treatment with enhanced stromal vascular fraction, PRP, and fat grafting demonstrated an enhancement in re-epithelization after regenerative surgery [131], and a novel autologous PRF matrix membrane showed significant potential for applicability [132].

Chronic wounds are unresponsive to conventional treatment methods, are quite common, and pose a challenge to clinicians. A systematic review and meta-analysis of PRP-therapy-based in vitro and in vivo studies reported improved healing of partial or complete, chronic, recalcitrant wounds [133,134], a combination of PRP injections and platelet-derived patches improved healing in patients, especially those with diabetes [135], the topical application of autologous-PRP owing to its antimicrobial properties and tissue-regenerative potential is recommended [136], especially in cases where conventional therapy is not sufficient, or surgery is not possible, local immunity is activated; while the pain and risk of infections are reduced [137,138], it significantly enhanced the re-epithelization process [139], demonstrated a considerable enhancement in the formation of healthy granulation tissue and healing edge; lesser pain, slough, bleeding on touch, discharge, and no superficial or deep infections [140–142]. PRP alone or combined with a powdered bioengineered skin substitute was used to synthesize a platelet-rich tissue graft, reducing the wound size and depth [143]. Autologous PRP, PPR-gel, and platelet-gel (PG) are safe with a wide range of applicability as tissue regenerative agents in a variety of postoperative procedures, especially in diabetic patients or those prone to surgical complications and as a replacement for connective tissues, activated PRP and fat tissues serves as a tissue matrix for enabling the cell migration, proliferation, differentiation, and granulation [144]. The short-term use of autologous PRP gel also enhanced the healing process consistently over time [145]. Homologous PRP gel reversed non-healing trends [146], induced granulation tissue formation, and reduced the size of cutaneous wounds [147]. Topical therapy with PG may be considered an adjuvant treatment to enhance the healing of cutaneous ulcers due to the formation of the granulation tissue in the initial stages, followed by complete re-epithelization [148]. As reported in a comprehensive review, PRP enhanced the healing of refractory pressure injuries and reduced the length of treatment and pain without any complications, all of which improved the quality of life in patients [149]. In a unique analysis, applying an algorithm developed by the study group before using PRP enhanced the number of successfully healed wounds, ensured that a higher proportion of acute skin wounds did not turn problematic, and allowed more predictable skin healing patterns [150].

Since PRP's application method has not been standardized, and the identification of the optimum conditions is complete, more controlled clinical studies are required, as only a few reports suggesting a positive role of PRP in the healing of burns are available [151,152]. The healing rate was prominently enhanced, and the healing time was markedly reduced in PRP-treated burn wounds [153]. PRP improved the healing of tendons, ligaments, muscles, and bones, and hence has been applied in treating sports-related injuries [154,155]. In systematic reviews, the efficacy of PRP in various musculoskeletal pathologies like tendinopathies, early osteoarthritis, and acute muscle injuries [156] and when applied to the bone-tendon interface during arthroscopic rotator cuff repair and wound healing has been addressed [157].

6. Role of Adipose Tissue-Derived Mesenchymal Stem Cells (ADSCs)

Stem cells like mesenchymal stem cells (MSCs) improve wound healing by expediting angiogenesis and re-epithelialization, leading to granulation tissue development. MSCs have a substantial role in the process mediated through paracrine interactions reducing wound inflammation and thus augmenting wound closure. As a result, ECM remodeling occurs, facilitating normal skin development and indicating a good therapeutic target [158,159]. MSCs isolated from the umbilical cord (fetal) and bone marrow (adult) tissues have been employed for the treatment of acute and chronic skin wounds [160]. Human adipose-derived stem cells (hADSCs) play crucial roles in the healing of cutaneous wounds by promoting cell proliferation, migration, differentiation, angiogenesis, matrix reconstruction, and regulation of the inflammatory response and collagen remodeling [161].

Stem cell classification can be based on their origin, such as (a) embryonic, (b) fetal (c) adult, and (d) induced pluripotent that can be designated as embryonic and adult mes enchymal stem cells (MSCs). Human embryonic stem cells (hESCs) and fetal mesenchymal stem cells (hfMSCs) are difficult to culture due to lack of supply and ethical concerns. The major limitation of employing induced pluripotent stem cells (iPSCs) is the laboratory procedure used to induce their differentiation into specific cell types requires certain disease action [162]. Due to these reasons, adult human stem cells have huge potential in clinical practice and basic research. From a clinical perspective, obtaining stem cells is both cost and time-intensive and involves the risk of contamination and loss. The source of stem cells should be easily accessible, which should cause minimal discomfort and provide enough cells without those time and cost-intensive processes. The sources of adult stem cells include the muscle, the bone marrow, the blood, the epidermis, the brain, the liver, and most recently, the adipose tissue [163–166].

In vitro and in vivo studies suggest that ADSCs are classified as mesenchymal cells having the capacity of self-renewal and differentiation into tri-germline ages (endoderm, mesoderm, and ectoderm) such as adipocytes, chondrocytes, myocytes, cardiomyocytes, hepatocytes, neurocytes, osteoblasts, vascular endothelial cells, and pancreatic cells [167,168] using specific triggers available in the laboratory [169–173]. The prominent benefits of ADSCs in comparison with other MSCs are easy availability and abundant sources for isolation, convenient tissue collection, and cell isolation methodologies. They can maintain their phenotype longer in culture, a greater proliferative capacity, and a demonstrated therapeutic potential; in addition, they secrete a wide range of cytokines, GFs, macromolecules, and miRNAs directly into the surrounding micro-environment or through the microvesicles [168,174]; these bioactive factors exert various 'trophic effects' such as suppressing the local immune system, inhibiting apoptosis and scar formation (fibrosis), enhancing angiogenesis, stimulating mitosis, and inducing the differentiation of tissue-intrinsic reparative or stem cells [175]. ADSCs can be isolated more easily, using a much safer approach, in considerably larger amounts, are not only equally effective but may be much better suited than BM-MSCs in certain cases, in clinical applications [176].

The quality of ADSCs varies among donors based on their demographic profiles, such as age, gender, ethnicity, disease status, and body mass index [168]. The yield of ADSCs is 40 times higher than that of BMSCs, with a success rate of 100%, which may not decrease with age, making this type of tissue attractive for isolating MSCs and progenitor cells (PCs) [177]. However, the number, proliferative capacity, and ability of these cells to differentiate into multiple lineages reduced with age while cell senescence increased [178]. ADSCs functions are not limited to tissue-specific PCs but have multiple therapeutic effects mediated through paracrine and regulating angiogenesis signaling, inflammation, cell survival, cell homing, and other processes regarded as action mechanisms [179]. ADSCs have been used as a therapeutic agent in treating diabetes mellitus, corneal, articular cutaneous lesions, and liver disease, and repair of damaged cardiac tissues, and for developing novel therapeutic methods useful in reconstructive or tissue engineering [180,181].

ADSCs are a valuable therapeutic alternative for tissue rescue and repair due to their easy availability, immunomodulatory effects, and capacities for secretion of pro-angiogenesis and anti-apoptotic factors, differentiation into multiline age cells, and expansion [182]. The ADSCs secretomes modify tissue biology. Thus, exciting tissue-resident stem cells change immune cell activity and facilitate therapeutic outcomes [168]. They participate in modulating the changes caused by macrophages in the inflammatory phenotype, endorsing neo-angiogenesis mediated through ECs increased differentiation and migration and augmenting granulation tissue formation, ECM, and skin cells at proliferation and remodeling stages of wound healing that is imperative and relevant in designing innovative therapeutic strategies in regenerative medicine domain [183]. The regenerative tissue effects of ADSCs in vivo rely on an interaction between the soluble factors released by them and the recipient's secretomes [184].

ADSCs may help repair tissue damage and help in neovascularization as a part of angiogenic therapy, as they can interact with and transform the wound-resident cells into matrix-building cells. This procedure is crucial for the dermal rebuilding course and epithelialization achieved through stimulating keratinocytes; a research study has elucidated ADSCs functioning as pericytes (in situ), facilitating vascular stability, and responding to environmental stimuli by communicating with ECs [107]. ADSCs may be vascular stem cells residing in a perivascular location and differentiate into smooth muscle and ECs used during angiogenesis and neo-vasculogenesis [185]. Coordination between ADSCs and ECs is required for network formation as ADSCs stabilize EC networks by enhancing pericyte-like characteristics. ADSCs induce vessel growth by secreting pro-angiogenic and regulatory proteins [186]. Induction in the expression of activin A is associated with new vessel formation. It directs the crosstalk between ADSCs and ECs, affecting these cell types of activity [187].

hADSCs produce exosomes that can induce cutaneous repair by regulating the remodeling of the ECM [188]. ADSCs-based cell therapies address wound healing of recalcitrant and chronic wounds by achieving full wound epithelialization rapidly and are safe without adverse effects for patients [107]. Various gene-modification approaches have been employed for manipulating genes and in vitro ADSCs preconditioning to increase the trophic factors production upon cell delivery in vivo [189]. In the past, ADSCs have been used to secrete VEGF in larger quantities to improve angiogenesis ability in therapeutic application in ischemic tissue [190].

7. Interactions between IL-2, IL-6, CD31, and CD34 with PRP and/or ADSCs in Use with Absorbable Meshes

Allogenic ADSCs and PRF combination can expedite full-thickness cartilage defect regeneration in the rabbit ear model devoid of any prominent immune trigger, as suggested by the lack of any prominent differences in the expression of the IL-2 gene in comparison with the control group [69]. IL-6 controls the healing process, especially in skin wounds, through migration, proliferation, and differentiation of stem cells, thus improving the healing process in skin wounds [191]. In response to inflammatory stimuli, ADSCs can produce IL-6 [192]. IL-6 released from ADSCs promoted the recovery of blood supply in the wounds [193]. The overexpression of S100A8, a calcium and zinc binding protein in ADSCs, significantly promoted their proliferation and differentiation, but the serum levels of IL-6 were significantly reduced, suggesting that S100A8 promoted the proliferation of ADSCs and inhibited inflammation to improve skin healing [194]. In in vivo studies, hematopoietic prostaglandin D synthase (HPGDS) was overexpressed to engineer hADSCs into hADSChpgds, and their effects on diabetic wound healing were evaluated using a full-thickness skin wound model in mice. The expression levels of IL-6 were prominently diminished. Still, the number of CD31+ ECs and scattered small blood vessels were significantly higher, indicating increased angiogenesis and vascularity in hADSChpgds group mice compared to the control [195]. In treating induced patellar tendon defects in rabbits with a PRP gel, the extent of neovascularization was significantly greater, as indicated by escalated expression of CD31 [196]. However, numerous studies have confirmed that ADSCs can express CD34 [197] but not CD31 [198]. Combined ADSCs and PRP therapy induced a strong angiogenic effect in diabetic albino rats as indicated by enhanced CD31 immuno-expression compared to control [199]. The in vitro co-culture of keloid tissue with ADSCs-CM brought a significant decrease in CD31+ and CD34+ vessels, thus exerting an anti-scarring effect [200]. Immuno-expression of CD31 in the endothelial cell lining of dermal blood vessels was enhanced in skin wounds in rats treated with ADSCs [201]. Wound healing studies in diabetic rats revealed that CD31+ cells were not only detected in the neo-capillaries, indicating spontaneous differentiation of engrafted ADSCs into vascular ECs, but also increased continuously and were detected in mature blood vessels, indicating a significant promotion of neovascularization of wounds [202]. In a study, topical application of ADSCs on excisional wounds on rabbit ears in full thickness resulted in enhanced expression of CD31 in granulation tissue CD31+ cells increased in the wound bed; however, CD31 expression in transplanted ADSCs was absently implicating a lack of ability to differentiate directly into ECs; similarly, CD34 expression was absent in AD-

SCs [203]. On the contrary, immuno-expression of CD31 in the endothelial cell lining of dermal blood vessels was enhanced in skin wounds in rats treated with ADSCs [188]. Wound healing studies in diabetic rats revealed that CD31+ cells were not only detected in the neo-capillaries, indicating spontaneous differentiation of engrafted ADSCs into vascular ECs, but also increased continuously and were detected in mature blood vessels, indicating a significant promotion of neovascularization of wounds [204]. In vitro co-culture of PRP and conditioned medium (CM) from ADSCs significantly stimulated the proliferation and migration of fibroblasts and keratinocytes, suggesting that PRP and ADSCs in combination may enhance healing and re-epithelialization of chronic wounds in vivo [205].

Alginate hydrogel containing EXOs derived from ADSCs productively increased wound closure, collagen synthesis, and vessel development, as demonstrated by the highest levels of CD31 expression compared to controls [206]. Velgraft®, a gelatin and chitosan biopolymer enhanced with ADSCs, improved wound healing by accelerating wound closure, rapid collagen synthesis, and deposition, thus leading to re-vascularization and re-epithelization. This was demonstrated through immunostaining, where CD31 positive expression was reported in ECs of neo-capillaries [207]. Three-dimensional scaffolds used in tissue engineering finely mimic the in vivo microenvironment and thus facilitate ADSCs' localization, attachment, proliferation, and differentiation, suggesting that tissue-engineered ADSCs can substitute tissue and organ transplantation [208]. Three-dimensional cultivation using a collagen sponge scaffold promoted the differentiation of CD34-hADSCs into ECs, which may be applied as an artificial dermis to heal skin wounds [209]. ADSCs differentiate rapidly into ECs to form simple vessel-like structures in Matrigel® substrates and thus may be crucial in regulating neo-vasculogenesis [210].

hADSCs stimulate wound healing in diabetic patients and function as a combined carrier scaffold for scar-less cutaneous repair [209]. For studying tissue repair in a murine skin injury model, two different sets of ECM scaffolds were used, namely-small intestinal submucosa (SIS) and acellular dermal matrix (ADM) and composite collagen–chondroitin sulfate–hyaluronic acid (Co–CS–HA) scaffold; the ADSCs-seeded scaffolds demonstrated enhanced wound healing capacity compared to non-seeded scaffolds; this suggested that ADSCs could be used as a source of cells to promote the vascularization capacities of scaffolds and that both ADSCs and the scaffolds exhibited synergistic effects in promoting angiogenesis; moreover, some ADSCs demonstrated GFP co-localization with CD31 implicating spontaneous differentiation into a vascular endothelial phenotype; ADSCs were negative for CD34 [210]. A bioactive PRP scaffold capable of releasing endogenous GFs, BMSCs, and ADSCs to differentiate into chondrocytes may be suitable for cell-based cartilage repair [211]. In a skin graft study in rats, the number of subcutaneous, neovascular CD31+ cells in the ADSCs embedded in the PRP gel scaffold-treated group was significantly greater than the control group, indicating that ADSCs+ PRP significantly induced early stage neovascularization after skin graft transplantation [212].

PRP stimulates the proliferation and differentiation, maintains the multipotency of MSCs, promotes their migration into the wound area, and enhances the wound-healing pathway; PRP or MSCs, and MSCs + PRP improved and accelerated wound healing represent a potential therapeutic approach [211]. PRP-gels can function as carriers for delivering both human MSCs and GFs in tissue engineering; the platelet concentration of PRP is crucial in providing the most favorable microenvironment for MSCs concerning the clinical application of PRP-gels [211].

8. Recent Advances and Challenges

Wound healing involving absorbable meshes constitutes a central area of focus in both surgical and medical research. This domain centers its endeavors on the manipulation of mesh materials to enhance and streamline tissue healing across a spectrum of wound types. These absorbable meshes are intentionally engineered to offer mechanical reinforcement during the initial phases of wound healing. As time progresses, they gradually degrade in synchronization with the tissue's recovery process. This property eliminates the necessity for subsequent removal procedures. In the course of research, significant attention has been directed toward understanding the intricate interaction between absorbable meshes and the body's intrinsic healing mechanisms. This interaction exerts a noticeable influence on the complex process of wound repair. Notable progress has been achieved in the design of absorbable mesh materials to ensure biocompatibility [213]. This ensures the seamless integration of these materials within the body, thereby preventing disruptive inflammatory reactions. Additionally, absorbable meshes that can integrate with neighboring tissues have provided insights into facilitating the formation of new blood vessels and promoting the migration of cells to the injury site. This integration is vital for enduring wound healing and the mitigation of potential complications. Furthermore, researchers have devoted their efforts to finely-tuning the controlled degradation of these meshes [214]. This controlled degradation allows for mechanical strength during the crucial early stages of wound healing.

However, these significant advancements have encountered challenges and variables that require thorough consideration. A prominent concern is the susceptibility to infections Absorbable meshes, being foreign elements, could exacerbate the risk of infections if not managed judiciously [215]. Striking a delicate balance between the mechanical properties of the mesh and its rate of degradation represents another challenge. If the degradation process occurs too rapidly, it could compromise essential support during critical phases of healing. Conversely, prolonged degradation might lead to complications or necessitate intervention. Furthermore, the variability in individual responses to absorbable meshes introduces complexity in predicting outcomes. This variability arises from distinct immune reactions, overall health statuses, and genetic compositions. Ensuring the sustained effectiveness of absorbable meshes in wound repair necessitates prolonged observation of patient outcomes. This extended observation is crucial to elucidate their effects on wound healing, scarring, and recurrence rates.

9. Conclusions

Wound healing is a multifaceted process involving intricate interactions among various elements. Cellular responses, molecular factors, and the introduction of biomaterials come together in a delicate interplay to orchestrate the repair of damaged tissue. The process of wound healing can be broken down into distinct phases: inflammation, proliferation, and remodeling. In the inflammatory phase, immune cells are recruited to the site of injury to manage any potential infections and begin the clean-up process. During proliferation, growth factors stimulate the production of new cells and blood vessels, aiding in the reconstruction of the damaged tissue. Remodeling involves refining the tissue's structure for improved strength and function.

- Immune cells, growth factors, and extracellular matrix components are central to the wound-healing process. Immune cells help clear debris and pathogens, while growth factors stimulate cell division and tissue regrowth. Extracellular matrix components provide the structural framework for new tissue formation.
- The involvement of cytoskeletal elements and proteins like the 'Formin' family shed light on the intricate cellular mechanisms driving wound healing. These mechanisms contribute to cell migration, proliferation, and tissue reorganization during the healing process.
- Incorporating absorbable meshes into wound repair strategies presents a promising avenue for enhancing healing outcomes. These meshes act as scaffolds that support the regeneration of tissue. They facilitate interactions with growth factors, cytokines, and various cellular components, such as interleukins, CD31, CD34, platelet-rich plasma (PRP), and adipose-derived stem cells (ADSCs). These interactions have the potential to expedite and optimize the healing process.

Particularly for individuals with diabetes, who often face compromised wound healing, absorbable meshes offer a renewed sense of optimism. These meshes can be engineered to release healing factors in a controlled manner, addressing the challenges that diabetic patients often encounter in the wound healing process.

Despite significant progress in wound healing research, several challenges persist. Ensuring the effective integration of meshes, maintaining biocompatibility, preventing infections, and managing postoperative complications are areas that continue to demand focused research and innovative solutions. Advances in mesh design, placement techniques, and personalized approaches are pivotal to shaping the field of wound healing interventions. Taking into account patient-specific factors ensures tailored solutions that can optimize outcomes and minimize risks. The ever-evolving nature of wound healing research necessitates collaboration among researchers, clinicians, and biomaterial scientists. By working together, they can unravel the complexities of wound healing processes and develop strategies that cater to diverse patient populations.

Funding: This research received no external funding.

Institutional Review Board Statement: Not applicable.

Informed Consent Statement: Not applicable.

Data Availability Statement: Not applicable.

Conflicts of Interest: The authors declare no conflict of interest.

References

1. Komi, D.E.A.; Khomtchouk, K.; Maria, P.L.S. A Review of the Contribution of MasT-cells in Wound Healing: Involved Molecular and Cellular Mechanisms. *Clin. Rev. Allergy Immunol.* **2020**, *58*, 298–312. [CrossRef] [PubMed]
2. Mills, S.J.; Hofma, B.R.; Cowin, A.J. Pathophysiology of Wound Healing. In *Mechanisms of Vascular Disease*; Springer: Berlin/Heidelberg, Germany, 2020; pp. 541–561.
3. Wang, P.H.; Huang, B.S.; Horng, H.C.; Yeh, C.C.; Chen, Y.J. Wound healing. *J. Chin. Med. Assoc.* **2018**, *81*, 94–101. [CrossRef] [PubMed]
4. Kiwanuka, E.; Junker, J.; Eriksson, E. Harnessing growth factors to influence wound healing. *Clin. Plast. Surg.* **2012**, *39*, 239–248. [CrossRef]
5. Reinke, J.M.; Sorg, H. Wound repair and regeneration. *Eur. Surg. Res.* **2012**, *49*, 35–43. [CrossRef]
6. Sorg, H.; Tilkorn, D.J.; Hager, S.; Hauser, J.; Mirastschijski, U. Skin Wound Healing: An Update on the Current Knowledge and Concepts. *Eur. Surg. Res.* **2017**, *58*, 81–94. [CrossRef] [PubMed]
7. Shah, J.M.; Omar, E.; Pai, D.R.; Sood, S. Cellular events and biomarkers of wound healing. *Indian J. Plast. Surg.* **2012**, *45*, 220–228.
8. Patel, S.; Maheshwari, A.; Chandra, A. Biomarkers for wound healing and their evaluation. *J. Wound Care* **2016**, *25*, 46–55. [CrossRef]
9. Ahangar, P.; Strudwick, X.L.; Cowin, A.J. Wound Healing from an Actin Cytoskeletal Perspective. *Cold Spring Harb. Perspect. Biol.* **2022**, *14*, a041235. [CrossRef]
10. Pegoraro, A.F.; Janmey, P.; Weitz, D.A. Mechanical Properties of the Cytoskeleton and Cells. *Cold Spring Harb. Perspect. Biol.* **2017**, *9*, a022038. [CrossRef]
11. Fletcher, D.A.; Mullins, R.D. Cell mechanics and the cytoskeleton. *Nature* **2010**, *463*, 485–492. [CrossRef]
12. Strudwick, X.L.; Cowin, A.J. Cytoskeletal Regulation of Dermal Regeneration. *Cells* **2012**, *1*, 1313–1327. [CrossRef] [PubMed]
13. Pollard, T.D. Actin and Actin-Binding Proteins. *Cold Spring Harb. Perspect. Biol.* **2016**, *8*, a018226. [CrossRef] [PubMed]
14. Huang, W.; Hickson, L.J.; Eirin, A.; Kirkland, J.L.; Lerman, L.O. Cellular senescence: The good, the bad and the unknown. *Nature* **2022**, *18*, 611–627. [CrossRef] [PubMed]
15. Baylón, K.; Rodríguez-Camarillo, P.; Elías-Zúñiga, A.; Díaz-Elizondo, J.A.; Gilkerson, R.; Lozano, K. Past, present and future of surgical meshes: A review. *Membranes* **2017**, *7*, 47. [CrossRef]
16. Öberg, S.; Andresen, K.; Rosenberg, J. Absorbable Meshes in Inguinal Hernia Surgery: A Systematic Review and Meta-Analysis. *Surg. Innov.* **2017**, *24*, 289–298. [CrossRef]
17. Renard, Y.; de Mestier, L.; Henriques, J.; de Boissieu, P.; de Mestier, P.; Fingerhut, A.; Palot, J.P.; Kianmanesh, R. Absorbable Polyglactin vs. Non-Cross-linked Porcine Biological Mesh for the Surgical Treatment of Infected Incisional Hernia. *J. Gastrointest. Surg.* **2020**, *24*, 435–443. [CrossRef]
18. Stoikes, N.F.N.; Scott, J.R.; Badhwar, A.; Deeken, C.R.; Voeller, G.R. Characterization of host response, resorption, and strength properties, and performance in the presence of bacteria for fully absorbable biomaterials for soft tissue repair. *Hernia* **2017**, *21*, 771–782. [CrossRef]
19. Mlodinow, A.S.; Yerneni, K.; Hasse, M.E.; Cruikshank, T.; Kuzycz, M.J.; Ellis, M.F. Evaluation of a Novel Absorbable Mesh in a Porcine Model of Abdominal Wall Repair. *Plast. Reconstr. Surg. Glob. Open* **2021**, *9*, e3529. [CrossRef]

20. Klinge, U.; Schumpelick, V.; Klosterhalfen, B. Functional assessment and tissue response of short-and long-term absorbable surgical meshes. *Biomaterials* **2001**, *22*, 1415–1424. [CrossRef]
21. Hjort, H.; Mathisen, T.; Alves, A.; Clermont, G.; Boutrand, J.P. Three-year results from a preclinical implantation study of a long-term resorbable surgical mesh with time-dependent mechanical characteristics. *Hernia* **2012**, *16*, 191–197. [CrossRef]
22. Ruiz-Jasbon, F.; Norrby, J.; Ivarsson, M.-L.; Björck, S. Inguinal hernia repair using a synthetic long-term resorbable mesh: Results from a 3-year prospective safety and performance study. *Hernia* **2014**, *18*, 723–730. [CrossRef] [PubMed]
23. Miserez, M.; Jairam, A.P.; Boersema, G.S.A.; Bayon, Y.; Jeekel, J.; Lange, J.F. Resorbable Synthetic Meshes for Abdominal Wall Defects in Preclinical Setting: A Literature Review. *J. Sur. Res.* **2019**, *237*, 67–75. [CrossRef] [PubMed]
24. Charleux-Muller, D.; Hurel, R.; Fabacher, T.; Brigand, C.; Rohr, S.; Manfredelli, S.; Passot, G.; Ortega-Deballon, P.; Dubuisson, V.; Renard, Y.; et al. Slowly absorbable mesh in contaminated incisional hernia repair: Results of a French multicenter study. *Hernia* **2021**, *25*, 1051–1059. [CrossRef] [PubMed]
25. Valverde, S.; Arbós, M.A.; Quiles, M.T.; Espín, E.; Sánchez-Garcia, J.L.; Rodrigues, V.; Pereira, J.A.; Villalobos, R.; García-Alamino, J.M.; Armengol, M.; et al. Use of a bioabsorbable mesh in midline laparotomy closure to prevent incisional hernia: Randomized controlled trial. *Hernia* **2022**, *26*, 1405–1406. [CrossRef] [PubMed]
26. Quesada, B.M.; Adelina, C.E. Use of absorbable meshes in laparoscopic paraesophageal hernia repair. *World J. Gastrointest. Surg.* **2019**, *11*, 388–394. [CrossRef]
27. Markar, S.R.; Karthikesalingam, A.; Alam, F.; Tang, T.Y.; Walsh, S.R.; Sadat, U. Partially or completely absorbable versus non-absorbable mesh repair for inguinal hernia: A systematic review and meta-analysis. *Surg. Laparosc. Endosc. Percutan Tech.* **2010**, *20*, 213–219. [CrossRef]
28. Brem, H.; Tomic-Canic, M. Cellular and molecular basis of wound healing in diabetes. *J. Clin. Investig.* **2007**, *117*, 1219–1222. [CrossRef]
29. Brown, C.N.; Finch, J.G. Which mesh for hernia repair? *Ann. R. Coll. Surg. Engl.* **2010**, *92*, 272–278. [CrossRef]
30. Kao, A.M.; Arnold, M.R.; Augenstein, V.A.; Heniford, B.T. Prevention and treatment strategies for mesh infection in abdominal wall reconstruction. *Plast. Reconst. Surg.* **2018**, *142*, 149S–155S. [CrossRef]
31. Mayagoitia, J.C.; Almaraz, A.; Diaz, C. Two cases of cystic seroma following mesh incisional hernia repair. *Hernia* **2006**, *10*, 83–86. [CrossRef]
32. Bendavid, R.; Lou, W.; Grischkan, D.; Koch, A.; Petersen, K.; Morrison, J.; Iakovlev, V. A mechanism of mesh-related post-herniorrhaphy neuralgia. *Hernia* **2016**, *20*, 357–365. [CrossRef] [PubMed]
33. Lima, H.V.; Rasslan, R.; Novo, F.C.; Lima, T.M.; Damous, S.H.; Bernini, C.O.; Montero, E.F.; Utiyama, E.M. Prevention of fascial dehiscence with onlay prophylactic mesh in emergency laparotomy: A randomized clinical trial. *J. Am. Coll. Surg.* **2020**, *230*, 76–87. [CrossRef] [PubMed]
34. Arenas-Ramirez, N.; Woytschak, J.; Boyman, O. Interleukin-2: Biology, Design and Application. *Trends Immunol.* **2015**, *36*, 763–777 [CrossRef] [PubMed]
35. Liao, W.; Lin, J.X.; Leonard, W.J. IL-2 family cytokines: New insights into the complex roles of IL-2 as a broad regulator of T helper cell differentiation. *Curr. Opin. Immunol.* **2011**, *23*, 598–604. [CrossRef]
36. Liao, W.; Lin, J.X.; Leonard, W.J. Interleukin-2 at the crossroads of effector responses, tolerance, and immunotherapy. *Immunity* **2013**, *38*, 13–25. [CrossRef]
37. Spolski, R.; Li, P.; Leonard, W.J. Biology, and regulation of IL-2: From molecular mechanisms to human therapy. *Nat. Rev. Immunol.* **2018**, *18*, 648–659. [CrossRef]
38. Byrd, V.M.; Ballard, D.W.; Miller, G.G.; Thomas, J.W. Fibroblast growth factor-1 (FGF-1) enhances IL-2 production and nuclear translocation of NF-kB in FGF receptor-bearing Jurkat T-cells. *J. Immunol.* **1999**, *162*, 5853–5859. [CrossRef]
39. Kang, R.; Tang, D.; Lotze, M.T.; Lii, H.J.Z. Autophagy is required for IL-2-mediated fibroblast growth. *Exp. Cell. Res.* **2013**, *319*, 556–565. [CrossRef]
40. Zhu, J.; Paul, W.E. CD4 T-cells: Fates, functions, and faults. *Blood* **2008**, *112*, 1557–1569. [CrossRef]
41. Kowal-Vern, A.; Walenga, J.M.; Hoppensteadt, D.; Sharp-Pucci, M.; Gamelli, R.L. Interleukin-2 and interleukin-6 in relation to burn wound size in the acute phase of thermal injury. *J. Am. Coll. Surg.* **1994**, *178*, 357–362.
42. Mikhal'chik, E.V.; Piterskaya, J.A.; Budkevich, L.Y.; Penkov, L.Y.; Facchiano, A.; De Luca, C. Comparative study of cytokine content in the plasma and wound exudate from children with severe burns. *Bull. Exp. Biol. Med.* **2009**, *148*, 771–775. [CrossRef] [PubMed]
43. Currie, H.N.; Loos, M.S.; Vrana, J.A.; Dragan, K.; Boyd, J.W. Spatial cytokine distribution following traumatic injury. *Cytokine* **2014**, *66*, 112–118. [CrossRef] [PubMed]
44. Han, A.A.; Currie, H.N.; Loos, M.S.; Vrana, J.A.; Fabyanic, E.B.; Prediger, M.S.; Boyd, J.W. Spatiotemporal phosphoprotein distribution and associated cytokine response of a traumatic injury. *Cytokine* **2016**, *79*, 12–22. [CrossRef] [PubMed]
45. Sakakibara, S.; Inouye, K.; Shudo, K.; Kishida, Y.; Kobayashi, Y.; Prockop, D.J. Synthesis of (Pro-Hyp-Gly) n of defined molecular weights. Evidence for the stabilization of collagen triple helix by hydroxyproline. *Biochem. Biophys. Acta.* **1973**, *303*, 198–202.
46. Barbul, A.; Knud-Hansen, J.; Wasserkrug, H.L.; Efron, G. Lnterleukin 2 Enhances Wound Healing in Rats. *J. Surg. Res.* **1986**, *40*, 315–319. [CrossRef]
47. Boyman, O.; Sprent, J. The role of interleukin-2 during homeostasis and activation of the immune system. *Nat. Rev. Immunol.* **2012**, *12*, 180–190. [CrossRef]

48. Boyman, O.; Kolios, A.G.A.; Raeber, M.E. Modulation of T cell responses by IL-2 and IL-2 complexes. *Clin. Exp. Rheumatol.* **2015**, *33*, S54–S57.
49. Doersch, K.M.; DelloStritto, D.J.; Newell-Rogers, M.K. The contribution of interleukin-2 to effective wound healing. *Exp. Biol. Med.* **2017**, *242*, 384–396. [CrossRef]
50. Febbraio, M.A.; Pedersen, B.K. Contraction-induced myokine production and release: Is skeletal muscle an endocrine organ? *Exerc. Sport Sci. Rev.* **2005**, *33*, 114–119. [CrossRef]
51. Ferguson-Smith, A.C.; Chen, Y.F.; Newman, M.S.; May, L.T.; Sehgal, P.B.; Ruddle, F.H. Regional localization of the interferon-beta 2/B-cell stimulatory factor 2/hepatocyte stimulating factor gene to human chromosome 7p15-p21. *Genomics* **1988**, *2*, 203–208. [CrossRef]
52. Van Snick, J.; Cayphas, S.; Szikora, J.-P.; Renauld, J.C.; Van Roost, E.; Boon, T.; Simpson, R.J. cDNA cloning of murine interleukin-HP1: Homology human interleukin 6. *Eur. J. Immunol.* **1988**, *18*, 193–200. [CrossRef]
53. May, L.T.; Santhanam, U.; Tatter, S.B.; Ghrayeb, J.; Sehgal, P.B. Multiple forms of human IL. *Ann. N. Y. Acad. Sci.* **1989**, *557*, 114–119. [CrossRef] [PubMed]
54. May, L.T.; Ghrayeb, J.; Santhanam, U.; Stoeger, Z.; Helfgott, D.C.; Chiorazzi, N.; Grieninger, G.; Sehgal, P.B. Synthesis and secretion of multiple forms of β2-interferon/B-cell differentiation factor 2/hepatocyte stimulating factor by human fibroblasts and monocytes. *J. Biol. Chem.* **1988**, *263*, 7760–7766. [CrossRef] [PubMed]
55. Biffl, W.L.; Moore, E.E.; Moore, F.A.; Peterson, V.M. Interleukin-6 in the Injured Patient Marker of Injury or Mediator of Inflammation? *Ann. Surg.* **1996**, *224*, 647–664. [CrossRef] [PubMed]
56. Barton, B.E. Interleukin-6 and new strategies for the treatment of cancer, hyperproliferative diseases and paraneoplastic syndromes. *Expert. Opin. Ther. Targets.* **2005**, *9*, 737–752. [CrossRef]
57. Li, Y.; Zhao, J.; Yin, Y.; Li, K.; Zhang, C.; Zheng, Y. The Role of IL-6 in Fibrotic Diseases: Molecular and Cellular Mechanisms. *Int. J. Biol. Sci.* **2022**, *18*, 5405–5414. [CrossRef]
58. Johnson, B.Z.; Stevenson, A.W.; Prêle, C.M.; Fear, M.W.; Wood, F.M. The Role of IL-6 in Skin Fibrosis and Cutaneous Wound Healing. *Biomedicines* **2020**, *8*, 101. [CrossRef]
59. Lin, Z.-Q.; Kondo, T.; Ishida, Y.; Takayasu, T.; Mukaida, N. Essential involvement of IL-6 in the skin wound-healing process as evidenced by delayed wound healing in IL-6-deficient mice. *J. Leukoc. Biol.* **2003**, *73*, 713–721. [CrossRef]
60. Kishimoto, T. The biology of interleukin 6. *Blood* **1989**, *74*, 1–10. [CrossRef]
61. Hirano, T. The biology of interleukin 6. *Chem. Immunol.* **1992**, *51*, 153–180.
62. Weissenbach, M.; Clahsen, T.; Weber, C.; Spitzer, D.; Wirth, D.; Vestweber, D.; Heinrich, P.C.; Schaper, F. Interleukin-6 is a direct mediator of T cell migration. *Eur. J. Immunol.* **2004**, *34*, 2895–2906. [CrossRef]
63. Wright, H.L.; Cross, A.L.; Edwards, S.W.; Moots, R.J. Effects of IL-6 and IL-6 blockade on neutrophil function in vitro and in vivo. *Rheumatology* **2014**, *53*, 1321–1331. [CrossRef] [PubMed]
64. Sunderkotter, C.; Goebeler, M.; Schulze-Osthoff, K.; Bhardwaj, R.; Sorg, C. Macrophage-derived angiogenesis factors. *Pharmacol.Ther.* **1991**, *51*, 195–216. [CrossRef] [PubMed]
65. Al-Jebouri, M.M.; Al-Mahmood, B.Y.R. Estimation of Cytokines Involved in Acute-Phase Wound Infection with Reference to Residence Time of Patients in Hospitals. *Mod. Res. Inflam.* **2019**, *8*, 1–10. [CrossRef]
66. Abraham, P.; Monard, C.; Schneider, A.; Rimmelé, T. Extracorporeal Blood Purification in Burns: For Whom, Why, and How? *Blood Purif.* **2023**, *52*, 17–24. [CrossRef] [PubMed]
67. Mateo, R.B.; Reichner, J.S.; Albina, J.E. Interleukin-6 activity in wounds. *Am. J. Physiol.* **1994**, *266*, R1840–R1844. [CrossRef] [PubMed]
68. Di Vita, G.; Patti, R.; D'Agostino, P.; Caruso, G.; Arcara, M.; Buscemi, S.; Bonventre, S.; Ferlazzo, V.; Arcoleo, F.; Cillari, E. Cytokines and growth factors in wound drainage fluid from patients undergoing incisional hernia repair. *Wound Rep. Reg.* **2006**, *14*, 259–264. [CrossRef]
69. Xiao, T.; Yan, Z.; Xiao, S.; Xia, Y. Pro-inflammatory cytokines regulate epidermal stem cells in wound epithelialization. *Stem Cell Res. Ther.* **2020**, *11*, 232. [CrossRef]
70. Chae, M.S.; Moon, K.U.; Chung, H.S.; Park, C.S.; Lee, J.; Choi, J.H.; Hong, S.H. Serum interleukin-6 and tumor necrosis factor-α are associated with early graft regeneration after living donor liver transplantation. *PLoS ONE* **2018**, *13*, e0195262. [CrossRef]
71. Patel, A.; Aslam, R.; Jamil, M.; Ansari, A.; Khan, S. The Effects of Growth Factors and Cytokines on Hepatic Regeneration: A Systematic Review. *Cureus* **2022**, *14*, e24539. [CrossRef]
72. Grellner, W.; Georg, T.; Wilske, J. Quantitative analysis of pro-inflammatory cytokines (IL-1beta, IL-6, TNF-alpha) in human skin wounds. *Forensic. Sci. Int.* **2000**, *113*, 251–264. [CrossRef] [PubMed]
73. Ligia, D.; Mostib, G.; Crocea, L.; Raffettoc, J.D.; Mannello, F. Chronic venous disease—Part I—Inflammatory biomarkers in wound healing. *BBA Mol. Basis Dis.* **2016**, *1862*, 1964–1974. [CrossRef] [PubMed]
74. Choi, J.-H.; Jun, J.H.; Kim, J.H.; Sung, H.J.; Lee, J.H. Synergistic Effect of Interleukin-6 and Hyaluronic Acid on Cell Migration and ERK Activation in Human Keratinocytes. *J. Korean Med. Sci.* **2014**, *29*, S210–S216. [CrossRef] [PubMed]
75. Liechty, K.W.; Adzick, N.S.; Crombleholme, T.M. Diminished interleukin 6 (IL-6) production during scarless human fetal wound repair. *Cytokine* **2000**, *12*, 671–676. [CrossRef]
76. Newman, P.J.; Berndt, M.C.; Gorski, J.; White, G.C.; Lyman, S.; Paddock, C.; Muller, W.A. PECAM-1 (CD31) cloning and relation to adhesion molecules of the immunoglobulin gene superfamily. *Science* **1990**, *247*, 1219–1222. [CrossRef] [PubMed]

77. Gumina, R.J.; Kirschbaum, N.E.; Rao, P.N.; vanTuinen, P.; Newman, P.J. The human PECAM1 gene maps to 17q23. *Genomics* **1996**, *34*, 229–232. [CrossRef] [PubMed]
78. Albelda, S.M.; Muller, W.A.; Buck, C.A.; Newman, P.J. Molecular and cellular properties of PECAM-1 (endoCAM/CD31): A novel vascular cell-cell adhesion molecule. *J. Cell Biol.* **1991**, *114*, 1059–1068. [CrossRef]
79. DeLisser, H.M.; Newman, P.J.; Albelda, S.M. Molecular and functional aspects of PECAM-1/CD31. *Immunol. Today* **1994**, *15*, 490–495. [CrossRef]
80. Novinska, M.S.; Rathore, V.; Newman, D.K.; Newman, P.J. *Pecam-Platelets*, 2nd ed.; Chapter 11,; Academin Press: Cambridge, MA, USA, 2007; pp. 221–230.
81. Elias, C.G.; Spellberg, J.P.; Karan-Tamir, B.; Lin, C.H.; Wang, Y.J.; McKenna, P.J.; Muller, W.A.; Zukowski, M.M.; Andrew, D.P. Ligation of CD31/PECAM-1 modulates the function of lymphocytes, monocytes and neutrophils. *Eur. J. Immunol.* **1998**, *28*, 1948–1958. [CrossRef]
82. Berman, M.E.; Xie, Y.; Muller, W.A. Roles of platelet/endothelial cell adhesion molecule-1 (PECAM-1, CD31) in natural killer cell transendothelial migration and beta 2 integrin activation. *J. Immunol.* **1996**, *156*, 1515–1524. [CrossRef]
83. Poggi, A.; Zocchi, M.R.; Carosio, R.; Ferrero, E.; Angelini, D.F.; Galgani, S.; Caramia, M.D.; Bernardi, G.; Borsellino, G.; Battistini, L. Transendothelial migratory pathways of V delta 1+TCR gamma delta+ and V delta 2+TCR gamma delta+ T lymphocytes from healthy donors and multiple sclerosis patients: Involvement of phosphatidylinositol 3 kinase and calcium calmodulin-dependent kinase II. *J. Immunol.* **2002**, *168*, 6071–6077. [CrossRef] [PubMed]
84. DeLisser, H.M.; Christofidou-Solomidou, M.; Strieter, R.M.; Burdick, M.D.; Robinson, C.S.; Wexler, R.S.; Kerr, J.S.; Garlanda, C.; Merwin, J.R.; Madri, J.A.; et al. Involvement of endothelial PECAM-1/CD31 in angiogenesis. *Am. J. Pathol.* **1997**, *151*, 671–677 [PubMed]
85. Eshaq, R.S.; Harris, N.R. Loss of Platelet Endothelial Cell Adhesion Molecule-1 (PECAM-1) in the Diabetic Retina: Role of Matrix Metalloproteinases. *Invest. Ophthalmol. Vis. Sci.* **2019**, *60*, 748–760. [CrossRef] [PubMed]
86. Lertkiatmongkol, P.; Liaoa, D.; Meib, H.; Hub, Y.; Newman, P.J. Endothelial functions of platelet/endothelial cell adhesion molecule-1 (CD31). *Curr. Opin. Hematol.* **2016**, *23*, 253–259. [CrossRef]
87. Kim, S.-J.; Kim, J.-S.; Papadopoulos, J.; Kim, S.W.; Maya, M.; Zhang, F.; He, J.; Fan, D.; Langley, R.; Fidler, I.J. Circulating Monocytes Expressing CD31-Implications for Acute and Chronic Angiogenesis. *Am. J. Pathol.* **2009**, *174*, 1972–1980. [CrossRef]
88. Satterthwaite, A.B.; Burn, T.C.; Le Beau, M.M.; Tenen, D.G. Structure of the gene encoding CD34, a human hematopoietic stem cell antigen. *Genomics* **1992**, *12*, 788–794. [CrossRef]
89. Civin, C.I.; Strauss, L.C.; Brovall, C.; Fackler, M.J.; Schwartz, J.F.; Shaper, J.H. Antigenic analysis of hematopoiesis. III. A hematopoietic progenitor cell surface antigen defined by a monoclonal antibody raised against KG-1a cells. *J. Immunol.* **1984**, *133*, 157–165. [CrossRef]
90. Tindle, R.W.; Katz, F.; Martin, H.; Watt, D.; Catovsky, D.; Janossy, G.; Greaves, M. BI-3C5 (CD34) defines multipotential and lineage restricted progenitor cells and their leukemic counterparts. In *Leucocyte Typing 111: White Cell Differentiation Antigens* Oxford University Press: Oxford, UK, 1987; pp. 654–655.
91. Sidney, L.E.; Branch, M.J.; Dunphy, S.E.; Dua, H.S.; Hopkinson, A. Concise review: Evidence for CD34 as a common marker for diverse progenitors. *Stem Cells* **2014**, *32*, 1380–1389. [CrossRef]
92. Nielsen, J.S.; McNagny, K.M. Novel functions of the CD34 family. *J. Cell Sci.* **2008**, *121*, 3683–3692. [CrossRef]
93. Ramsfjell, V.; Bryder, D.; Björgvinsdóttir, H.; Kornfält, S.; Nilsson, L.; Borge, O.J.; Jacobsen, S.E. Distinct requirements for optimal growth and In vitro expansion of human CD34(+) CD38(−) bone marrow long-term culture-initiating cells (LTC-IC), extended LTC-IC, and murine in vivo long-term reconstituting stem cells. *Blood* **1999**, *94*, 4093–4102. [CrossRef]
94. Hogan, C.J.; Shpall, E.J.; Keller, G. Differential long-term and multilineage engraftment potential from subfractions of human CD34+ cord blood cells transplanted into NOD/SCID mice. *Proc. Natl. Acad. Sci. USA* **2002**, *99*, 413–418. [CrossRef] [PubMed]
95. Kapoor, S.; Shenoy, S.P.; Bose, B. CD34 cells in somatic, regenerative and cancer stem cells: Developmental biology, cell therapy and omics big data perspective. *J. Cell. Biochem.* **2020**, *121*, 3058–3069. [CrossRef]
96. Smane-Filipova, L.; Pilmane, M.; Akota, I. Immunohistochemical analysis of nestin, CD34 and TGFβ3 in facial tissue of children with complete unilateral and bilateral cleft lip and palate. *Stomatol. Balt. Dent. Maxillofac. J.* **2016**, *18*, 98–104.
97. Madonna, R.; Renna, F.V.; Cellini, C.; Cotellese, R.; Picardi, N.; Francomano, F.; Innocenti, P.; De Caterina, R. Age-dependent impairment of number and angiogenic potential of adipose tissue-derived progenitor cells. *Eur. J. Clin. Invest.* **2011**, *41*, 126–133. [CrossRef] [PubMed]
98. Stzepourginski, I.; Nigrod, G.; Jacoba, J.-M.; Dulauroy, S.; Sansonettid, P.J.; Eberl, G.; Peduto, L. CD34+ mesenchymal cells are a major component of the intestinal stem cells niche at homeostasis and after injury. *Proc. Natl. Acad. Sci. USA* **2017**, *114*, E506–E513. [CrossRef] [PubMed]
99. Katori, Y.; Kiyokawa, H.; Kawase, T.; Murakami, G.; Cho, B.H.; Ide, Y. CD34-positive primitive vessels and other structures in human fetuses: An immunohistochemical study. *Acta Otolaryngol.* **2011**, *131*, 1086–1090. [CrossRef] [PubMed]
100. Bucala, R.; Spiegel, L.A.; Chesney, J.; Hogan, M.; Cerami, A. Circulating fibrocytes define a new leukocyte subpopulation that mediates tissue repair. *Mol. Med.* **1994**, *1*, 71–81. [CrossRef]
101. Abe, R.; Donnelly, S.C.; Peng, T.; Bucala, R.; Christine, N. Peripheral Blood Fibrocytes: Differentiation Pathway and Migration to Wound Sites. *Met. J. Immunol.* **2001**, *166*, 7556–7562. [CrossRef]

102. Ishida, Y.; Kimura, A.; Nosaka, M.; Kuninaka, Y.; Shimada, E.; Yamamoto, H.; Nishiyama, K.; Inaka, S.; Takayasu, T.; Eisenmenger, W.; et al. Detection of endothelial progenitor cells in human skin wounds and its application for wound age determination. *Int. J. Legal. Med.* **2015**, *129*, 1049–1054. [CrossRef]
103. Le, A.D.K.; Enweze, L.; DeBaun, M.R.; Dragoo, J.L. Current Clinical Recommendations for Use of Platelet-Rich Plasma. *Curr. Rev. Musculoskelet. Med.* **2018**, *11*, 624–634. [CrossRef]
104. Alves, R.; Grimalt, R. A Review of Platelet-Rich Plasma: History, Biology, Mechanism of Action, and Classification. *Ski. Appendage Disord.* **2018**, *4*, 18–24. [CrossRef] [PubMed]
105. Everts, P.A. Autologous Platelet-Rich Plasma and Mesenchymal Stem Cells for the Treatment of Chronic Wounds. In *Wound Healing-Current Perspectives*; IntechOpen: London, UK, 2018; pp. 149–179.
106. Andia, I. Platelet-rich plasma biology. In *Clinical Indications and Treatment Protocols with Platelet-Rich Plasma in Dermatology*; Alves, R., Grimalt, R., Eds.; Ediciones Mayo: Barcelona, Spain, 2016; pp. 3–15.
107. Conde Montero, E.; Fernández Santos, M.E.; Suárez Fernández, R. Platelet-rich plasma: Applications in dermatology. *Actas Dermo Sifiliogr.* **2015**, *106*, 104–111. [CrossRef] [PubMed]
108. Lynch, M.D.; Bashir, S. Applications of platelet-rich plasma in dermatology: A critical appraisal of the literature. *J. Dermatolog. Treat.* **2016**, *27*, 285–289. [CrossRef] [PubMed]
109. Pavlovic, V.; Ciric, M.; Jovanovic, J.; Stojanovic, P. Platelet Rich Plasma: A short overview of certain bioactive components. *Open Med.* **2016**, *11*, 242–247. [CrossRef] [PubMed]
110. Hara, G.R.; Basu, T. Platelet-rich plasma in regenerative medicine. *Biomed. Res. Ther.* **2014**, *1*, 25–31. [CrossRef]
111. Moroz, A.; Deffune, E. Platelet-rich plasma and chronic wounds: Remaining fibronectin may influence matrix remodeling and regeneration success. *Cytotherapy* **2013**, *15*, 1436–1439. [CrossRef]
112. Parrish, W.R.; Roides, B. Physiology of Blood Components in Wound Healing: An Appreciation of Cellular Co-Operativity in Platelet Rich Plasma Action. *J. Exerc. Sports. Orthop.* **2017**, *4*, 1–14. [CrossRef]
113. Lai, H.; Chen, G.; Zhang, W.; Wu, G.; Xia, Z. Research trends on platelet-rich plasma in the treatment of wounds during 2002—A 20-year bibliometric analysis. *Int. Wound. J.* **2021**, *20*, 1882–1892. [CrossRef]
114. Lang, S.; Loibl, M.; Herrmann, M. Platelet-Rich Plasma in Tissue Engineering: Hype and Hope. *Eur. Surg. Res.* **2018**, *59*, 265–275. [CrossRef]
115. Lacci, K.M.; Dardik, A. Platelet-Rich Plasma: Support for Its Use in Wound Healing. *Yale J. Biol. Med.* **2010**, *83*, 1–9.
116. Chicharro-Alcántara, D.; Rubio-Zaragoza, M.; Damiá-Giménez, E.; Carrillo-Poveda, J.M.; Cuervo-Serrato, B.; Peláez-Gorrea, P.; Sopena-Juncosa, J.J. Platelet Rich Plasma: New Insights for Cutaneous Wound Healing Management. *J. Funct. Biomater.* **2018**, *9*, 10. [CrossRef] [PubMed]
117. Davis, V.L.; Abukabda, A.B.; Radio, N.M.; Witt-Enderby, P.A.; Clafshenkel, W.P.; Cairone, J.V.; Rutkowski, J.L. Platelet-Rich Preparations to Improve Healing. Part I: Workable Options for Every Size Practice. *J. Oral. Implantol.* **2014**, *40*, 500–510. [CrossRef] [PubMed]
118. Miron, R.J.; Fujioka-Kobayashi, M.; Bishara, M.; Zhang, Y.; Hernandez, M.; Choukroun, J. Platelet-Rich Fibrin and Soft Tissue Wound Healing: A Systematic Review. *Tissue Eng. Part B Rev.* **2017**, *23*, 83–99. [CrossRef] [PubMed]
119. Zhang, W.; Guo, Y.; Kuss, M.; Shi, W.; Aldrich, A.L.; Untrauer, J.; Kielian, T.; Duan, B. Platelet-Rich Plasma for the Treatment of Tissue Infection: Preparation and Clinical Evaluation. *Tissue Eng. Part B Rev.* **2019**, *25*, 225–236. [CrossRef] [PubMed]
120. Sethi, D.; Martin, K.E.; Shrotriya, S.; Brown, B.L. Systematic literature review evaluating evidence and mechanisms of action for platelet-rich plasma as an antibacterial agent. *J. Cardiothorac. Surg.* **2021**, *16*, 277. [CrossRef]
121. Cieslik-Bieleckaa, A.; Skowronskib, R.; Jedrusik-Pawłowskac, M.; Pierchała, M. The application of L-PRP in AIDS patients with crural chronic ulcers: A pilot study. *Adv. Med. Sci.* **2018**, *63*, 140–146. [CrossRef]
122. Lovisolo, F.; Carton, F.; Gino, S.; Migliario, M.; Renò, F. Platelet rich plasma-derived microvesicles increased in vitro wound healing. *Eur. Rev. Med. Pharmacol. Sci.* **2020**, *24*, 9658–9664.
123. Jain, N.K.; Gulati, M. Platelet-rich plasma: A healing virtuoso. *Blood Res.* **2016**, *51*, 3–5. [CrossRef]
124. Cho, J.-W.; Kim, A.-E.; Lee, K.-S. Platelet-rich plasma induces increased expression of G1 cell cycle regulators, type I collagen, and matrix metalloproteinase-1 in human skin fibroblasts. *Int. J. Mol. Med.* **2012**, *29*, 32–36.
125. Andia, I.; Rubio-Azpeitia, E.; Martin, I.; Abate, M. Current concepts and translational uses of platelet-rich plasma biotechnology. In *Biotechnology*; Ekinci, D., Ed.; InTech: London, UK, 2015.
126. Motolese, A.; Vignati, F.; Antelmi, A.; Saturni, V. Effectiveness of platelet-rich plasma in healing necrobiosis lipoidica diabeticorum ulcers. *Clin. Exp. Dermatol.* **2015**, *40*, 39–41. [CrossRef]
127. Bharathi, M.S.; Tarun. Role of Platelet Rich Plasma [PRP] in the Treatment of Chronic Wounds. *Int. J. Contemp. Med. Res.* **2018**, *5*, E13–E16. [CrossRef]
128. Kacker, N. Surgical Management of Diabetic Foot Ulcers with Platelet Rich Plasma. *Ann. Int. Med. Dent. Res.* **2020**, *6*, 1–4.
129. Suthar, M.; Gupta, S.; Bukhari, S.; Ponemone, V. Treatment of chronic non-healing ulcers using autologous platelet rich plasma: A case series. *J. Biomed. Sci.* **2017**, *24*, 16. [CrossRef] [PubMed]
130. Arora, K.K.; Kapila, R.; Chaudhary, A.; Singhal, A.; Patra, A.; Kapila, S. Proficiency of topical platelet-rich plasma with vacuum-assisted closure over platelet-rich plasma alone in diabetic foot ulcers—A clinical, prospective, comparative study. *Arch. Trauma. Res.* **2022**, *11*, 37–43. [CrossRef]

131. Shan, G.-Q.; Zhang, Y.-N.; Ma, J.; Li, Y.-H.; Zuo, D.-M.; Qiu, J.-L.; Cheng, B.; Chen, Z.-L. Evaluation of the Effects of Homologous Platelet Gel on Healing Lower Extremity Wounds in Patients with Diabetes. *Int. J. Low. Extrem. Wounds* **2013**, *12*, 22–29. [CrossRef]
132. Sakata, J.; Sasaki, S.; Handa, K.; Uchino, T.; Sasaki, T.; Higashita, R.; Tsuno, N.; Hiyoshi, T.; Imakado, S.; Morimoto, S.; et al. A Retrospective, Longitudinal Study to Evaluate Healing Lower Extremity Wounds in Patients with Diabetes Mellitus and Ischemia Using Standard Protocols of Care and Platelet-Rich Plasma Gel in a Japanese Wound Care Program. *Ostomy Wound Manag.* **2012**, *58*, 36–49.
133. Salazar-Álvarez, A.E.; Riera-del-Moral, L.F.; García-Arranz, M.; Álvarez-García, J.; Concepción-Rodriguez, N.A.; Riera-de-Cubas, L. Use of Platelet-Rich Plasma in the Healing of Chronic Ulcers of the Lower Extremity. *Actas Dermo-Sifiliográficas* **2014**, *105*, 597–604. [CrossRef]
134. Cervelli, V.; Gentile, P.; De Angelis, B.; Calabrese, C.; Di Stefani, A.; Scioli, M.G.; Curcio, B.; Marco Felici, B.C.; Orland, A. Application of enhanced stromal vascular fraction and fat grafting mixed with PRP in post-traumatic lower extremity ulcers. *Stem Cell Res.* **2011**, *6*, 103–111. [CrossRef]
135. Tsai, H.-C.; Lehman, C.W.; Chen, C.-M. Use of platelet-rich plasma and platelet derived patches to treat chronic wounds. *J. Wound Care* **2019**, *28*, 15–21. [CrossRef]
136. O'Connell, S.M.; Impeduglia, T.; Karen Hessler, R.N.; Wang, X.-J.; Carroll, R.J.; Dardik, H. Autologous platelet-rich fibrin matrix as cell therapy in the healing of chronic lower-extremity ulcers. *Wound Rep. Reg.* **2008**, *16*, 749–756. [CrossRef]
137. Putrantyo, I.I.; Mosahebi, A.; Smith, O.; De Vega, B. Investigating Effectiveness of Topical Autologous Platelet-rich Plasma as Prophylaxis to Prevent Wound Infection: A Systematic Review and Meta-analysis. *Malays. J. Med. Health Sci.* **2021**, *17*, 72–82.
138. Conde-Montero, E.; de la Cueva Dobao, P.; González, J.M.M. Platelet-rich plasma for the treatment of chronic wounds: Evidence to date. *Chronic Wound Care Manag. Res.* **2017**, *4*, 107–120. [CrossRef]
139. Carter, M.J.; Fylling, C.P.; Parnell, L.K.S. Use of platelet rich plasma gel on wound healing: A systematic review and meta-analysis *Eplasty* **2011**, *11*, e38.
140. Sokolov, T.; Valentinov, B.; Andonov, J.; Angelov, S.; Kosev, P. Platelet-Rich plasma (PRP) and its application in the treatment of chronic and hard-to-heal skin wounds—A Review. *J. IMAB Annu. Proc. Sci. Pap.* **2015**, *21*, 982–986. [CrossRef]
141. Smith, R.G.; Gassmann, C.J.; Campbell, M.S. Platelet-rich Plasma: Properties and Clinical Applications. *J. Lanc. Gen. Hosp.* **2007**, *2*, 73–77.
142. Kim, S.-A.; Ryu, H.-W.; Lee, K.-S.; Cho, J.-W. Application of platelet-rich plasma accelerates the wound healing process in acute and chronic ulcers through rapid migration and upregulation of cyclin A and CDK4 in HaCaT-cells. *Mol. Med. Rep.* **2013**, *7*, 476–480. [CrossRef]
143. Hall, M.P.; Band, P.A.; Meislin, R.J.; Jazrawi, L.M.; Cardone, D.A. Platelet-Rich Plasma: Current Concepts and Application in Sports Medicine. *J. Am. Acad. Orthop. Surg.* **2009**, *17*, 602–608. [CrossRef]
144. Everts, P.A.M.; Hoogbergen, M.M.; Weber, T.A.; Devilee, R.J.J.; van Monfort, G.; de Hingh, I.H.J.T. Is the Use of Autologous Platelet-Rich Plasma Gels in Gynecologic, Cardiac, and General, Reconstructive Surgery Beneficial? *Curr. Pharm. Biotechnol.* **2012**, *13*, 1163–1172. [CrossRef]
145. de Leon, J.M.; Driver, V.R.; Fylling, C.P.; Carter, M.J.; Anderson, C.; Wilson, J.; Dougherty, R.M.; Fuston, D.; Trigilia, D.; Valenski, V.; et al. The Clinical Relevance of Treating Chronic Wounds with an Enhanced Near-Physiological Concentration of Platelet-Rich Plasma Gel. *Adv. Ski. Wound Care* **2011**, *24*, 357–368. [CrossRef]
146. Frykberg, R.G.; Driver, V.R.; Carman, D.; Lucero, B.; Borris-Hale, C.; Fylling, C.P.; Rappl, L.M.; Clausen, P.A. Chronic Wounds Treated with a Physiologically Relevant Concentration of Platelet-rich Plasma Gel: A Prospective Case Series. *Ostomy Wound Manag.* **2010**, *56*, 36–44.
147. Palumbo, V.D.; Rizzuto, S.; Damiano, G.; Fazzotta, S.; Gottardo, A.; Mazzola, G.; Lo Monte, A.I. Use of platelet concentrate gel in second-intention wound healing: A case report. *J. Med. Case. Rep.* **2021**, *15*, 85. [CrossRef]
148. Crovetti, G.; Martinelli, G.; Issi, M.; Barone, M.; Guizzardi, M.; Campanati, B.; Moroni, M.; Carabelli, A. Platelet gel for healing cutaneous chronic wounds. *Transfus. Apher. Sci.* **2004**, *30*, 145–151. [CrossRef] [PubMed]
149. Gupta, A.; Shrivastava, S. Study of PRP assisted wound repair and regeneration in chronic non-healing wounds. *Orthop. JMPC* **2018**, *24*, 14–20.
150. Sokolov, T.; Manukova, A.; Kovachev, V.; Kovachev, K. Treatment of problematic skin wounds based on the Platelet-rich plasma method. *J. IMAB Annu. Proc. Sci. Pap.* **2020**, *26*, 3436–3442.
151. Upadhyay, S.; Varma, H.S.; Yadav, S. Potential therapeutic effects of autologous platelet rich plasma on impaired wound healing: A prospective clinical study. *Int. J. Res. Orthop.* **2018**, *4*, 820–825. [CrossRef]
152. Pallua, N.; Wolter, T.; Markowicz, M. Platelet-rich plasma in burns. *Burns* **2010**, *36*, 4–8. [CrossRef]
153. Zheng, W.; Zhao, D.-L.; Zhao, Y.-Q.; Li, Z.-Y. Effectiveness of platelet rich plasma in burn wound healing: A systematic review and meta-analysis. *J. Dermatolog. Treat.* **2022**, *33*, 131–137. [CrossRef]
154. Foster, T.E.; Puskas, B.L.; Mandelbaum, B.R.; Gerhardt, M.B.; Rodeo, S.A. Platelet-Rich Plasma: From Basic Science to Clinical Applications. *Am. J. Sports Med.* **2009**, *37*, 2259–2272. [CrossRef]
155. Chen, X.; Jones, I.A.; Park, C.; Vangsness, C.T., Jr. The Efficacy of Platelet-Rich Plasma on Tendon and Ligament Healing: A Systematic Review and Meta-Analysis with Bias Assessment. *Am. J. Sports Med.* **2018**, *46*, 2020–2032. [CrossRef]
156. Yang, F. -A.; Liao, C.-D.; Wu, C.-W.; Shih, Y.-C.; Wu, L.-C.; Chen, H-C. Effects of applying platelet-rich plasma during arthroscopic rotator cuff repair: A systematic review and meta-analysis of randomized controlled trials. *Sci. Rep.* **2020**, *10*, 17171. [CrossRef]

157. Mahmoudian-Sani, M.-R.; Rafeei, F.; Amini, R.; Saidijam, M. The effect of mesenchymal stem cells combined with platelet-rich plasma on skin wound healing. *J. Cosmet. Dermatol.* **2018**, *17*, 650–659. [CrossRef] [PubMed]
158. Dehkordi, A.N.; Babaheydari, F.M.; Chehelgerdi, M.; Dehkordi, S.R. Skin tissue engineering: Wound healing based on stem-cell-based therapeutic strategies. *Stem Cell Res. Ther.* **2019**, *10*, 111. [CrossRef] [PubMed]
159. Azari, Z.; Nazarnezhad, S.; Webster, T.J.; Hoseini, S.J.; Milan, P.B.; Baino, F.; Kargozar, S. Stem cell-mediated angiogenesis in skin tissue engineering and wound healing. *Wound Rep. Reg.* **2022**, *30*, 421–435. [CrossRef]
160. Goodson, H.V.; Jonasson, E.M. Microtubules and Microtubule-Associated Proteins. *Cold Spring Harb. Perspect. Biol.* **2018**, *10*, a022608. [CrossRef] [PubMed]
161. Charvet, H.J.; Orbay, H.; Harrison, L.; Devi, K.; Sahar, D.E. In vitro effects of adipose-derived stem cells on breast cancer cells harvested from the same patient. *Ann. Plast. Surg.* **2016**, *76*, S241–S245. [CrossRef]
162. Moore, K.E.; Mills, J.F.; Thornton, M.M. Alternative sources of adult stem cells: A possible solution to the embryonic stem cell debate. *Gend. Med.* **2006**, *3*, 161–168. [CrossRef]
163. Zuk, P.A.; Zhu, M.; Mizuno, H.; Huang, J.; Futrell, J.W.; Katz, A.J.; Benhaim, P.; Lorenz, H.P.; Hedrick, M.H. Multilineage cells from human adipose tissue: Implications for cell-based therapies. *Tissue Eng.* **2001**, *7*, 211–228. [CrossRef]
164. Lazar, M.A. Developmental biology. How now, brown fat? *Science* **2008**, *321*, 1048–1049. [CrossRef]
165. Psaltis, P.J.; Zannettino, A.C.; Worthley, S.G.; Gronthos, S. Concise review: Mesenchymal stromal cells: Potential for cardiovascular repair. *Stem Cells* **2008**, *26*, 2201–2210. [CrossRef]
166. Thomson, J.A.; Itskovitz-Eldor, J.; Shapiro, S.S.; Waknitz, M.A.; Swiergiel, J.J.; Marshall, V.S.; Jones, J.M. Embryonic stem cell lines derived from human blastocysts. *Science* **2011**, *5391*, 1145–1147. [CrossRef]
167. Bunnell, B.A. Adipose Tissue-Derived Mesenchymal Stem Cells. *Cells* **2021**, *10*, 3433. [CrossRef] [PubMed]
168. Gimble, J.; Katz, A.; Bunnell, B. Adipose-derived stem cells for regenerative medicine. *Circ. Res.* **2009**, *100*, 1249–1260. [CrossRef] [PubMed]
169. Kim, E.Y.; Kim, W.K.; Oh, K.J.; Han, B.S.; Lee, S.C.; Bae, K.H. Recent advances in proteomic studies of adipose tissues and adipocytes. *Int. J. Mol. Sci.* **2015**, *16*, 4581–4599. [CrossRef] [PubMed]
170. Coelho, M.; Oliveira, T.; Fernandez, R. Biochemistry of adipose tissue: An endocrine organ. *Arch. Med. Sci.* **2013**, *9*, 191–200. [CrossRef]
171. Zimmerlin, L.; Donnenberg, V.S.; Rubin, J.P.; Donnenberg, A.D. Mesenchymal markers on human adipose stem/progenitor cells. *Cytom. A* **2013**, *83*, 134–140. [CrossRef]
172. Lindroos, B.; Suuronen, R.; Miettinen, S. The potential of adipose stem cells in regenerative medicine. *Stem Cell Rev.* **2011**, *7*, 269–291. [CrossRef]
173. Kunze, K.N.; Burnett, R.A.; Wright-Chisem, J.; Frank, R.M.; Chahla, J. Adipose-derived mesenchymal stem cell treatments and available formulations. *Curr. Rev. Musculoskelet. Med.* **2020**, *13*, 264–280. [CrossRef]
174. Caplan, A.I.; Dennis, J.E. Mesenchymal Stem Cells as Trophic Mediators. *J. Cell Biochem.* **2006**, *98*, 1076–1084. [CrossRef]
175. Strioga, M.; Viswanathan, S.; Darinskas, A.; Slaby, O.; Michalek, J. Same or Not the Same? Comparison of Adipose Tissue-Derived versus Bone Marrow-Derived Mesenchymal Stem and Stromal Cells. *Stem Cells Dev.* **2012**, *21*, 2724–2752. [CrossRef]
176. Zuttion, M.S.S.R.; Wenceslau, C.V.; Lemos, P.A.; Takimura, C.; Kerkis, I. Adipose Tissue-Derived Stem Cells and the Importance of Animal Model Standardization for Pre-Clinical Trials. *Rev. Bras. Cardiol. Invasiva* **2013**, *21*, 281–287. [CrossRef]
177. Alt, E.U.; Senst, C.; Murthy, S.N.; Slakey, D.P.; Dupin, C.L.; Chaffin, A.E.; Kadowitz, P.J.; Izadpanah, R. Aging alters tissue resident mesenchymal stem cell properties. *Stem Cell Res.* **2012**, *8*, 215–225. [CrossRef]
178. Frese, L.; Dijkman, P.E.; Simon, P. Adipose Tissue-Derived Stem Cells in Regenerative Medicine. *Transfus. Med. Hemother.* **2016**, *43*, 268–274. [CrossRef]
179. Madonna, R.; De Caterina, R. Adipose tissue: A new source for cardiovascular repair. *J. Cardiovasc. Med.* **2010**, *11*, 71–80. [CrossRef] [PubMed]
180. Miana, V.V.; González, E.A.P. Adipose tissue stem cells in regenerative medicine. *Ecancermedicalscience* **2018**, *12*, 822. [CrossRef] [PubMed]
181. Hong, S.J.; Traktueva, D.O.; March, K.L. Therapeutic potential of adipose-derived stem cells in vascular growth and tissue repair. *Curr. Opin. Organ Transplant.* **2010**, *15*, 86–91. [CrossRef]
182. Mazini, L.; Rochette, L.; Admou, B.; Amal, S.; Malka, G. Hopes and Limits of Adipose-Derived Stem Cells (ADSCs) and Mesenchymal Stem Cells (MSCs) in Wound Healing. *Int. J. Mol. Sci.* **2020**, *21*, 1306. [CrossRef] [PubMed]
183. Yiou, R.; Mahrouf-Yorgov, M.; Trebeau, C.; Zanaty, M.; Lecointe, C.; Souktani, R.; Zadigue, P.; Figeac, F.; Rodriguez, A.M. Delivery of human mesenchymal adipose-derived stem cells restores multiple urological dysfunctions in a rat model mimicking radical prostatectomy damages through tissue-specific paracrine mechanisms. *Stem Cells* **2016**, *34*, 392–404. [CrossRef]
184. Lin, C.S.; Xin, Z.C.; Deng, C.H.; Ning, H.; Lin, G.; Lue, T.F. Defining adipose tissue-derived stem cells in tissue and in culture. *Histol. Histopathol.* **2010**, *25*, 807–815.
185. Rohringer, S.; Hofbauer, P.; Schneider, K.H.; Husa, A.-M.; Feichtinger, G.; Peterbauer-Scherb, A.; Redl, H.; Holnthoner, W. Mechanisms of vasculogenesis in 3D fibrin matrices mediated by the interaction of adipose-derived stem cells and endothelial cells. *Angiogenesis* **2014**, *17*, 921–933. [CrossRef]
186. Merfeld-Clauss, S.; Lupov, I.P.; Lu, H.; March, K.L.; Traktuev, D.O. Adipose Stromal Cell Contact with Endothelial Cells Results in Loss of Complementary Vasculogenic Activity Mediated by Induction of Activin A. *Stem Cells* **2015**, *33*, 3039–3051. [CrossRef]

187. Wang, L.; Hu, L.; Zhou, X.; Zhang, C.; Shehada, H.M.A.; Hu, B.; Song, J.; Chen, L. Exosomes secreted by human adipose mesenchymal stem cells promote scarless cutaneous repair by regulating extracellular matrix remodelling. *Sci. Rep.* **2017**, *7*, 13321 [CrossRef] [PubMed]
188. Stessuk, T.; Puzzi, M.B.; Chaim, E.A.; Alves, P.C.M.; de Paula, E.V.; Forte, A.; Izumizawa, J.M.; Oliveira, C.C.; Frei, F.; Ribeiro-Paes, J.T. Platelet-rich plasma (PRP) and adipose-derived mesenchymal stem cells: Stimulatory effects on proliferation and migration of fibroblasts and keratinocytes in vitro. *Arch. Dermatol. Res.* **2016**, *308*, 511–520. [CrossRef] [PubMed]
189. Phillips, M.I.; Tang, Y.L. Genetic modification of stem cells for transplantation. *Adv. Drug Deliv. Rev.* **2008**, *60*, 160–172. [CrossRef] [PubMed]
190. Shevchenko, E.K.; Makarevich, P.I.; Tsokolaeva, Z.I.; Boldyreva, M.A.; Sysoeva, V.Y.; Tkachuk, V.A.; Parfyonova, Y.V. Transplantation of modified human adipose derived stromal cells expressing VEGF165 results in more efficient angiogenic response in ischemic skeletal muscle. *J. Transl. Med.* **2013**, *11*, 138. [CrossRef] [PubMed]
191. Xu, F.; Yang, Y.; Yang, T.; Dai, T.; Shao, X.; Xu, H.; An, R.; Liu, Y.; Liu, B. The use of allogenic adipose-derived stem cells in combination with platelet-rich fibrin for the treatment of cartilage defects in rabbit ear. *Am. J. Transl. Res.* **2018**, *10*, 1900–1907.
192. Rad, F.; Ghorbani, M.; Roushandeh, A.M.; Roudkenar, M.H. Mesenchymal stem cell-based therapy for autoimmune diseases: Emerging roles of extracellular vesicles. *Mol. Biol. Rep.* **2019**, *46*, 1533–1549. [CrossRef]
193. Li, P.; Guo, X. A review: Therapeutic potential of adipose-derived stem cells in cutaneous wound healing and regeneration. *Stem Cell Res. Ther.* **2018**, *9*, 302. [CrossRef]
194. Su, W.G.; Wang, P.L.; Dong, Q.Q.; Li, S.; Hu, S.W. S100A8 accelerates wound healing by promoting adipose stem cell proliferation and suppressing inflammation. *Regen. Ther.* **2022**, *21*, 166–174. [CrossRef]
195. Ouyang, L.; Qiu, D.; Fu, X.; Wu, A.; Yang, P.; Yang, Z.; Wang, Q.; Yan, L.; Xiao, R. Overexpressing HPGDS in adipose-derived mesenchymal stem cells reduces inflammatory state and improves wound healing in type 2 diabetic mice. *Stem Cell Res. Ther.* **2022**, *13*, 395. [CrossRef]
196. Lyras, D.; Kazakos, K.; Verettas, D.; Polychronidis, A.; Simopoulos, C.; Botaitis, S.; Agrogiannis, G.; Kokka, A.; Patsouris, E. Immunohistochemical study of angiogenesis after local administration of platelet-rich plasma in a patellar tendon defect. *Int. Orthop.* **2010**, *34*, 143–148. [CrossRef]
197. Suzuki, E.; Fujita, D.; Takahashi, M.; Oba, S.; Nishimatsu, H. Adipose tissue-derived stem cells as a therapeutic tool for cardiovascular disease. *World J. Cardiol.* **2015**, *7*, 454–465. [CrossRef] [PubMed]
198. Barba, M.; Cicione, C.; Bernardini, C.; Michetti, F.; Lattanzi, W. Adipose-derived mesenchymal cells for bone regeneration: State of the art. *Biol. Med. Res. Int.* **2013**, *2013*, 416391. [CrossRef] [PubMed]
199. Ebrahim, N.; Dessouky, A.A.; Mostafa, O.; Hassouna, A.; Yousef, M.M.; Seleem, Y.; El Gebaly, E.A.E.A.M.; Allam, M.M.; Farid, A.S.; Saffaf, B.A.; et al. Adipose mesenchymal stem cells combined with platelet-rich plasma accelerate diabetic wound healing by modulating the Notch pathway. *Stem Cell Res. Ther.* **2021**, *12*, 392. [CrossRef] [PubMed]
200. Wang, X.; Ma, Y.; Gao, Z.; Yang, J. Human adipose-derived stem cells inhibit bioactivity of keloid fibroblasts. *Stem Cell Res. Ther.* **2018**, *9*, 40. [CrossRef]
201. Hashem, H.E.; Mobasher, M.O.I.; Mohamed, M.Z.; Alkhodary, A.A.M. Efficiency of Adipose-Derived versus Bone Marrow-Derived Stem Cells in Modulation of Histopathological Changes and CD31 Immunoexpression during Wound Healing in Rats. *J. Biochem. Cell Biol.* **2018**, *1*, 106.
202. Nie, C.; Yang, D.; Xu, J.; Si, Z.; Jin, X.; Zhang, J. Locally Administered Adipose-Derived Stem Cells Accelerate Wound Healing through Differentiation and Vasculogenesis. *Cell Transplant.* **2011**, *20*, 205–216. [CrossRef]
203. Hong, S.J.; Jia, S.X.; Xie, P.; Xu, W.; Leung, K.P.; Mustoe, T.A.; Galiano, R.D. Topically delivered adipose derived stem cells show an activated-fibroblast phenotype and enhance granulation tissue formation in skin wounds. *PLoS ONE* **2013**, *8*, e55640. [CrossRef]
204. Shafei, S.; Khanmohammadi, M.; Heidari, R.; Ghanbari, H.; Nooshabadi, V.T.; Farzamfar, S.; Akbariqomi, M.; Sanikhani, N.S.; Absalan, M.; Tavoosidana, G. Exosome loaded alginate hydrogel promotes tissue regeneration in full-thickness skin wounds: An in vivo study. *J. Biomed. Mater. Res.* **2020**, *108A*, 545–556. [CrossRef]
205. Shukla, A.; Choudhury, S.; Chaudhary, G.; Singh, V.; Prabhu, S.N.; Pandey, S.; Garg, S.K. Chitosan and gelatin biopolymer supplemented with Mesenchymal Stem cells (Velgraft®) enhanced wound healing in goats (*Capra hircus*): Involvement of VEGF TGF and CDJ. *Tissue Viability* **2021**, *30*, 59–66. [CrossRef]
206. Dai, R.; Wang, Z.; Samanipour, R.; Koo, K.-I.; Kim, K. Adipose-Derived Stem Cells for Tissue Engineering and Regenerative Medicine Applications. *Stem Cells Int.* **2016**, *2016*, 6737345. [CrossRef]
207. Li, M.; Ma, J.; Gao, Y.; Dong, M.; Zheng, Z.; Li, Y.; Tan, R.; She, Z.; Yang, L. Epithelial differentiation of human adipose derived stem cells (hASCs) undergoing three-dimensional (3D) cultivation with collagen sponge scaffold (CSS) via an indirect co-culture strategy. *Stem Cell Res. Ther.* **2020**, *11*, 141. [CrossRef] [PubMed]
208. Colazzo, F.; Chester, A.H.; Taylor, P.M.; Yacoub, M.H. Induction of mesenchymal to endothelial transformation of adipose-derived stem cells. *J. Heart Valve Dis.* **2010**, *19*, 736–744. [PubMed]
209. Breitsprecher, D.; Goode, B.L. Formins at a glance. *J. Cell Sci.* **2013**, *126*, 1–7. [CrossRef] [PubMed]
210. Liu, S.; Zhang, H.; Zhang, X.; Lu, W.; Huang, X.; Xie, H.; Zhou, J.; Wang, W.; Zhang, Y.; Liu, Y.; et al. Synergistic Angiogenesis Promoting Effects of Extracellular Matrix Scaffolds and Adipose-Derived Stem Cells during Wound Repair. *Tissue Eng. Part A* **2011**, *17*, 725–739. [CrossRef] [PubMed]

211. Xie, X.; Wang, Y.; Zhao, C.; Guo, S.; Liu, S.; Jia, W.; Tuan, R.S.; Zhang, C. Comparative evaluation of MSCs from bone marrow and adipose tissue seeded in PRP-derived scaffold for cartilage regeneration. *Biomaterials* **2012**, *33*, 7008–7018. [CrossRef]
212. Gao, Y.; Gao, B.; Zhu, H.; Yu, Q.; Xie, F.; Cheng, C.; Li, Q. Adipose-derived stem cells embedded in platelet-rich plasma scaffolds improve the texture of skin grafts in a rat full-thickness wound model. *Burns* **2020**, *46*, 377–385. [CrossRef]
213. Lucchina, A.G.; Radica, M.K.; Costa, A.L.; Mortellaro, C.; Soliani, G.; Zavan, B. Mesh-tissue integration of synthetic and biologic meshes in wall surgery: Brief state of art. *Eur. Rev. Med. Pharmacol. Sci.* **2022**, *26*, 21–25.
214. Khandaker, M.; Alkadhem, N.; Progri, H.; Nikfarjam, S.; Jeon, J.; Kotturi, H.; Vaughan, M.B. Glutathione immobilized polycaprolactone nanofiber mesh as a dermal drug delivery mechanism for wound healing in a diabetic patient. *Processes* **2022**, *10*, 512. [CrossRef]
215. Xu, D.; Fang, M.; Wang, Q.; Qiao, Y.; Li, Y.; Wang, L. Latest trends on the attenuation of systemic foreign body response and infectious complications of synthetic hernia meshes. *ACS Appl. Bio. Mater.* **2021**, *5*, 1–9. [CrossRef]

Disclaimer/Publisher's Note: The statements, opinions and data contained in all publications are solely those of the individual author(s) and contributor(s) and not of MDPI and/or the editor(s). MDPI and/or the editor(s) disclaim responsibility for any injury to people or property resulting from any ideas, methods, instructions or products referred to in the content.

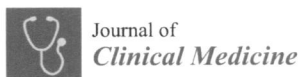 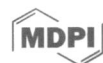

Article

Factors Influencing Postoperative Complications Following Minimally Invasive Ivor Lewis Esophagectomy: A Retrospective Cohort Study

Antje K. Peters [1,2,3,†], Mazen A. Juratli [1,†], Dhruvajyoti Roy [4], Jennifer Merten [1], Lukas Fortmann [1], Andreas Pascher [1] and Jens Peter Hoelzen [1,*]

1. Department of General, Visceral and Transplant Surgery, University Hospital Muenster, 48149 Muenster, Germany; antje.peters@uni-muenster.de (A.K.P.); mazen.juratli@ukmuenster.de (M.A.J.)
2. Institute of Medical Psychology and Systems Neuroscience, University of Muenster, 48149 Muenster, Germany
3. Otto Creutzfeldt Center for Cognitive and Behavioral Neuroscience, University of Muenster, 48149 Muenster, Germany
4. Department of Surgical Oncology, University of Texas MD Anderson Cancer Center, Houston, TX 77030, USA
* Correspondence: jenspeter.hoelzen@ukmuenster.de; Tel.: +49-251-83-56361; Fax: +49-251-83-56414
† These authors contributed equally to this work.

Abstract: Background: Complications arising following minimally invasive Ivor Lewis esophagectomy often result from inadequate enteral nutrition, highlighting the need for proactive measures to prevent such issues. One approach involves identifying high-risk cases prone to complications and implementing percutaneous endoscopic jejunostomy (PEJ) tube placement during esophageal resection to ensure timely enteral nutrition. Methods: In this single-center, retrospective cohort study, we examined patients who underwent minimally invasive esophagectomy for esophageal cancer at a high-volume center. The dataset encompassed demographic information, comorbidities, laboratory parameters, and intraoperative details. Our center utilized the EndoVac system pre-emptively to safeguard the anastomosis from harmful secretions and to enhance local oxygen partial pressure. All patients received pre-emptive EndoVac therapy and underwent esophagogastroduodenoscopy in the early postoperative days. The need for multiple postoperative EndoVac cycles indicated complications, including anastomotic insufficiency and subsequent requirement for a PEJ. The primary objectives were identifying predictive factors for anastomotic insufficiency and the need for multi-cycle EndoVac therapy, quantifying their effects, and assessing the likelihood of postoperative complications. Results: 149 patients who underwent minimally invasive or hybrid Ivor Lewis esophagectomy were analyzed and 21 perioperative and demographic features were evaluated. Postoperative complications were associated with the body mass index (BMI) category, the use of blood pressure medication, and surgery duration. Anastomotic insufficiency as a specific complication was correlated with BMI and the Charlson comorbidity index. The odds ratio of being in the high-risk group significantly increased with higher BMI (OR = 1.074, p = 0.048) and longer surgery duration (OR = 1.005, p = 0.004). Conclusions: Based on our findings, high BMI and longer surgery duration are potential risk factors for postoperative complications following minimally invasive esophagectomy. Identifying such factors can aid in pre-emptively addressing nutritional challenges and reducing the incidence of complications in high-risk patients.

Keywords: minimally invasive Ivor Lewis esophagectomy; RAMIE; enteral nutrition; percutaneous endoscopic jejunostomy (PEJ); anastomotic insufficiency

Citation: Peters, A.K.; Juratli, M.A.; Roy, D.; Merten, J.; Fortmann, L.; Pascher, A.; Hoelzen, J.P. Factors Influencing Postoperative Complications Following Minimally Invasive Ivor Lewis Esophagectomy: A Retrospective Cohort Study. *J. Clin. Med.* 2023, 12, 5688. https://doi.org/10.3390/jcm12175688

Academic Editor: Orestis Ioannidis

Received: 30 July 2023
Revised: 29 August 2023
Accepted: 30 August 2023
Published: 31 August 2023

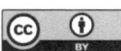

Copyright: © 2023 by the authors. Licensee MDPI, Basel, Switzerland. This article is an open access article distributed under the terms and conditions of the Creative Commons Attribution (CC BY) license (https://creativecommons.org/licenses/by/4.0/).

1. Introduction

Esophageal carcinomas are the sixth leading cause of cancer mortality worldwide [1], and their incidence in the Western population is increasing [2]. Minimally invasive Ivor

Lewis esophagectomy is a surgical procedure commonly performed to treat esophageal cancer [3–6]. While this technique offers numerous benefits, including reduced postoperative pain and shorter hospital stays, post-surgery complications, such as anastomotic insufficiency (AI), remain a significant concern, with an incidence of 11.4–21.2 percent [7]. Among the key challenges is the inability to provide adequate enteral nutrition during recovery, leading to potential complications and delayed healing of anastomotic sites. One approach for mitigating these issues involves identifying cases at high risk of complications and implementing feeding tubes, such as percutaneous endoscopic jejunostomy (PEJ) tubes, during esophageal resection. This strategy ensures timely enteral nutrition delivery, hence reducing the likelihood of postoperative complications.

Our high-volume center has adopted a pioneering approach over the past decade by utilizing a pre-emptive EndoVac sponge, following each esophagectomy with intrathoracic anastomosis. After each esophageal resection, esophagogastroduodenoscopy is performed and a diameter-matched sponge is positioned on the anastomosis under visualization using a retraction technique. After 5 days, the EndoVac sponge is removed and a control endoscopy is performed. In case of irregularities, an individually trimmed sponge is placed again. This proactive measure has proven beneficial in preventing potential complications. In certain cases, extended EndoVac therapy is required, particularly in instances of AI. When postoperative complications necessitate the prolonged use of EndoVac therapy, enteral therapy is recommended as a complementary intervention [8]. As parenteral nutrition carries the potential risks of hyperglycemia, hypertriglyceridemia, electrolyte imbalances, and long-term hepatobiliary and bone diseases [9], alternative nutritional strategies are sought to ensure optimal patient outcomes. Among these, enteral nutrition is preferred [10], and PEJ is mainly considered for patients at high risk of AI [11]. However, the lack of a standardized postoperative PEJ insertion procedure raises concerns about the timing and necessity of this intervention, as the process can be burdensome for patients: On the one hand, inserting a PEJ tube has risks, including potential complications such as aspiration pneumonia, wound infection, and bleeding [12]. These risks argue against an overly generous use of a tube. On the other hand, if a patient develops postoperative complications, a separate surgery is required for PEJ tube insertion, adding to the overall complexity of their care. This consideration would argue for the simultaneous insertion of a probe.

To address this ambiguity, there is a growing interest in predicting the likelihood of post-esophagectomy complications based on perioperative and demographic patient data. By identifying patients at high risk of complications, healthcare professionals can make informed decisions and potentially perform PEJ tube insertion during the esophagectomy, streamlining the process and minimizing the need for additional surgeries. Such predictive tools offer the potential to enhance patient care by optimizing nutritional support and reducing the impact of complications, ultimately leading to improved postoperative outcomes.

This single-center, retrospective cohort study investigated factors influencing postoperative complications such as AI following minimally invasive Ivor Lewis esophagectomy. This study was unique because it was able to draw conclusions from a local population in which pre-emptive EndoVac therapy and regular endoscopy were performed. We hypothesized that the data collected would identify risk factors associated with postoperative complications. The study aimed to identify predictors of AI as a specific and very common complication. However, AI affects only a few cases of the total sample, which makes the evaluation challenging. Therefore, we introduced the need for multiple cycles of EndoVac therapy as a surrogate parameter for a complicative course. This event occurs more often and is more straightforward to address.

2. Materials and Methods

Patients: This retrospective cohort study comprised 149 patients who underwent either minimally invasive or hybrid Ivor Lewis esophagectomy for esophageal cancer at Münster University Hospital between February 2012 and March 2022. We included all patients aged 18 years or older with thoracic or abdominal esophagus carcinoma that was both histologically diagnosed and resectable. In the case of neoadjuvant therapy, respectability after therapy was decisive. Cases where surgery could not be completed or where laparoscopic intervention became necessary were excluded. The study also excluded patients with evidence of COVID-19 infection and those undergoing two-stage operations. All included patients had undergone postoperative pre-emptive EndoVac insertion. For this purpose, at the end of the operation, and before removing the double-lumen tube for ventilation, an esophagogastroduodenoscopy was performed and the anastomosis was examined. An EndoVac sponge was then cut to fit the diameter of the gastric tube and positioned at the level of the anastomosis using the retraction technique under visual control. The tube was then fed out of the nose, connected to a suction generator with a suction of -125 mmHg, and fixed to the nose. After 5 days, the sponge was removed and control endoscopy was performed under short-term anesthesia. In case of irregularities in anastomosis healing, for example, a widened anastomosis or visible staples, prophylactic therapy was continued in 5-day cycles. EndoVac therapy was continued in the event of an anastomotic leak, albeit not as a prevention but as a therapy. Where this therapeutical approach was used, esophagogastroduodenoscopy was performed and repeated every 5 days. Diagnostics for cancer staging were performed based on physical and nutritional assessments, endoscopy (including biopsy), endoscopic ultrasound and computer tomography scan. A multidisciplinary cancer board decided on surgery and neoadjuvant treatments were administered following the German Cancer Society (DKG) guidelines for esophageal adenocarcinoma and squamous cell carcinoma, using FLOT (fluorouracil/leucovorin/oxaliplatin/docetaxel) or CROSS (carboplatin/paclitaxel) treatment schemes [13,14].

All procedures were conducted using minimally invasive techniques, either as hybrid esophagectomy (laparoscopic gastric mobilization and open right thoracotomy) or robot-assisted minimally invasive esophagectomies (RAMIEs) utilizing the da Vinci Surgery System (Intuitive Surgical Inc., Sunnyvale, CA, USA). As a high-volume center with many years of experience in esophageal surgery, surgical methods were changed to minimally invasive procedures after the publication of the Time Study [15]. In 2018, the robot-assisted technique (RAMIE) was introduced. The MIRO Trial [16], ROBOT Trial [17], and RAMIE Trial [18] showed the advantages of robot-assisted procedures. All procedures had the minimally invasive approach in common. Resection and anastomosis were the same, with different access routes, and, therefore, had comparable risks. In this regard, our sample represents a homogeneous collective. Gastrolysis, gastric tube formation, and D2 lymphadenectomy were performed in all surgical procedures. At the end of the abdominal phase, an initial vascularization check of the gastric tube was performed with ICG. In the thoracic part, an en bloc esophagectomy with lymphadenectomy and appropriate safety margin was performed and checked using frozen sections. Anastomosis of the gastric tube with the remaining esophagus was performed using an end-to-side technique using a 29 mm circular stapler. After completing the anastomosis, another vascularization check was performed with ICG. For more details on the surgical procedures (hybrid esophagectomy and RAMIE), refer to Ref [4].

Clinical characteristics, surgery details, and preoperative laboratory parameters were extracted from hospital records. Patients were followed up for at least 30 days to monitor postoperative complications. The dataset contained 21 features, as listed in Table 1. All procedures adhered to the Declaration of Helsinki with Good Clinical Practice (GCP) and the STROCSS 2019 Guideline [19–21]. Ethical approval was obtained from the combined ethics committee of the University of Muenster (Muenster, Germany) and the Medical Association of Westphalia-Lippe (reference number: 2022-123-f-S), and written general consent for the scientific use of medical data was obtained from all patients.

Table 1. Pre- and perioperative characteristics: Number of cases with the respective conditions with respect to the two endpoints investigated in this study. *p*-values correspond to a chi-square test and * denotes statistical significance. AI = anastomotic insufficiency, BMI = body mass index, ASA = American Society of Anesthesiologists, CRP = C-reactive protein.

	Endpoint: AI			Endpoint: Multi-Cycle EndoVac Therapy		
Preoperative characteristics	No AI	AI	*p*-value	Single-cycle	Multi-cycle	*p*-value
Demographic data						
Age in years						
<65	67	14	0.842	36	45	0.882
65–75	33	8		20	21	
>75	21	6		13	14	
Sex						
male	94	26	0.118	54	66	0.657
female	27	2		15	14	
BMI in kg/m^2						
<25	53	6	0.092	37	22	0.004 *
25–30	41	13		21	33	
>30	27	9		11	25	
Preoperative diagnostics and therapy						
ASA score						
<2	4	0	0.744	4	0	0.094
≥2	117	28		65	80	
Tumor localization						
upper or middle third	0	1	0.423	0	1	0.625
gastroesophageal junction	121	27		79	69	
Neoadjuvant therapy						
chemotherapy	47	6	0.335	29	24	0.244
chemoradiotherapy	65	19		34	50	
none	9	3		6	6	
Charlson comorbidity index						
<3	28	1	0.036	12	17	0.709
≥3	93	27		57	63	
T-status pretherapy						
T1	8	5		8	5	
T2	25	4	0.234	16	13	0.281
T3	86	19		59	46	
T4	2	0		0	2	
N-status pretherapy						
N0	27	6	0.999	13	20	0.491
N+	94	22		56	60	
Medication						
Blood pressure medication						
yes	69	21	0.124	35	55	0.038 *
no	52	7		34	25	
Cortisone medication						
yes	2	0	0.999	0	2	0.542
no	119	28		69	78	
Immunosuppression						
yes	1	2	0.162	0	3	0.298
no	120	26		69	77	
Anticoagulant						
yes	27	9	0.395	13	23	0.224
no	94	19		56	57	

Table 1. Cont.

	Endpoint: AI			Endpoint: Multi-Cycle EndoVac Therapy		
Laboratory parameters						
Preoperative CRP in mg/dl						
<0.5	33	6	0.999	23	16	0.999
≥0.5	23	4		16	11	
Preoperative leucocytes						
<10,000	81	14	0.473	64	70	0.679
≥10,000	33	9		4	7	
Preoperative hemoglobin in mg/dL						
<12	37	10	0.763	22	25	0.999
≥12	84	18		47	55	
Perioperative characteristics						
Treatment group						
full-robotic	54	10	0.518	27	37	0.478
hybrid-robotic	67	18		42	43	
Surgery duration (complete procedure) in minutes						
<360	33	5	0.430	25	13	0.009 *
≥360	88	23		44	67	
Surgery duration (thoracic part) in minutes						
<240	81	14	0.473	52	43	0.004 *
≥240	33	9		11	31	
Intraoperative blood loss in mL						
<100	37	11	0.597	24	24	0.081
≥100	49	10		27	32	
R status						
R0	115	26	0.999	65	76	0.999
R1	6	2		4	4	

Endpoints: At Münster University Hospital, a proactive approach is implemented to minimize postoperative complications after esophagectomy. Patients undergo pre-emptive EndoVac therapy, which involves the placement of an EndoVac intraoperatively. This approach contrasts with the standard procedure, where the EndoVac is used only in case of complications [22]. The EndoVac is a standard therapy for postoperative treatment [23–25]. The pre-emptive EndoVac therapy is a novel technology for reducing AI rate and postoperative morbidity. The approach has also been used successfully in other centers [26–28]. Following surgery, patients are closely monitored in the Intensive Care Unit (ICU) for at least one night, with extended stay if necessary. Once there are no complications, patients are transferred to the general ward, where they receive standardized postoperative care.

All patients undergo esophagogastroduodenoscopy on the fifth day after surgery to check for AI and identify any defects based on the Esophagectomy Complications Consensus Group standards [29]. If the findings are normal, the EndoVac is removed and the patient is started on an oral diet. The occurrence of AI is defined as the first endpoint in this investigation. However, in cases where complications—including but not limited to AI—arise, EndoVac therapy is continued. If the EndoVac probe remains in place beyond the fifth day, enteral nutrition is given using a PEJ tube (Freka FCJ FR 9, Fresenius Kabi, Bad Homburg, Germany). Note that, in principle, a feeding tube can be placed along the sponge of the EndoVac. However, this is disadvantageous because pressure points and concomitant local reduced blood flow delay the healing of the surgical area. In this regard, a PEJ tube is chosen to provide nutrition via enteral feeding, which is the standard after esophagectomy [30,31]. During laparotomic esophagectomy, PEJ tube insertion is recommended for patients regardless of complications [32].

The need for one or more EndoVac changes beyond the single prophylactic EndoVac cycle indicates a complicated course and defines the second endpoint. Based on the number of EndoVac cycles required, patients can be categorized into low-risk or high-risk groups, allowing for further risk stratification. This proactive approach aims to optimize patient outcomes by promptly identifying and managing complications, ultimately enhancing the success of esophagectomy procedures.

Statistical analysis: Statistical analyses were performed in Python 3 to explore the different feature expressions within the two classes defined by the endpoints. Statistical significance was determined using the chi-square test to compare two proportions to test the hypothesis that proportions do not differ between the high and low-risk groups. The test was performed with Scipy using the statsmodels toolbox [33]. We performed Welch's t-test to test two independent samples' average (expected) values for equality. We chose Welch's t-test as it is less biased compared with the Student's t-test in cases of non-equal variance in the compared datasets [34]. The t-test was performed using Python's Pingouin package [35]. Binomial logistic regression was performed to determine the ability of certain correlated features to predict the dichotomous variable of the investigated cases' group membership (high or low-risk group). These features are the laboratory and patient data specified in the results section. The logistic regression assigns weights to the respective features. It also assigns the odds of being in the high-risk group based on the features. We used the statsmodels' Logit function to perform logistic regression. All reported p-values are two-sided. The significance level was set to $p = 0.05$.

3. Results

3.1. Preoperative Characteristics

Between September 2017 and March 2022, 149 patients underwent minimally invasive surgery for resectable esophageal cancer, followed by prophylactic EndoVac treatment. Of these, 124 patients were treated via RAMIE and 25 were treated via hybrid surgery. Cases were divided based on two endpoints: endpoint 1, division based on the event of an AI (cases with AI: $n = 28$, 18.8%), and endpoint 2, division based on the number of postoperative EndoVac cycles required (cases with multi-cycle EndoVac therapy: $n = 80$, 53.7%). An overview of the data and endpoints can be found in Figure 1. Common clinical cutoff values were chosen for the quantitative variables to realize group division.

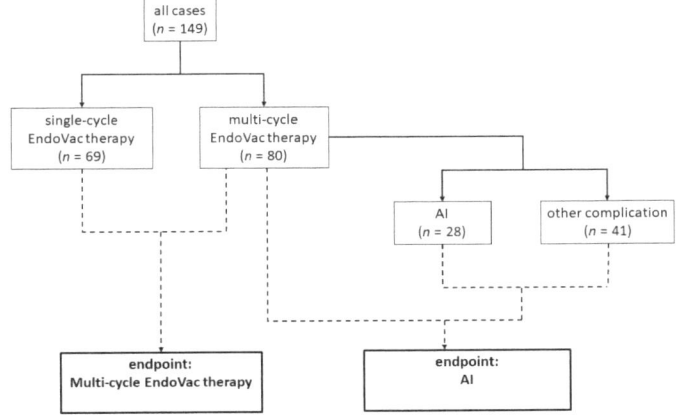

Figure 1. Overview of the data used in this study and the two endpoints. AI = anastomotic insufficiency.

We found the correlation between BMI category (<25 kg/m^2 (normal), 25–30 kg/m^2 (overweight), >30 kg/m^2 (obesity)) and AI to be significant ($p = 0.049$). The correlation between Charlson comorbidity index category (<3 (moderate), ≥3 (severe)) and AI was also significant ($p = 0.036$). Additionally, we found the correlation between BMI category and multi-cycle EndoVac therapy to be significant ($p = 0.004$). Moreover, the relationship between blood pressure medication and multi-cycle EndoVac therapy was also significant ($p = 0.038$). Other patient characteristics were not statistically significant (see Table 1).

3.2. Perioperative Characteristics

Perioperative characteristics comprised surgery type and duration, intraoperative blood loss, and R status. The correlation between surgery duration (<360 min (short), ≥360 min (long)) and multi-cycle EndoVac therapy was significant, with $p = 0.009$ for the complete procedure and $p = 0.004$ for the thoracic part of the procedure (here <240 min (short), ≥240 min (long)). Other correlations were not statistically significant. Perioperative parameters are presented in Table 1.

We also computed Welch's t-test for continuous variables to test the averages of the two groups for equality for each endpoint. Details can be found in Table 2. We found a significant difference in BMI for cases with and without AI ($p = 0.05$) and cases with single- and multi-cycle EndoVac therapy ($p = 0.002$). We also found a significant difference between single- and multi-cycle EndoVac therapy for the complete ($p < 0.001$) and thoracic ($p = 0.001$) surgery durations (Figure 2).

Table 2. Details of continuous variables and results of Welch's t-test based on the AI and multi-cycle EndoVac therapy endpoints. * denotes statistical significance. AI = anastomotic insufficiency, BMI = body mass index, CRP = C-reactive protein.

	No AI		AI		
	mean	SD	mean	SD	p-value
Age in years	64.23	9.89	66.19	9.29	0.33
BMI in kg/m^2	26.44	5.52	28.36	4.30	0.05 *
Preoperative CRP in mg/dL	0.85	1.86	0.68	1.09	0.71
Preoperative leucocytes	6640	2120	6400	1460	0.50
Preoperative hemoglobin in mg/dL	12.56	1.45	12.77	2.20	0.64
Surgery duration (complete procedure) in minutes	436.80	107.37	473.07	137.17	0.20
Surgery duration (thoracic part) in minutes	214.69	80.92	240.91	91.59	0.22
Intraoperative blood loss in mL	246.51	358.69	304.76	470.03	0.60
	Single-cycle		Multi-cycle		
	mean	SD	mean	SD	p-value
Age in years	65.17	9.32	64.10	10.19	0.508
BMI in kg/m^2	25.34	4.80	28.07	5.50	0.002 *
Preoperative CRP in mg/dL	0.90	2.14	0.70	1.01	0.621
Preoperative leucocytes	6350	1960	6810	2060	0.174
Preoperative hemoglobin in mg/dL	12.49	1.49	12.70	1.72	0.417
Surgery duration (complete procedure) in minutes	405.90	100.92	476.15	115.43	<0.001 *
Surgery duration (thoracic part) in minutes	195.13	61.11	239.50	93.74	0.001 *
Intraoperative blood loss in mL	230.39	373.78	283.04	391.02	0.482

3.3. Modeling the Likelihood of an AI and a Multi-Cycle EndoVac Therapy

We used the variables that were correlated with the endpoints to model the likelihood of the respective events. We performed a binomial logistic regression to determine the ability of BMI and the Charlson comorbidity index to predict the likelihood of an AI; the model was not significant ($p = 0.107$). Additionally, we performed a binomial logistic regression analysis to determine the ability of BMI, blood pressure medication, and surgery duration to predict the likelihood of multi-cycle EndoVac therapy. We performed a similar analysis using the duration of surgery on the thoracic part instead of the duration of the full surgery and found similar results. The binomial logistic regression model was statistically significant ($p < 0.001$). Balanced accuracy in classification was 66.7%, with a sensitivity of 72.5% and a specificity of 60.9%. Of the three variables input into the regression model, two, BMI ($p = 0.048$) and surgery duration ($p = 0.004$), contributed significantly to predicting multi-cycle EndoVac therapy, while the third variable, blood pressure medication, showed no significant effect ($p = 0.090$). For every unit increase in BMI, the odds of the patient being in the high-risk group were 1.074 times larger than the odds of the patient not being in the high-risk group when all other variables were held constant. For every unit increase in surgery duration, the odds of the patient being in the high-risk group were 1.005 times larger than the odds of the patient not being in the high-risk group when all other variables were held constant. Thus, both BMI and surgery duration had small but significant negative effects. For all model coefficients and odds, see Table 3.

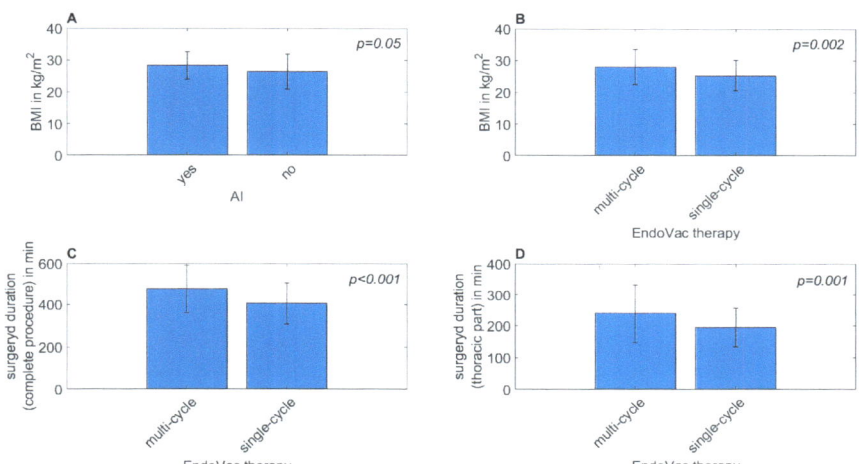

Figure 2. Bar plots of continuous variables with mean values of the different endpoints. The error bars denote standard deviations. (**A**) BMI for the AI endpoint, (**B**) BMI for the multi-cycle EndoVac therapy endpoint, (**C**) surgery duration of the complete procedure for the multi-cycle EndoVac therapy endpoint, (**D**) surgery duration of the thoracic part for the multi-cycle EndoVac therapy endpoint. Pairwise p-values comparing the distributions of variables for different event groups were computed using Welch's t-test.

Table 3. Model coefficients of the logistic regression used to determine the ability of BMI, blood pressure medication, and surgery duration to predict the likelihood of multi-cycle EndoVac therapy. * denotes statistical significance. CI = confidence interval, BMI = body mass index.

	Coefficient	Standard Error	*p*-Value	Odds Ratio	Lower 95% CI	Upper 95% CI
Intercept	−4.381	1.143	<0.001 *	0.013	0.001	0.118
BMI in kg/m^2	0.072	0.036	0.048 *	1.074	1.001	1.15
Blood pressure medication	0.617	0.364	0.090	1.854	0.909	3.783
Surgery duration (complete procedure) in minutes	0.005	0.002	0.004 *	1.005	1.002	1.009

3.4. Subgroup Analysis

We performed a subgroup analysis using only cases in which the variables above had values that defined the high-risk group. Significant results are presented in Table 4. Note that, unless otherwise specified, we used the cutoff values defined in Table 1. The subgroup analysis underlies the differences in BMI and surgery duration across differently defined high-risk and low-risk groups.

Table 4. Subgroup analysis investigating variables in the multi-cycle EndoVac therapy endpoint Subgroups are defined by cutoffs resulting in subgroup sizes given in the left column. Only significant results are shown. AI = anastomotic insufficiency, BMI = body mass index, ASA = American Society of Anesthesiologists.

Subgroup Definition	Variable	p-Value
Endpoint: Multi-cycle EndoVac therapy		
BMI ≥ 25 (n = 90)	ASA score	0.018
	Blood pressure medication	0.038
	BMI category	0.003
Blood pressure medication (n = 90)	Hemoglobin preoperative	0.047
	Surgery duration (thoracic part)	0.005
Surgery duration (thoracic part) ≥ 240 min (n = 41)	Neoadjuvant surgery radiochemotherapy vs. chemotherapy or none	0.035
Surgery duration (full surgery) ≥ 360 min (n = 110)	BMI > 25	0.014
	ASA score	0.041
Charlson comorbidity index ≥ 3 (n = 120)	BMI category	0.021
Endpoint: AI		
Surgery duration (thoracic part) ≥ 240 min (n = 41)	Neoadjuvant surgery radiochemotherapy vs. chemotherapy or none	0.024

4. Discussion

Esophagectomy is a complex surgical procedure that involves removing and reconnecting parts of the esophagus to the stomach. There has been considerable technical progress in the field of esophagectomy in the last decade [6,15,17,18,36–38]. While minimally invasive techniques offer several advantages, including reduced postoperative pain and shorter hospital stays, there is still a risk of complications that can affect patient outcomes. Unlike other complications, the rate of AI has not substantially decreased with the transition from surgical approaches to minimally invasive surgery. It is expected that this will improve in the future through the use of modern technologies and artificial intelligence methods [39]. At present, AI is still a complication that needs to be addressed. One of the critical challenges in managing postoperative complications is the provision of adequate enteral nutrition to support the healing process and prevent complications such as AI, where the surgical connection between the esophagus and stomach does not heal properly. This study investigated risk factors for a complicated postoperative course and the subsequent need for PEJ tube supply for enteral nutrition. The high-volume center at Münster University Hospital implements pre-emptive EndoVac therapy after esophagectomy, which ensures uniform postoperative access and control. Therefore, this study provides a unique opportunity to examine risk factors using a limited but high-quality dataset.

The findings of this study reveal that BMI and the Charlson comorbidity index are significantly correlated with the occurrence of AI. These results are consistent with previous experiences of anastomotic healing [40–43]. Additionally, the surrogate parameter, multi-cycle EndoVac therapy, is correlated with BMI, blood pressure medication use, and the duration of surgery. High BMI and longer surgery durations were identified as potential risk factors for multi-cycle EndoVac therapy and a complicated postoperative course. A subgroup analysis hints at the importance of BMI and surgery duration, as well as ASA score, blood pressure medication, hemoglobin level, and neoadjuvant therapy type as indicators of a high-risk subgroup. BMI, surgery duration, ASA score, hemoglobin level, cardiovascular comorbidities, and neoadjuvant therapy are known risk factors for AI following gastrointestinal surgery [44–46]. Future studies of more extensive samples might confirm these features as risk factors for AI following esophagectomy.

The study's results offer valuable insights into managing postoperative complications after minimally invasive esophagectomy. We found evidence that high BMI and prolonged surgery duration increase the risk of postoperative complications.

By identifying predictive factors, healthcare professionals can proactively address the nutritional needs of high-risk patients, potentially reducing the incidence of complications and improving overall postoperative outcomes. Pre-emptive placement of a PEJ tube can be justified in cases involving the factors we identified in this study. Despite these valuable findings, the study has limitations that need to be acknowledged. The study was conducted at a single center; therefore, the generalizability of the results may be limited, and multi-center studies are suggested for future research. The use of machine learning methods may allow the exploration of interactions between variables and the generation of more generalizable predictive models.

5. Conclusions

In conclusion, understanding and identifying risk factors associated with postoperative complications following minimally invasive esophagectomy can help improve patient care. The study's findings emphasize the importance of personalized approaches in managing post-surgery complications and highlight potential areas for intervention to optimize patient outcomes. Ultimately, this research contributes to the ongoing efforts to enhance the safety and effectiveness of minimally invasive esophagectomy procedures.

Author Contributions: Conceptualization, A.K.P., M.A.J., A.P. and J.P.H.; methodology, A.K.P., J.M. and L.F.; software A.K.P.; validation, A.K.P.; formal analysis, A.K.P.; investigation, A.K.P., M.A.J. and J.P.H.; resources, A.P. and J.P.H.; data curation, A.K.P.; writing—original draft preparation, A.K.P., M.A.J. and J.P.H.; writing—review and editing, A.K.P., M.A.J., D.R., A.P. and J.P.H.; visualization, A.K.P., M.A.J., A.P. and J.P.H.; supervision, M.A.J., A.P. and J.P.H.; project administration, A.P. and J.P.H.; funding acquisition, A.P. and J.P.H. All authors have read and agreed to the published version of the manuscript.

Funding: This research received no specific grant from any funding agency in the public, commercial, or not-for-profit sectors.

Institutional Review Board Statement: This study was conducted in line with the principles of the Declaration of Helsinki. Approval was granted by the Ethics Committee of the University of Muenster (Muenster, Germany) and the Medical Association of Westphalia-Lippe (11 March 2022/2022-123-f-S).

Informed Consent Statement: Informed consent was obtained from all subjects involved in the study.

Data Availability Statement: All data are available in the main text.

Acknowledgments: We thank Brooke Frankauer for her help with editing and improving the language in the manuscript. We thank the Institute of Medical Informatics in Muenster for their help with data retrieval.

Conflicts of Interest: Jens P. Hoelzen is a proctor for Intuitive Surgical Inc. (Sunnyvale, CA, USA). Other authors have no conflict of interest to declare.

References

1. Bray, F.; Ferlay, J.; Soerjomataram, I.; Siegel, R.L.; Torre, L.A.; Jemal, A. Global Cancer Statistics 2018: GLOBOCAN Estimates of Incidence and Mortality Worldwide for 36 Cancers in 185 Countries. *CA A Cancer J. Clin.* **2018**, *68*, 394–424. [CrossRef]
2. Simard, E.P.; Ward, E.M.; Siegel, R.; Jemal, A. Cancers with Increasing Incidence Trends in the United States: 1999 through 2008. *CA A Cancer J. Clin.* **2012**, *62*, 118–128. [CrossRef]
3. Banks, K.C.; Hsu, D.S.; Velotta, J.B. Outcomes of Minimally Invasive and Robot-Assisted Esophagectomy for Esophageal Cancer. *Cancers* **2022**, *14*, 3667. [CrossRef] [PubMed]
4. Hoelzen, J.P.; Sander, K.J.; Sesia, M.; Roy, D.; Rijcken, E.; Schnabel, A.; Struecker, B.; Juratli, M.A.; Pascher, A. Robotic-Assisted Esophagectomy Leads to Significant Reduction in Postoperative Acute Pain: A Retrospective Clinical Trial. *Ann. Surg. Oncol.* **2022**, *29*, 7498–7509. [CrossRef]
5. Straatman, J.; van der Wielen, N.; Cuesta, M.A.; Daams, F.; Roig Garcia, J.; Bonavina, L.; Rosman, C.; van Berge Henegouwen, M.I.; Gisbertz, S.S.; van der Peet, D.L. Minimally Invasive Versus Open Esophageal Resection: Three-Year Follow-up of the Previously Reported Randomized Controlled Trial: The TIME Trial. *Ann. Surg.* **2017**, *266*, 232. [CrossRef]
6. Mariette, C.; Markar, S.R.; Dabakuyo-Yonli, T.S.; Meunier, B.; Pezet, D.; Collet, D.; D'Journo, X.B.; Brigand, C.; Perniceni, T.; Carrère, N.; et al. Hybrid Minimally Invasive Esophagectomy for Esophageal Cancer. *N. Engl. J. Med.* **2019**, *380*, 152–162. [CrossRef]

7. Fabbi, M.; Hagens, E.R.C.; van Berge Henegouwen, M.I.; Gisbertz, S.S. Anastomotic Leakage after Esophagectomy for Esophageal Cancer: Definitions, Diagnostics, and Treatment. *Dis. Esophagus* **2021**, *34*, doaa039. [CrossRef]
8. Steenhagen, E.; van Vulpen, J.K.; van Hillegersberg, R.; May, A.M.; Siersema, P.D. Nutrition in Peri-Operative Esophageal Cancer Management. *Expert Rev. Gastroenterol. Hepatol.* **2017**, *11*, 663–672. [CrossRef]
9. Berlana, D. Parenteral Nutrition Overview. *Nutrients* **2022**, *14*, 4480. [CrossRef]
10. Wobith, M.; Weimann, A. Oral Nutritional Supplements and Enteral Nutrition in Patients with Gastrointestinal Surgery. *Nutrients* **2021**, *13*, 2655. [CrossRef]
11. Zhuang, W.; Wu, H.; Liu, H.; Huang, S.; Wu, Y.; Deng, C.; Tian, D.; Zhou, Z.; Shi, R.; Chen, G.; et al. Utility of Feeding Jejunostomy in Patients with Esophageal Cancer Undergoing Esophagectomy with a High Risk of Anastomotic Leakage. *J. Gastrointest. Oncol.* **2021**, *12*, 433–445. [CrossRef]
12. Lim, A.H.; Schoeman, M.N.; Nguyen, N.Q. Long-Term Outcomes of Direct Percutaneous Endoscopic Jejunostomy: A 10-Year Cohort. *Endosc. Int. Open* **2015**, *3*, E610–E614. [CrossRef]
13. Al-Batran, S.-E.; Hofheinz, R.D.; Pauligk, C.; Kopp, H.-G.; Haag, G.M.; Luley, K.B.; Meiler, J.; Homann, N.; Lorenzen, S.; Schmalenberg, H.; et al. Histopathological Regression after Neoadjuvant Docetaxel, Oxaliplatin, Fluorouracil, and Leucovorin versus Epirubicin, Cisplatin, and Fluorouracil or Capecitabine in Patients with Resectable Gastric or Gastro-Oesophageal Junction Adenocarcinoma (FLOT4-AIO): Results from the Phase 2 Part of a Multicentre, Open-Label, Randomised Phase 2/3 Trial. *Lancet Oncol.* **2016**, *17*, 1697–1708. [CrossRef]
14. van Hagen, P.; Hulshof, M.C.C.M.; van Lanschot, J.J.B.; Steyerberg, E.W.; van Berge Henegouwen, M.I.; Wijnhoven, B.P.L.; Richel, D.J.; Nieuwenhuijzen, G.A.P.; Hospers, G.A.P.; Bonenkamp, J.J.; et al. Preoperative Chemoradiotherapy for Esophageal or Junctional Cancer. *N. Engl. J. Med.* **2012**, *366*, 2074–2084. [CrossRef]
15. Biere, S.S.A.Y.; van Berge Henegouwen, M.I.; Maas, K.W.; Bonavina, L.; Rosman, C.; Garcia, J.R.; Gisbertz, S.S.; Klinkenbijl, J.H.G.; Hollmann, M.W.; de Lange, E.S.M.; et al. Minimally Invasive versus Open Oesophagectomy for Patients with Oesophageal Cancer: A Multicentre, Open-Label, Randomised Controlled Trial. *Lancet* **2012**, *379*, 1887–1892. [CrossRef]
16. Mariette, C.; Markar, S.; Dabakuyo-Yonli, T.S.; Meunier, B.; Pezet, D.; Collet, D.; D'Journo, X.B.; Brigand, C.; Perniceni, T.; Carrere, N.; et al. Health-Related Quality of Life Following Hybrid Minimally Invasive Versus Open Esophagectomy for Patients With Esophageal Cancer, Analysis of a Multicenter, Open-Label, Randomized Phase III Controlled Trial: The MIRO Trial. *Ann. Surg.* **2020**, *271*, 1023. [CrossRef]
17. Van der Sluis, P.C.; van der Horst, S.; May, A.M.; Schippers, C.; Brosens, L.A.A.; Joore, H.C.A.; Kroese, C.C.; Haj Mohammad, N.; Mook, S.; Vleggaar, F.P.; et al. Robot-Assisted Minimally Invasive Thoracolaparoscopic Esophagectomy Versus Open Transthoracic Esophagectomy for Resectable Esophageal Cancer: A Randomized Controlled Trial. *Ann. Surg.* **2019**, *269*, 621–630. [CrossRef]
18. Yang, Y.; Li, B.; Yi, J.; Hua, R.; Chen, H.; Tan, L.; Li, H.; He, Y.; Guo, X.; Sun, Y.; et al. Robot-Assisted Versus Conventional Minimally Invasive Esophagectomy for Resectable Esophageal Squamous Cell Carcinoma: Early Results of a Multicenter Randomized Controlled Trial: The RAMIE Trial. *Ann. Surg.* **2022**, *275*, 646–653. [CrossRef]
19. EMA ICH E6 (R2) Good Clinical Practice–Scientific Guideline. Available online: https://www.ema.europa.eu/en/ich-e6-r2-good-clinical-practice-scientific-guideline (accessed on 23 August 2023).
20. World Medical Association. World Medical Association Declaration of Helsinki: Ethical principles for medical research involving human subjects. *JAMA* **2013**, *310*, 2191–2194. [CrossRef]
21. Mathew, G.; Agha, R.; Albrecht, J.; Goel, P.; Mukherjee, I.; Pai, P.; D'Cruz, A.K.; Nixon, I.J.; Roberto, K.; Enam, S.A.; et al STROCSS 2021: Strengthening the Reporting of Cohort, Cross-Sectional and Case-Control Studies in Surgery. *Int. J. Surg.* **2021**, *96*, 106165. [CrossRef]
22. Min, Y.W.; Kim, T.; Lee, H.; Min, B.-H.; Kim, H.K.; Choi, Y.S.; Lee, J.H.; Rhee, P.-L.; Kim, J.J.; Zo, J.I.; et al. Endoscopic Vacuum Therapy for Postoperative Esophageal Leak. *BMC Surg.* **2019**, *19*, 37. [CrossRef] [PubMed]
23. Maier, J.; Kandulski, A.; Donlon, N.E.; Werner, J.M.; Mehrl, A.; Müller, M.; Doenecke, A.; Schlitt, H.J.; Hornung, M.; Weiss, A.R.R Endoscopic Vacuum Therapy Significantly Improves Clinical Outcomes of Anastomotic Leakages after 2-Stage, 3-Stage, and Transhiatal Esophagectomies. *Langenbecks Arch Surg.* **2023**, *408*, 90. [CrossRef] [PubMed]
24. Satoskar, S.; Kashyap, S.; Benavides, F.; Jones, R.; Angelico, R.; Singhal, V. Success of Endoscopic Vacuum Therapy for Persistent Anastomotic Leak after Esophagectomy—A Case Report. *Int. J. Surg. Case Rep.* **2021**, *80*, 105342. [CrossRef] [PubMed]
25. El-Sourani, N.; Miftode, S.; Bockhorn, M. Endoscopic Vacuum Therapy for Anastomotic Leakage after Esophagectomy: A Retrospective Analysis at a Tertiary University Center. *Surg. Open Sci.* **2022**, *11*, 69–72. [CrossRef]
26. Gubler, C.; Vetter, D.; Schmidt, H.M.; Müller, P.C.; Morell, B.; Raptis, D.; Gutschow, C.A. Preemptive Endoluminal Vacuum Therapy to Reduce Anastomotic Leakage after Esophagectomy: A Game-Changing Approach? *Dis. Esophagus* **2019**, *32*, doy126. [CrossRef]
27. Müller, P.C.; Morell, B.; Vetter, D.; Raptis, D.A.; Kapp, J.R.; Gubler, C.; Gutschow, C.A. Preemptive Endoluminal Vacuum Therapy to Reduce Morbidity After Minimally Invasive Ivor Lewis Esophagectomy: Including a Novel Grading System for Postoperative Endoscopic Assessment of GI-Anastomoses. *Ann. Surg.* **2021**, *274*, 751–757. [CrossRef]
28. Müller, P.C.; Vetter, D.; Kapp, J.R.; Gubler, C.; Morell, B.; Raptis, D.A.; Gutschow, C.A. Pre-Emptive Endoluminal Negative Pressure Therapy at the Anastomotic Site in Minimally Invasive Transthoracic Esophagectomy (the PreSPONGE Trial): Study Protocol for a Multicenter Randomized Controlled Trial. *Int. J. Surg. Protoc.* **2021**, *25*, 7–15. [CrossRef]

29. Low, D.E.; Alderson, D.; Cecconello, I.; Chang, A.C.; Darling, G.E.; D'Journo, X.B.; Griffin, S.M.; Hölscher, A.H.; Hofstetter, W.L.; Jobe, B.A.; et al. International Consensus on Standardization of Data Collection for Complications Associated With Esophagectomy: Esophagectomy Complications Consensus Group (ECCG). *Ann. Surg.* **2015**, *262*, 286. [CrossRef]
30. Berkelmans, G.H.; van Workum, F.; Weijs, T.J.; Nieuwenhuijzen, G.A.; Ruurda, J.P.; Kouwenhoven, E.A.; van Det, M.J.; Rosman, C.; van Hillegersberg, R.; Luyer, M.D. The Feeding Route after Esophagectomy: A Review of Literature. *J. Thorac. Dis.* **2017**, *9*, S785–S791. [CrossRef]
31. Delany, H.M.; Carnevale, N.J.; Garvey, J.W. Jejunostomy by a Needle Catheter Technique. *Surgery* **1973**, *73*, 786–790. [CrossRef]
32. Wani, M.L.; Ahangar, A.G.; Lone, G.N.; Singh, S.; Dar, A.M.; Bhat, M.A.; Lone, R.A.; Irshad, I. Feeding Jejunostomy: Does the Benefit Overweight the Risk (a Retrospective Study from a Single Centre). *Int. J. Surg.* **2010**, *8*, 387–390. [CrossRef]
33. Seabold, S.; Perktold, J. *Statsmodels: Econometric and Statistical Modeling with Python*; SCIPY: Austin, TX, USA, 2010; pp. 92–96.
34. Delacre, M.; Lakens, D.; Leys, C. Why Psychologists Should by Default Use Welch's t-Test Instead of Student's t-Test. *Int. Rev. Soc. Psychol.* **2017**, *30*, 92. [CrossRef]
35. Vallat, R. Pingouin: Statistics in Python. *J. Open Source Softw.* **2018**, *3*, 1026. [CrossRef]
36. Capovilla, G.; Uzun, E.; Scarton, A.; Moletta, L.; Hadzijusufovic, E.; Provenzano, L.; Salvador, R.; Pierobon, E.S.; Zanchettin, G.; Tagkalos, E.; et al. Minimally Invasive Ivor Lewis Esophagectomy in the Elderly Patient: A Multicenter Retrospective Matched-Cohort Study. *Front. Oncol.* **2023**, *13*, 1104109. [CrossRef]
37. Mann, C.; Berlth, F.; Hadzijusufovic, E.; Lang, H.; Grimminger, P.P. Minimally Invasive Esophagectomy: Clinical Evidence and Surgical Techniques. *Langenbecks Arch Surg.* **2020**, *405*, 1061–1067. [CrossRef]
38. Berlth, F.; Hadzijusufovic, E.; Mann, C.; Fetzner, U.K.; Grimminger, P. Minimally Invasive Esophagectomy for Esophageal Cancer. *Ther. Umsch.* **2022**, *79*, 181–187. [CrossRef]
39. Wagner, M.; Schulze, A.; Bodenstedt, S.; Maier-Hein, L.; Speidel, S.; Nickel, F.; Berlth, F.; Müller-Stich, B.P.; Grimminger, P. Technical innovations and future perspectives. *Chirurg* **2022**, *93*, 217–222. [CrossRef]
40. Mengardo, V.; Pucetti, F.; Mc Cormack, O.; Chaudry, A.; Allum, W.H. The Impact of Obesity on Esophagectomy: A Meta-Analysis. *Dis. Esophagus* **2018**, *31*, dox149. [CrossRef]
41. Nugent, T.S.; Kelly, M.E.; Donlon, N.E.; Fahy, M.R.; Larkin, J.O.; McCormick, P.H.; Mehigan, B.J. Obesity and Anastomotic Leak Rates in Colorectal Cancer: A Meta-Analysis. *Int. J. Color. Dis.* **2021**, *36*, 1819–1829. [CrossRef]
42. Kassis, E.S.; Kosinski, A.S.; Ross, P.; Koppes, K.E.; Donahue, J.M.; Daniel, V.C. Predictors of Anastomotic Leak After Esophagectomy: An Analysis of The Society of Thoracic Surgeons General Thoracic Database. *Ann. Thorac. Surg.* **2013**, *96*, 1919–1926. [CrossRef]
43. Vasiliu, E.C.Z.; Zarnescu, N.O.; Costea, R.; Neagu, S. Review of Risk Factors for Anastomotic Leakage in Colorectal Surgery. *Chirurgia* **2015**, *110*, 319–326. [PubMed]
44. Kryzauskas, M.; Bausys, A.; Degutyte, A.E.; Abeciunas, V.; Poskus, E.; Bausys, R.; Dulskas, A.; Strupas, K.; Poskus, T. Risk Factors for Anastomotic Leakage and Its Impact on Long-Term Survival in Left-Sided Colorectal Cancer Surgery. *World J. Surg. Oncol.* **2020**, *18*, 205. [CrossRef] [PubMed]
45. Liedman, B.; Johnsson, E.; Merke, C.; Ruth, M.; Lundell, L. Preoperative Adjuvant Radiochemotherapy May Increase the Risk in Patients Undergoing Thoracoabdominal Esophageal Resections. *Dig. Surg.* **2001**, *18*, 169–175. [CrossRef]
46. Bosset, J.F.; Gignoux, M.; Triboulet, J.P.; Tiret, E.; Mantion, G.; Elias, D.; Lozach, P.; Ollier, J.C.; Pavy, J.J.; Mercier, M.; et al. Chemoradiotherapy Followed by Surgery Compared with Surgery Alone in Squamous-Cell Cancer of the Esophagus. *N. Engl. J. Med.* **1997**, *337*, 161–167. [CrossRef] [PubMed]

Disclaimer/Publisher's Note: The statements, opinions and data contained in all publications are solely those of the individual author(s) and contributor(s) and not of MDPI and/or the editor(s). MDPI and/or the editor(s) disclaim responsibility for any injury to people or property resulting from any ideas, methods, instructions or products referred to in the content.

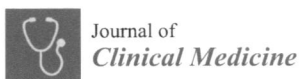

Article

Postoperative Hiatal Hernia after Ivor Lewis Esophagectomy—A Growing Problem in the Age of Minimally Invasive Surgery

Jasmina Kuvendjiska [1,2,*], Robert Jasinski [2], Julian Hipp [1,2], Mira Fink [1,2], Stefan Fichtner-Feigl [1,2], Markus K. Diener [1] and Jens Hoeppner [2,3]

1 Department of General and Visceral Surgery, University Medical Center, 79106 Freiburg, Germany
2 Faculty of Medicine, Albert-Ludwigs-University of Freiburg, 79085 Freiburg, Germany
3 Department of Surgery, University Medical Center Schleswig-Holstein, 23538 Lübeck, Germany
* Correspondence: jasmina.kuvendjiska@uniklinik-freiburg.de

Abstract: Background: Even though minimally invasive esophagectomy is a safe and oncologically effective procedure, several authors have reported an increased risk of postoperative hiatal hernia (PHH). This study evaluates the incidence and risk factors of PHH after hybrid minimally invasive (HMIE) versus open esophagectomy (OE). Methods: A retrospective single-center analysis was performed on patients who underwent Ivor Lewis esophagectomy between January 2009 and April 2018. Computed tomography scans and patient files were reviewed to identify the PHH. Results: 306 patients were included (152 HMIE; 154 OE). Of these, 23 patients (8%) developed PHH. Most patients (13/23, 57%) were asymptomatic at the time of diagnosis and only 4 patients (17%) presented in an emergency setting with incarceration. The rate of PHH was significantly higher after HMIE compared to OE (13.8% vs. 1.3%, $p < 0.001$). No other risk factors for the development of PHH were identified in uni- or multi-variate analysis. Surgical repair of PHH was performed in 19/23 patients (83%). The recurrence rate of PHH after surgical repair was 32% (6/19 patients). Conclusions: The development of PHH is a relevant complication after hybrid minimally invasive esophagectomy. Although most patients are asymptomatic, surgical repair is recommended to avoid incarceration with potentially fatal outcomes. Innovative techniques for the prevention and repair of PHH are urgently needed.

Keywords: esophagectomy; esophageal cancer; hiatal hernia; minimally invasive surgery; postoperative complication

1. Introduction

Esophageal carcinoma is the eighth most common cancer in the world and the sixth most common cause of cancer death worldwide [1]. Although multimodal treatment protocols are progressively applied, surgery remains the central part of curative treatment for most patients. Different techniques of esophagectomy with variations in terms of resection and reconstruction are performed internationally. Established techniques include a transhiatal, two-field transthoracic (Ivor Lewis) and tri-incisional resection (abdominal incision, right thoracotomy and left neck incision.). The two-field Ivor Lewis procedure is the technique most used in the Western world today. It includes an abdominal part as well as a thoracic part of the resection via right thoracotomy. The reconstruction is performed with intrathoracic anastomosis. For most patients, a gastric sleeve is used for reconstruction and esophageal replacement, whereas reconstruction with jejunum or colon is far less commonly performed. Esophagectomy is associated with significant surgical morbidity. Postoperative morbidity has been reduced by the use of minimally invasive techniques, regardless of the respective technique, e.g., complete minimally invasive or hybrid techniques [2–4]. The main benefit of minimally invasive esophagectomy is a

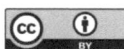

reduction in pulmonary morbidity [2,3]. Since the oncological outcome remains comparable to open esophagectomy, totally and hybrid minimally invasive esophagectomy has become the standard procedure.

At the Medical Centre of the University of Freiburg, hybrid minimally invasive esophagectomy (HMIE) and open esophagectomy (OE) are both applied as highly standardized procedures [5,6]. Over the years, HMIE has become the gold standard technique for esophageal resections in our center. However, with the consecutive clinical implementation of HMIE as the standard technique, an increased occurrence of postoperative paraconduit hiatal hernia (PHH) has been observed. The occurrence of PHH after totally minimally invasive esophagectomy (TMIE) was recently reported to be more frequent than after open esophagectomy [7–9]. Although there are several studies on the occurrence of PHH after a TMIE procedure, there are very few studies on the HMIE procedure. Although PHHs are often asymptomatic, there is a risk of ischemia of the herniated intestine, with potentially fatal consequences [10].

Overall, the literature on PHH is still quite limited, including mostly retrospective studies and two meta-analyses based on retrospective data. A further problem in the existing literature on this topic is the frequent use of heterogeneous patient collectives with diverse operating techniques such as gastrectomy, transhiatal esophagectomy, Ivor Lewis or McKeown esophagectomy. However, research on the comparison between HMIE and OE in terms of PHH occurrence is still limited.

This study aims to determine and compare the incidence, potential risk factors and outcome of PHH after OE and HMIE.

2. Materials and Methods

2.1. Study Design

We conducted a single-center retrospective study with the objective of determining incidence and outcomes of PHH after esophagectomy. We included patients operated between January 2009 and April 2018. The included patients underwent either a fully open Ivor Lewis esophagectomy (OE) or hybrid minimally invasive esophagectomy (HMIE). The applied technique of HMIE included a laparoscopic abdominal and open thoracic part via right thoracotomy as described in prior reports [11,12]. All patients were reconstructed using a gastric sleeve, and patients with other forms of reconstruction were excluded from the analysis. In both groups, a widening of the hiatus by intraoperative hiatotomy of the right crura and prophylactic colopexy of the transverse colon to the abdominal wall were sometimes performed based on the surgeon's preference. Clinical follow-up of all patients was conducted routinely in our specialized outpatient department for Upper GI Surgery. Occurrence of PHH was identified by a computed tomography (CT) performed in all patients either during the regular oncological follow-up or due to specific symptoms. PHH was defined as herniation of abdominal organs (excluding the gastric conduit) through the esophageal hiatus. Anatomical details about PHH were identified through evaluation of CT scans. Patient data, including medical history, disease symptoms and management of the hiatal hernia, were extracted from patient charts. The study was approved by the Medical Ethics Committee of the University of Freiburg (File No. 253/19).

2.2. Statistical Analysis

Descriptive statistics were applied for the patient characteristics and postoperative complications. Univariate analysis was performed to assess the role of potential risk factors for the occurrence of PHH. All parameters with a significance of $p < 0.1$ were subsequently entered into a binary logistic regression analysis with backwards stepwise variable selection. A statistical significance level of 0.05 was used and statistical analysis was performed using IBM SPSS Statistics version 28.0 (IBM Corp, Armonk, NY, USA).

3. Results

3.1. Study Population

Overall, 387 patients underwent an esophagectomy between January 2009 and April 2018. Seventy-four of these patients underwent a transhiatal distal esophagectomy with gastrectomy and were excluded from the analysis. One patient underwent an emergency esophagectomy without reconstruction and a further six patients received an esophagectomy with a reconstruction other than gastric pull-up (colonic interposition (n = 3); jejunal interposition (n = 3)), and were also excluded in the analysis. Finally, 306 patients who underwent esophagectomy and reconstruction with gastric conduit were included. HMIE was performed in 152 patients (49.67%) and OE in 154 patients (50.3%) (Figure 1). There were no conversions to open surgery in the HMIE group. Overall, 295 procedures were performed for esophageal cancer, with esophageal adenocarcinoma being the most frequent diagnosis (n = 215, 70.3%). Most of the patients received neoadjuvant treatment in the form of chemoradiation (n = 104, 34%) or chemotherapy alone (n = 140, 45.6%), in accordance with national guidelines. Demographic data are shown in Table 1.

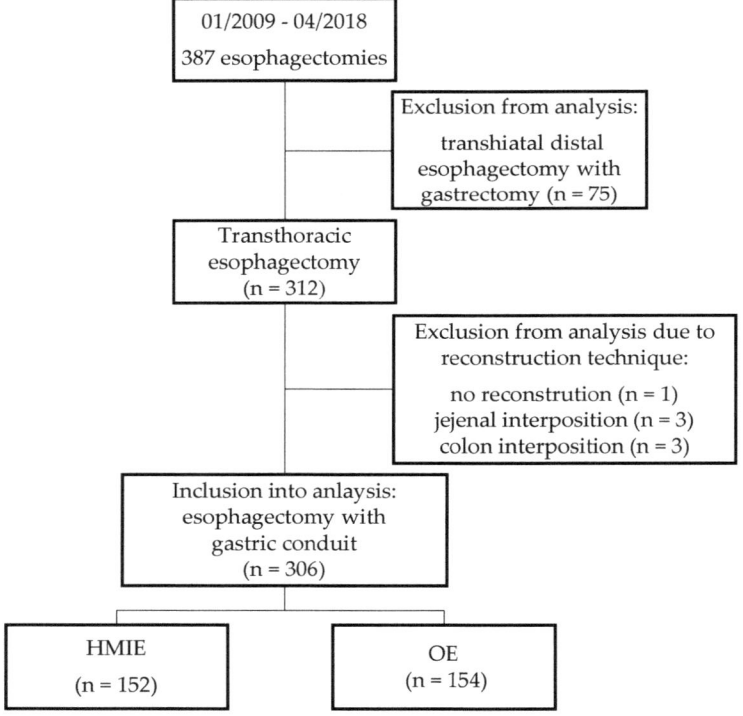

Figure 1. Flowchart of the study population selection. OE = open esophagectomy, HMIE = hybrid minimally invasive esophagectomy.

Table 1. Clinicopathological characteristics of the study population.

	HMIE	OE
Patients (*n*)	152	154
Male gender (*n*, %)	117 (77%)	133 (86.4%)
Age (median, years)	62	63
BMI (median, kg/m^2)	26.5	25
ASA-score (*n*, %)		
I	1 (0.7%)	2 (1.3%)
II	75 (49.3%)	76 (49.4%)
III	72 (47.4%)	73 (47.4%)
IV	4 (2.6%)	3 (1.9%)
Tumor histology (*n*, %)		
Adenocarcinoma	114 (75%)	101 (65.6%)
Squamouscell carcinoma	33 (21.7%)	47 (30.5%)
Others	5 (3.3%)	6 (3.9%)
Neoadjuvant treatment (*n*, %)		
None	34 (22.4%)	27 (17.7%)
Chemotherapy	68 (44.7%)	72 (46.7%)
Chemoradiation	49 (32.2%)	55 (35.7%)
Radiotherapy	1	0
Comorbidity (*n*, %)		
Nicotine abuse	57 (37.5%)	67 (43.5%)
CHD	16 (10.5%)	18 (11.7%)
Diabetes	20 (13.2%)	21 (13.6%)
Adipositas	25 (16.4%)	21 (13.6%)
COPD	22 (14.5%)	19 (12.3%)

BMI = body mass index; ASA = American Society of Anaesthesiologists; CHD = coronary heart disease; COPD = chronic obstructive pulmonary disease.

3.2. Postoperative Hiatal Hernia

Overall, 23 of the patients (7.5%) developed PHH in the postoperative course. The median follow-up time was 21 months. The occurrence of PHH was significantly increased after HMIE (*n* = 21, 13.8%) compared to OE (*n* = 2, 1.3%, *p* < 0.001). The median time to diagnosis after HMIE was 14 months, and it was 75.5 months after OE. In every analyzed case, the transverse colon was the herniated organ, with additional herniation of the small intestine in three cases. Most frequently, the hiatal hernia occurred on the left thoracic side (*n* = 18, 78.3%) (Figure 2), followed by small mediastinal hernias in the middle (*n* = 3, 13%). In one case, the hernia occurred on the right side (4.4%) (Figure 3) and in another case bilaterally (4.4%).

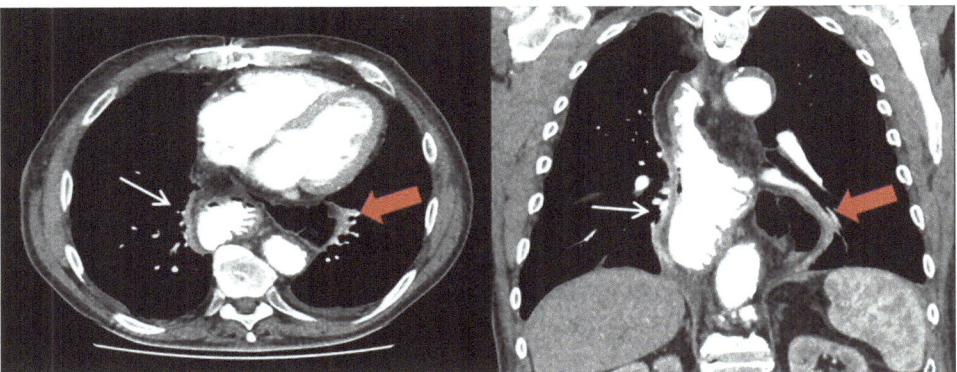

Figure 2. Exemplary CT-scan of a hiatal hernia on the left thoracic side after HMIE. Gastric conduit marked with thin white arrow; herniated colon marked with thick red arrow.

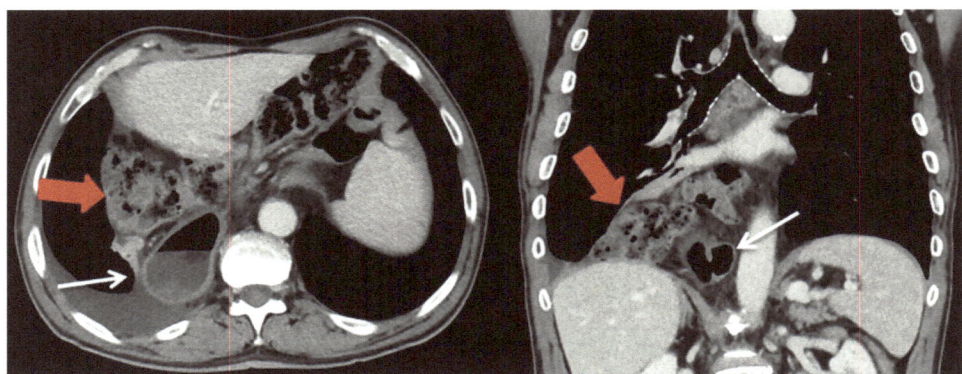

Figure 3. Exemplary CT-scan of a hiatal hernia on the right thoracic side after HMIE. Gastric conduit marked with thin white arrow; herniated colon marked with thick red arrow.

Univariate analysis was performed to assess the role of potential risk factors for the occurrence of PHH. The examined factors included patient characteristics, surgical technique factors and postoperative complications. The following parameters were included in the univariate analysis: age, gender, ASA, operating technique (HMIE vs. OE), T and N stadium, intraoperative hiatotomy, prophylactic colopexy, preexisting hiatal hernia, BMI, nicotine abuse, COPD, CHD, diabetes mellitus, use and type of neoadjuvant treatment, postoperative pneumonia, postoperative mediastinitis, anastomotic leakage, anastomotic stricture and delayed gastric emptying (Table 2). Five parameters showed a significance $p < 0.1$ and were entered into a binary logistic regression analysis. Using backwards stepwise variable selection, the following variables were excluded from the equation: prophylactic colopexy, intraoperative hiatotomy, T-stage and N-stage, leaving HMIE as the only significant factor related to an increased development of PHH after esophagectomy (Table 3).

Table 2. Univariate analysis of risk factors for postoperative hiatal hernia.

Variable	Hiatal Hernia (n, %)	No Hiatal Hernia (n, %)	p-Value
Patients	23	283	
Male gender	16 (69.6%)	234 (82.7%)	0.118
Age (years)			
<65	12 (52.2%)	157 (55.5%)	0.759
≥65	11 (47.8%)	126 (44.5%)	
BMI (kg/m^2)			
<25	9 (39.1%)	124 (43.8%)	0.66
≥25	14 (60.9%)	159 (56.2%)	
ASA-score			
I + II	14 (60.9%)	140 (49.5%)	0.29
III + IV	9 (39.1%)	143 (50.5%)	
Comorbidity			
Nicotine abuse	10 (43.5%)	114 (40.3%)	0.76
CHD	2 (8.7%)	32 (11.3%)	0.7
Diabetes	2 (8.7%)	39 (13.8%)	0.49
COPD	3 (13%)	38 (13.4%)	0.96
Preexisting hiatal hernia	2 (8.7%)	30 (10.6%)	0.78
T stadium			
T 0–2	20 (87%)	183 (66.8%)	0.046
T 3–4	3 (13%)	91 (33.2%)	

Table 2. Cont.

Variable	Hiatal Hernia (n, %)	No Hiatal Hernia (n, %)	p-Value
N- stadium			
N0	18 (78.3%)	166 (61%)	0.1
N+	5 (21.7%)	106 (39%)	
Neoadjuvant treatment			
Chemotherapy	18 (78.3%)	226 (79.9%)	0.86
Radiochemotherapy	8 (34.8%)	97 (34.3%)	0.96
Operation technique			
HMIE	21 (91.3%)	131 (46.3%)	<0.001
OE	2 (8.7%)	152 (53.7%)	
Hiatotomy	20 (87%)	196 (69.3%)	0.073
Colopexy	19 (82.6%)	171 (60.4%)	0.035
Postoperative complications			
Pneumonia	6 (26.1%)	62 (21.9%)	0.64
Mediastinitis	0	6 (2.1%)	0.48
Anastomotic leakage	1 (4.3%)	17 (6%)	0.75
Anastomotic stenosis	3 (13%)	15 (5.3%)	0.13
Delayed gastric emptying	2 (8.7%)	28 (9.9%)	0.85

BMI = body mass index; ASA = American Society of Anaesthesiologists; CHD = coronary heart disease; COPD = chronic obstructive pulmonary disease, OE = open esophagectomy, HMIE = hybrid minimally invasive esophagectomy.

Table 3. Multivariate analysis of risk factors for postoperative hiatal hernia.

Variable		Odds Ratio	95%-CI	p-Value
HMIE vs. OE	OE	Reference	Reference	<0.001
	HMIE	11.812	2.717–51.366	

In most cases, PHH were asymptomatic (n = 13, 56.5%) and were diagnosed coincidentally by CT scans performed as part of the routine oncologic follow-up (Table 4). The remaining patients (n = 10, 43.5%) were symptomatic, with four patients (17.4%) presenting as an emergency (one ileus and three incarcerations of intestine) (Figure 4). The most common symptom was abdominal pain and discomfort. Surgical repair was strongly recommended to every patient with diagnosed PHH. Out of 23 patients, 4 patients declined surgical intervention despite the strong recommendation. Meanwhile, 19 patients underwent surgical repair (82.6%), of which 4 (21%) were in emergency settings. One of the patients operated in an emergency setting died in the ICU due to septic shock.

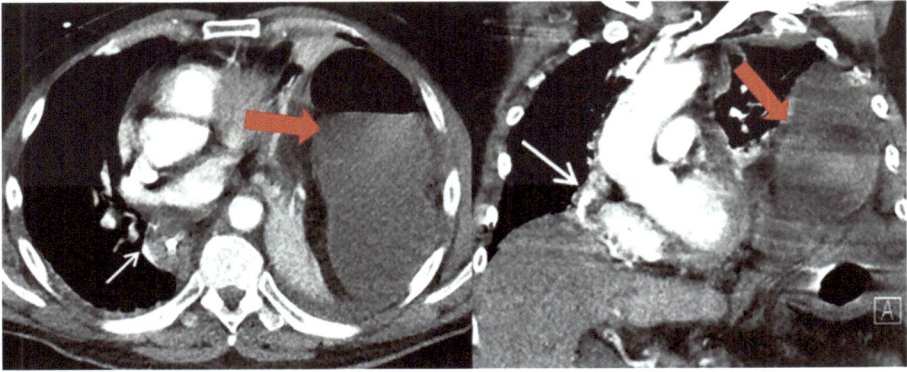

Figure 4. Exemplary CT-scan of an incarcerated hiatal hernia on the left thoracic side with a clear mediastinal shift to the right. Gastric conduit marked with thin white arrow; herniated colon marked with thick red arrow.

Table 4. Characteristics of the hiatal hernia and surgical repair technique.

Characteristics	HH (n = 23) (%)
Content of HH, n (%)	
Colon	23 (100)
Additionally small bowel	3 (13)
Position of the HH n (%)	
Left thoracic side	18 (78.3)
Right thoracic side	1 (4.4)
Both sides	1 (4.4)
Lower mediastinum	3 (13)
Symptoms n (%)	
None	13 (56.5)
Abdominal pain and discomfort	10 (43.5)
Ileus/incarceration	4 (17.4)
Surgical repair, n (%)	
Laparoscopic	16 (84.2)
Conversion	2 (12.5)
Open	3 (15.8)
Gastropexy	8 (42)
Hiatoplasty	9 (47.4)
Mesh augmentation	4 (21)
Colopexy	15 (78.9)
Recurrence rate, n (%)	6 (31.6)

The operation on the PHH was usually performed laparoscopically (n = 16, 84.2%) with only two conversions to open surgery (Table 4). The standard procedure involved a repositioning of the intestine and colopexy. In 42%, a gastropexy to the hiatus was performed to minimize the hiatal opening. If feasible, a suture hiatoplasty was also performed (47.4%). Since this is not always possible due to wide and scarified hiatus (Figure 5), different procedures were used like mesh augmentation of the hiatus (21%) or a curtain-like suspension of the mesocolon in front of the hiatus by a wide colopexy to the abdominal wall (31.6%). We observed a significant recurrence of the hiatal hernia after repair (n = 6, 31.6%). Here, again, the transverse colon was always involved, with additional herniation of small intestine in one case. The surgical repair of the hernia was repeated in five of the cases. One patient did not undergo surgical treatment due to tumor progression

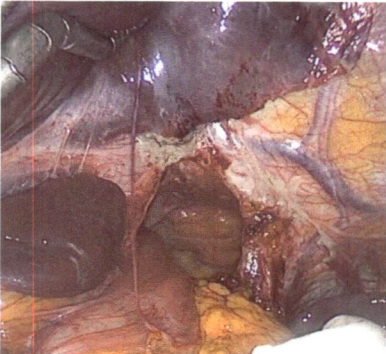

Figure 5. Exemplary picture of extremely enlarged, scarified and inflexible hiatus after HMIE. The herniated intestine (colon) has already been removed from the thorax.

4. Discussion

HMIE with gastric pull-up is performed with high safety as a standardized operative technique for patients with esophageal cancer, as reported previously [5]. Reduction in the intraoperative and postoperative complications can be achieved by the use of minimally invasive techniques like HMIE or TMIE [2–4]. Despite the great advantages over the years with the implementation of minimally invasive techniques in esophageal surgery, one complication seemed to increase: the PHH [13]. The literature on this growing problem is limited since only retrospective studies and two meta-analyses based on retrospective data [13–17] are available. Most of the studies focus on totally minimally invasive esophagectomy or use a heterogeneous patient collective with diverse operating techniques such as gastrectomy, transhiatal distal esophagectomy, Ivor Lewis or McKeown esophagectomy (Table 5).

Table 5. Literature review on post-esophagectomy PHH.

Study	Year	Patients (n)	Included Operations	PHH Overall (%)	PHH OE (%)	PHH TMIE (%)	PHH HMIE (%)	PHH Recurrence (%)
Vallböhmer et al. [18]	2007	355	OE Ivor Lewis HMIE (two-stage)	2.5	2.4	/	2.7	/
Kent et al. [19]	2008	1075	OE and TMIE Ivor Lewis OE and TMIE McKeown	4	0.8	2.8	/	29
Price et al. [20]	2011	2182	OE Ivor Lewis OE transhiatal	0.7	0.7	/	/	13.3
Ganeshan et al. [21]	2013	440	OE Ivor Lewis OE McKeown OE transhiatal TMIE	15	12 17 24	10	/	44
Bronson et al. [13]	2014	114	TMIE Transhiatal TMIE McKeown	8	/	8	/	12.5
Benjamin et al. [22]	2015	120	MIE	5.8	/	5.8	/	20
Messenger et al. [23]	2015	273	OE, TMIE and HMIE Ivor Lewis	4	1	13.2	/	18
Severino et al. [24]	2016	390	HMIE	8.2	/	/	8.2	19
Matthews et al. [25]	2016	631	OE and TMIE Ivor Lewis OE and TMIE McKeown HMIE	5.5	2	7	10	26
Andreou et al. [26]	2017	471	Gastrectomy OE Ivor Lewis Open gastrectomy Open extended gastrectomy	2.8	2.7 0.7 6.1	/	/	N/A
Brenkman et al. [27]	2017	657	OE and TMIE Ivor Lewis OE and TMIE McKeown OE and TMIE transhiatal	7	4 4 11	10 7 4	/	15
Gooszen et al. [28]	2018	851	OE and TMIE Ivor Lewis OE and TMIE McKeown OE and TMIE transhiatal	2.5	0 1.4 1.3	9.4 1.6 2.3	/	19
Gust et al. [9]	2019		OE, HMIE or TMIE Ivor Lewis OE or TMIE McKeown OE and MIE transhiatal	1.2	0.7	1.4	/	/
Takeda et al. [29]	2019	328	TMIE McKeown HMIE McKeown RAMIE McKeown	2.4	/	2.4	/	0
Iwasaki et al. [16]	2020	113	TMIE McKeown	9.7	/	9.7	/	/
Fuchs et al. [30]	2020		HMIE Ivor Lewis	/	/	/	N/A.	7.7
Hanna et al. [17]	2020	258	OE and MIE Ivor Lewis, transhiatal and McKeown	31	N/A	N/A	N/A	17
Lubbers et al. [10]	2021	307	TMIE Ivor Lewis TMIE McKeown	2.6	/	2.6	/	38
Puccetti et al. [8]	2021	414	OE, TMIE and HMIE Ivor Lewis	5.3	2.9	8.3	5.4	13.6
Chung et al. [31]	2021	49	MIE	14	/	14	/	80

PHH = paraconduit hiatal hernia, OE = open esophagectomy, TMIE = totally minimally invasive esophagectomy, MIE = minimally invasive esophagectomy, HMIE = hybrid minimally invasive esophagectomy, N/A = not applicable.

In the present study, we investigated the occurrence of PHH after an Ivor Lewis esophagectomy performed in the period from January 2009 to April 2018. The patient collective involved only patients with Ivor Lewis esophagectomies performed either as open or hybrid minimally invasive. We observed a significantly higher rate of hiatal hernia after HMIE in comparison with OE (13.8% vs. 1.3%, $p < 0.001$). The transverse colon was herniated in every case of PHH and 78.3% of the PHHs were on the left thoracic side, similar to the study results of Brenkman et al. [27].

A recently published meta-analysis reports 2.6% PHHs after OE and 6.3% after TMIE including Ivor Lewis, McKeown and transhiatal esophagectomies [15]. Regarding HMIE, 6.7% of PHHs were reported based only on two studies [15,18,25]. The mentioned studies report different outcomes. While Vallböhmer et al. report a low incidence of 2.7% PHHs after HMIE, the incidence reported by Mathews et al. estimates 10% PHHs after HMIE [18,25] Here, we have to take into account that the operating technique used in the study by Vallböhmer et al. was a two-stage HMIE consisting of a laparoscopic mobilization of the stomach followed by a second operation (open transthoracic esophagectomy) with a mean delay of 4 days [18]. In a mixed collective of 414 patients operated, including different techniques of Ivor Lewis esophagectomy, Pucceti et al. report 5.4% PHHs after HMIE but no significant association between minimally invasive surgery and the occurrence of PHH [8]

The suspected mechanism for the higher incidence of PHH after HMIE or TMIE is the presence of less adhesion after minimally invasive surgery, which allows a higher mobility of the intestine. Also, it is suggested that the surgical widening of the hiatus is larger in minimally invasive techniques. However, in our study, there was no significant impact of a hiatotomy on the development of PHH. Regarding the extension of the widening of the hiatus, a comparison between the groups was not possible due to the retrospective nature of our study.

Although most patients are asymptomatic, surgical repair is recommended since a significant percentage of patients develop unpredictable incarceration of the herniated intestine. This can easily lead to perforation of the intestine with consecutive mediastinitis, septic shock and high morbidity and mortality. In order to prevent such potentially fatal complications, we recommend elective surgical repair regardless of whether the patient is symptomatic or not. Besides the minimally invasive operating technique, no other risk factors could be identified for the development of PHH. This should not discourage the use of minimally invasive techniques, since their advantages have already been proven [2,3] Nevertheless, this new risk factor for postoperative complications must raise awareness in postoperative follow-up. Since a large part of the patients do not report any clear symptoms, care must be given in the process of reviewing the follow-up imaging, to not miss possible PHH. Furthermore, the occurrence of PHH after HMIE demands further refinement of the technique. Until now, no prophylactic measures during esophagectomy have been shown to significantly reduce the occurrence of PHH. In our study, there was also no significant impact of prophylactic colopexy of the transverse colon to the abdominal wall performed during the esophagectomy in terms of PHH.

A further problem regarding the treatment of PHH is the high recurrence rate after surgical repair. We observed a PHH recurrence in 31.6% of the operated patients. Price et al. analyzed over 2000 patients with PHH after MIE who underwent a hiatoplasty with or without mesh reinforcement and reported morbidity rates of up to 60% and recurrence rates of 13.3%, similar to the recently published data by Oppelt et al. [20,32]. Kent et al. also analyzed the PHH repair with or without the use of mesh and reported recurrence rates of up to 29%, which is comparable to our results [19]. The main reason for the high recurrence rates is probably the technical difficulty of covering/closing the often extremely wide hiatal opening and thinned crura. Depending on the large hiatal opening, it is sometimes not possible to approximate the crura and an alternative solution for the closure of the gap may be needed, such as the use of Goretex mesh or ligamentum teres hepatis, as previously reported by our group [33]. Regardless of the technique used, maximum care must be taken not to damage the feeding gastroepiploic vessels of the conduit.

The current study has several limitations, including the retrospective design. Particularly technical details, such as hiatal widening during operations, cannot be evaluated in a retrospective setting. Furthermore, some learning curve bias cannot be excluded due to the implementation of HMIE during the course of the study. Also, since there is no standard treatment for PHH, the surgical treatment chosen was based on the surgeon's preferences. Loss to follow-up is minimized due to the close routine oncological follow-up in our outpatient setting.

Prospective studies are needed to examine possible prophylactic measures during the esophagectomy such as cruroplasty or wide colopexy, in order to reduce the occurrence of PHH. Furthermore, in the absence of a standardized repair technique for PHH, only prospective randomized studies comprising comparisons of different techniques and mesh grafts can help us find the optimal repair solution in the case of PHH and reduce recurrences.

5. Conclusions

PHH is a relevant complication after HMIE, with frequent herniation of the transverse colon in the left thoracic side. Even though it is mostly asymptomatic, PHH can lead to incarceration of the intestine with a potentially fatal outcome and should undergo surgical repair. Surgeons must be aware of this complication and remain vigilant in the postoperative radiological follow-up. Further refinement of the minimally invasive esophagectomy technique as well as the PHH repair technique is needed to reduce the occurrence of PHH and recurrence after repair.

Author Contributions: Conceptualization, J.K. and J.H. (Jens Hoeppner); formal analysis, J.H. (Julian Hipp); investigation, J.K. and R.J.; resources, S.F.-F.; data curation, R.J.; writing—original draft preparation, J.K.; writing—review and editing, J.H. (Julian Hipp), R.J., S.F.-F., M.F., M.K.D. and J.H. (Jens Hoeppner); supervision, J.H. (Jens Hoeppner). All authors have read and agreed to the published version of the manuscript.

Funding: The article processing charge was funded by the Albert Ludwigs University Freiburg in the funding program Open Access Publishing. Beyond that this research received no external funding.

Institutional Review Board Statement: The study was approved by the Medical Ethics Committee of the University of Freiburg (File No. 253/19 June 2019).

Informed Consent Statement: Informed consent was obtained from all subjects involved in the study.

Data Availability Statement: The data presented in this study are available on request from the corresponding author.

Conflicts of Interest: The authors declare no conflict of interest.

References

1. Ferlay, J.; Shin, H.-R.; Bray, F.; Forman, D.; Mathers, C.; Parkin, D.M. Estimates of worldwide burden of cancer in 2008: GLOBOCAN 2008. *Int. J. Cancer* **2010**, *127*, 2893–2917. [CrossRef] [PubMed]
2. Biere, S.S.A.Y.; van Berge Henegouwen, M.I.; Maas, K.W.; Bonavina, L.; Rosman, C.; Garcia, J.R.; Gisbertz, S.S.; Klinkenbijl, J.H.G.; Hollmann, M.W.; de Lange, E.S.M.; et al. Minimally invasive versus open oesophagectomy for patients with oesophageal cancer: A multicentre, open-label, randomised controlled trial. *Lancet* **2012**, *379*, 1887–1892. [CrossRef] [PubMed]
3. Mariette, C.; Markar, S.R.; Dabakuyo-Yonli, T.S.; Meunier, B.; Pezet, D.; Collet, D.; D'Journo, X.B.; Brigand, C.; Perniceni, T.; Carrère, N.; et al. Hybrid Minimally Invasive Esophagectomy for Esophageal Cancer. *N. Engl. J. Med.* **2019**, *380*, 152–162. [CrossRef]
4. Ben-David, K.; Sarosi, G.A.; Cendan, J.C.; Howard, D.; Rossidis, G.; Hochwald, S.N. Decreasing morbidity and mortality in 100 consecutive minimally invasive esophagectomies. *Surg. Endosc.* **2012**, *26*, 162–167. [CrossRef] [PubMed]
5. Kuvendjiska, J.; Marjanovic, G.; Glatz, T.; Kulemann, B.; Hoeppner, J. Hybrid Minimally Invasive Esophagectomy-Surgical Technique and Results. *J. Clin. Med.* **2019**, *8*, 978. [CrossRef] [PubMed]
6. Glatz, T.; Marjanovic, G.; Kulemann, B.; Sick, O.; Hopt, U.T.; Hoeppner, J. Hybrid minimally invasive esophagectomy vs. open esophagectomy: A matched case analysis in 120 patients. *Langenbeck's Arch. Surg.* **2017**, *402*, 323–331. [CrossRef]
7. Lung, K.; Carroll, P.A.; Rogalla, P.; Yeung, J.; Darling, G. Paraconduit Hernia in the Era of Minimally Invasive Esophagectomy: Underdiagnosed? *Ann. Thorac. Surg.* **2021**, *111*, 1812–1819. [CrossRef]
8. Puccetti, F.; Cossu, A.; Parise, P.; Barbieri, L.; Elmore, U.; Carresi, U.; de Pascale, S.; Fumagalli Romario, U.; Rosati, R. Diaphragmatic hernia after Ivor Lewis esophagectomy for cancer: A retrospective analysis of risk factors and post-repair outcomes. *J. Thorac. Dis.* **2021**, *13*, 160–168. [CrossRef] [PubMed]
9. Gust, L.; Nafteux, P.; Allemann, P.; Tuech, J.-J.; El Nakadi, I.; Collet, D.; Goere, D.; Fabre, J.-M.; Meunier, B.; Dumont, F.; et al. Hiatal hernia after oesophagectomy: A large European survey. *Eur. J. Cardio-Thorac. Surg.* **2019**, *55*, 1104–1112. [CrossRef] [PubMed]
10. Lubbers, M.; Kouwenhoven, E.A.; Smit, J.K.; van Det, M.J. Hiatal Hernia with Acute Obstructive Symptoms After Minimally Invasive Oesophagectomy. *J. Gastrointest. Surg.* **2021**, *25*, 603–608. [CrossRef]

11. Hoeppner, J.; Marjanovic, G.; Glatz, T.; Kulemann, B.; Hopt, U.T. Hybrid laparoscopic thoracotomic esophagectomy with intrathoracic esophagogastric anastomosis. *Chir. Z. Alle Geb. Oper. Medizen* **2014**, *85*, 628–635. [CrossRef]
12. Hoeppner, J. Hybrid Minimally Invasive Esophagectomy: How I Teach It. *Ann. Thorac. Surg.* **2021**, *112*, 10–15. [CrossRef] [PubMed]
13. Bronson, N.W.; Luna, R.A.; Hunter, J.G.; Dolan, J.P. The incidence of hiatal hernia after minimally invasive esophagectomy. *J. Gastrointest. Surg.* **2014**, *18*, 889–893. [CrossRef]
14. Oor, J.E.; Wiezer, M.J.; Hazebroek, E.J. Hiatal Hernia After Open versus Minimally Invasive Esophagectomy: A Systematic Review and Meta-analysis. *Ann. Surg. Oncol.* **2016**, *23*, 2690–2698. [CrossRef] [PubMed]
15. Murad, H.; Huang, B.; Ndegwa, N.; Rouvelas, I.; Klevebro, F. Postoperative hiatal herniation after open vs. minimally invasive esophagectomy; A systematic review and meta-analysis. *Int. J. Surg.* **2021**, *93*, 106046. [CrossRef] [PubMed]
16. Iwasaki, H.; Tanaka, T.; Miyake, S.; Yoda, Y.; Noshiro, H. Postoperative hiatal hernia after minimally invasive esophagectomy for esophageal cancer. *J. Thorac. Dis.* **2020**, *12*, 4661–4669. [CrossRef] [PubMed]
17. Hanna, A.N.; Guajardo, I.; Williams, N.; Kucharczuk, J.; Dempsey, D.T. Hiatal Hernia after Esophagectomy: An Underappreciated Complication? *J. Am. Coll. Surg.* **2020**, *230*, 700–707. [CrossRef]
18. Vallböhmer, D.; Hölscher, A.H.; Herbold, T.; Gutschow, C.; Schröder, W. Diaphragmatic hernia after conventional or laparoscopic-assisted transthoracic esophagectomy. *Ann. Thorac. Surg.* **2007**, *84*, 1847–1852. [CrossRef] [PubMed]
19. Kent, M.S.; Luketich, J.D.; Tsai, W.; Churilla, P.; Federle, M.; Landreneau, R.; Alvelo-Rivera, M.; Schuchert, M. Revisional surgery after esophagectomy: An analysis of 43 patients. *Ann. Thorac. Surg.* **2008**, *86*, 975–983; discussion 967–974. [CrossRef] [PubMed]
20. Price, T.N.; Allen, M.S.; Nichols, F.C., 3rd; Cassivi, S.D.; Wigle, D.A.; Shen, K.R.; Deschamps, C. Hiatal hernia after esophagectomy: Analysis of 2,182 esophagectomies from a single institution. *Ann. Thorac. Surg.* **2011**, *92*, 2041–2045. [CrossRef]
21. Ganeshan, D.M.; Correa, A.M.; Bhosale, P.; Vaporciyan, A.A.; Rice, D.; Mehran, R.J.; Walsh, G.L.; Iyer, R.; Roth, J.A.; Swisher, S.G.; et al. Diaphragmatic hernia after esophagectomy in 440 patients with long-term follow-up. *Ann. Thorac. Surg.* **2013**, *96*, 1138–1145. [CrossRef] [PubMed]
22. Benjamin, G.; Ashfaq, A.; Chang, Y.-H.; Harold, K.; Jaroszewski, D. Diaphragmatic hernia post-minimally invasive esophagectomy: A discussion and review of literature. *Hernia J. Hernias Abdom. Wall Surg.* **2015**, *19*, 635–643. [CrossRef] [PubMed]
23. Messenger, D.E.; Higgs, S.M.; Dwerryhouse, S.J.; Hewin, D.F.; Vipond, M.N.; Barr, H.; Wadley, M.S. Symptomatic diaphragmatic herniation following open and minimally invasive oesophagectomy: Experience from a UK specialist unit. *Surg. Endosc.* **2015**, *29*, 417–424. [CrossRef] [PubMed]
24. Ulloa Severino, B.; Fuks, D.; Christidis, C.; Denet, C.; Gayet, B.; Perniceni, T. Laparoscopic repair of hiatal hernia after minimally invasive esophagectomy. *Surg. Endosc.* **2016**, *30*, 1068–1072. [CrossRef] [PubMed]
25. Matthews, J.; Bhanderi, S.; Mitchell, H.; Whiting, J.; Vohra, R.; Hodson, J.; Griffiths, E. Diaphragmatic herniation following esophagogastric resectional surgery: An increasing problem with minimally invasive techniques?: Post-operative diaphragmatic hernias. *Surg. Endosc.* **2016**, *30*, 5419–5427. [CrossRef]
26. Andreou, A.; Pesthy, S.; Struecker, B.; Dadras, M.; Raakow, R.; Knitter, S.; Duwe, G.; Sauer, I.M.; Beierle, A.S.; Denecke, C.; et al. Incidence and Risk Factors of Symptomatic Hiatal Hernia Following Resection for Gastric and Esophageal Cancer. *Anticancer Res.* **2017**, *37*, 7031–7036. [CrossRef] [PubMed]
27. Brenkman, H.J.F.; Parry, K.; Noble, F.; van Hillegersberg, R.; Sharland, D.; Goense, L.; Kelly, J.; Byrne, J.P.; Underwood, T.J.; Ruurda, J.P. Hiatal Hernia After Esophagectomy for Cancer. *Ann. Thorac. Surg.* **2017**, *103*, 1055–1062. [CrossRef]
28. Gooszen, J.A.H.; Slaman, A.E.; van Dieren, S.; Gisbertz, S.S.; van Berge Henegouwen, M.I. Incidence and Treatment of Symptomatic Diaphragmatic Hernia After Esophagectomy for Cancer. *Ann. Thorac. Surg.* **2018**, *106*, 199–206. [CrossRef]
29. Takeda, F.R.; Tustumi, F.; Filho, M.A.S.; Silva, M.O.; Júnior, U.R.; Sallum, R.A.A.; Cecconello, I. Diaphragmatic Hernia Repair After Esophagectomy: Technical Report and Lessons After a Series of Cases. *J. Laparoendosc. Adv. Surg. Tech. Part A* **2020**, *30*, 433–437. [CrossRef]
30. Fuchs, H.F.; Knepper, L.; Müller, D.T.; Bartella, I.; Bruns, C.J.; Leers, J.M.; Schröder, W. Transdiaphragmatic herniation after transthoracic esophagectomy: An underestimated problem. *Dis. Esophagus* **2020**, *33*, doaa024. [CrossRef] [PubMed]
31. Chung, S.K.; Bludevich, B.; Cherng, N.; Zhang, T.; Crawford, A.; Maxfield, M.W.; Whalen, G.; Uy, K.; Perugini, R.A. Paraconduit Hiatal Hernia Following Esophagectomy: Incidence, Risk Factors, Outcomes and Repair. *J. Surg. Res.* **2021**, *268*, 276–283. [CrossRef] [PubMed]
32. Oppelt, P.U.; Askevold, I.; Hörbelt, R.; Roller, F.C.; Padberg, W.; Hecker, A.; Reichert, M. Trans-hiatal herniation following esophagectomy or gastrectomy: Retrospective single-center experiences with a potential surgical emergency. *Hernia J. Hernias Abdom. Wall Surg.* **2022**, *26*, 259–278. [CrossRef] [PubMed]
33. Runkel, M.; Kuvendjiska, J.; Marjanovic, G.; Fichtner-Feigl, S.; Diener, M.K. Ligamentum teres augmentation (LTA) for hiatal hernia repair after minimally invasive esophageal resection: A new use for an old structure. *Langenbeck's Arch. Surg.* **2021**, *406*, 2521–2525. [CrossRef] [PubMed]

Disclaimer/Publisher's Note: The statements, opinions and data contained in all publications are solely those of the individual author(s) and contributor(s) and not of MDPI and/or the editor(s). MDPI and/or the editor(s) disclaim responsibility for any injury to people or property resulting from any ideas, methods, instructions or products referred to in the content.

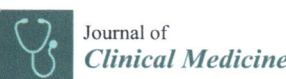

Article

The Role of Adipose Tissue Mesenchymal Stem Cells in Colonic Anastomosis Healing in Inflammatory Bowel Disease: Experimental Study in Rats

Georgios Ntampakis [1], Manousos-Georgios Pramateftakis [1], Orestis Ioannidis [1,*], Stefanos Bitsianis [1], Panagiotis Christidis [1], Savvas Symeonidis [1], Georgios Koliakos [2], Maria Karakota [2], Chrysanthi Bekiari [3,4], Anastasia Tsakona [5], Angeliki Cheva [5] and Stamatios Aggelopoulos [1]

[1] 4th Department of General Surgery, Aristotle University of Thessaloniki, 54124 Thessaloniki, Greece; gntampak@auth.gr (G.N.)
[2] Laboratory of Biochemistry, Aristotle University of Thessaloniki, 54124 Thessaloniki, Greece
[3] Experimental and Research Center, Papageorgiou General Hospital of Thessaloniki, 56403 Thessaloniki, Greece
[4] Laboratory of Anatomy and Histology, Veterinary School, Aristotle University of Thessaloniki, 54124 Thessaloniki, Greece
[5] Pathology Department, Faculty of Medicine, Aristotle University of Thessaloniki, 54124 Thessaloniki, Greece
* Correspondence: iorestis@auth.gr; Tel.: +30-6979790968

Abstract: (1) Background: A surgical operation on an inflamed bowel is, diachronically, a challenge for the surgeon, especially for patients with inflammatory bowel disease. Adipose tissue-derived mesenchymal stromal cells are already in use in clinical settings for their anti-inflammatory properties. The rationale of the current study was to use AdMSCs in high-risk anastomoses to monitor if they attenuate inflammation and prevent anastomotic leak. (2) Methods: a total of 4 groups of rats were subjected to a surgical transection of the large intestine and primary anastomosis. In two groups, DSS 5% was administered for 7 days prior to the procedure, to induce acute intestinal inflammation. After the anastomosis, 5×10^6 autologous AdMSCs or an acellular solution was injected locally. Macroscopic evaluation, bursting pressure, hydroxyproline, and inflammatory cytokine expression were the parameters measured on the 8th post-operative day. (3) Results: Significantly less intra-abdominal complications, higher bursting pressures, and a decrease in pro-inflammatory markers were found in the groups that received AdMSCs. No difference in VEGF expression was observed on the 8th post-operative day. (4) Conclusions: AdMSCs attenuate inflammation in cases of acutely inflamed anastomosis.

Keywords: adipose tissue mesenchymal stromal cells; inflammatory bowel disease; bowel anastomosis; anastomotic leak; colorectal surgery; dextran sodium sulfate

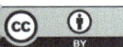

1. Introduction

Inflammatory bowel disease (IBD) is an immunological disease of the gastrointestinal tract which is caused by an uncontrollable immunological response of the body. There are two distinct clinical types of IBD, Crohn's disease (CD) and ulcerative colitis (UC), the incidence of which is significantly high in Europe compared to the rest of the world [1]. Demographically, CD affects younger patients in their 20s or 30s, while UC is more common in the 3rd–4th decade of life, even though their presence in all age groups (0–90) is not excluded [2]. As an illness that primarily affects young populations, which constitute the working power of society, IBD has a significant socio-economic impact in the modern world. Therapeutic costs, absence from work, and emotional disturbances are a great burden for society and the individuals suffering from these diseases. In addition, these patients suffer from a low quality of life after a surgical procedure that might require an ostomy, as well as the high inpatient costs due to prolonged hospitalization and perioperative complications [3].

With regards to the phenotype of the disease, one third of patients with CD are diagnosed with terminal ileitis; in another third of the patients, the disease is localized in the colon only; and the final third of patients present with ileocolic disease. Approximately 10–20% of the patients present with perianal disease (abscesses, fistulae). Approximately one third of patients with UC present with inflammation below the rectosigmoid junction, another third present with a diseased colon up to the splenic flexure; and the final third of patients present with extensive colitis [2].

The use of biological factors in the therapeutic arsenal of IBD has resulted in less surgical operations, offering patients a better quality of life, with longer disease-free intervals. Nevertheless, complications requiring surgical intervention can still occur, leading to extended bowel resections and stomas [4]. The selection of the most appropriate operation for each individual patient is tailored according to the characteristics of the individual patient's disease. In all disease phenotypes, the operations include limited or extended resections with or without diverting stoma creation, and complex procedures to restore the continuity of the gastrointestinal tract [5,6].

In the last few years, in addition to other therapeutic approaches that utilize biological agents, mesenchymal stromal cells (MSC) have been utilized as an adjunct therapy. MSCs are multipotent cells that are considered to have immunomodulatory and anti-inflammatory properties. These cells can be harvested from bone marrow, placenta, or adipose tissue and be used either systematically or locally [7].

Recent studies have aimed to investigate the metabolic and molecular pathways through which the MSCs affect the inflammatory response; it is thought that MSCs affect the inflammatory response by regulating the expression of certain inflammation-related cytokines and reprogramming M1 macrophages [8–16]. Small molecules derived from the MSCs, called exosomes, might affect intracellular communication by altering the inflammatory response. This constitutes another experimental field which already shows promising results in the pre-clinical studies [12,17–26].

Currently, the use of MSCs in extraluminal CD (fistulae, abscesses) shows good results in clinical trials regarding their efficacy and safety. In addition, the literature shows that adipose tissue-derived mesenchymal stromal cells (AdMSC) are the best choice for fistulae therapy in CD [27–32]. Other MSC clinical trials target the recurrence of CD and UC with the systematic administration of MSCs; this approach has promising results, as the meta-analysis of Dave et al. shows [33].

Only a few studies have been designed to show the efficacy of MSCs in high-risk gastrointestinal anastomoses, but the experimental protocols used, and the variables measured, are very diverse between the studies. Van de Putte et al. have shown that MSCs have the ability to attenuate inflammation caused by preoperative radiotherapy, and ameliorate the quality of the anastomosis [34]. Pascual et al. have shown increased medium bursting pressure in a high-risk anastomosis with biological stromal cell embedded sutures [35]. A few studies have shown reduced leak rates and increased medium bursting pressure with MSCs in the ischemic anastomosis model [36–39]. Alvarenga et al. have shown, using an experimental high-risk anastomosis model, that the use of AdMSCs resulted in reduced local complication rates, the attenuation of the inflammation, and reduced tissue damage, as well as the downregulation of pro-inflammatory cytokines [40].

The objective of the current study is to experimentally confirm that AdMSCs can be applied on an acutely inflamed colonic anastomosis and decrease the risk of anastomotic complications and its derivatives (dehiscence, leak, abscess formation, peritonitis, adhesions, and sepsis).

2. Materials and Methods

2.1. Ethics Statement

All animal manipulations were in line with the current national laws for experimentation (PD 56/2013). The license number for this experimental study is #810556(3269) and granted by the prefecture of Central Macedonia. The ethical committee of Aristotle University of Thessaloniki (license no. 07/2020/07.02.2020) co-signed the approval of the current study. Compliance with ARRIVE guidelines was ensured during the approval process [41].

2.2. Experimental Design

For the purpose of the experiment, young Wistar rats (Rattus norvegicus) were used, and were 10–14 weeks old, with an average weight of 250–300 g. The rats were bred in the Research and Experimental Centre of the Papageorgiou General Hospital of Thessaloniki (license no. EL54BIOsup43), where they were hosted throughout the entire experimental process. The rats were living in pairs in their cages, with access to standard chaw and water ad libitum. Room temperature was stable at 22 °C and humidity was between 55% and 65%, while the cycle of light (12 h of light and 12 h of darkness) was maintained with an automatic switch.

Twelve rats received dextran sodium sulfate (DSS) 5% with water ad libitum to induce acute colitis [42]. The rest of the animals drank water without DSS.

After power analysis, 24 rats were used and were equally assigned randomly to the following experimental groups. Group A (Op): laparotomy with colonic anastomosis only. Group B (Op + AdMSCs): laparotomy with colonic anastomosis and local injection of 5×10^6 AdMSCs in 70 µL power buffer saline (PBS) [34,43,44]. Group C (Op + DSS + Sal): DSS 5%, laparotomy with colonic anastomosis, and local injection of 70 µL power buffer saline (PBS). Group D (Op + DSS + AdMSC): DSS 5%, laparotomy with colonic anastomosis, and local injection of 5×10^6 AdMSCs in 70 µL PBS.

All the animals were sacrificed on the 8th post-operative day according to local euthanasia protocols (CO_2 cage).

After euthanasia, all animals were subjected to laparotomy. The abdominal cavity was then assessed, and a macroscopic complication score was calculated. After careful dissection, a 2.5 cm specimen was retrieved, and bursting pressure was measured. Finally, the specimen was split into two pieces, one for hydroxyproline measurement and the other for real-time PCR to measure IL-6, TNF-a, and VEGF.

2.3. Adipose Tissue-Derived Mesenchymal Stromal Cells

Fat tissue was washed with normal saline after harvesting from the rats' right inguinal fold and cut into smaller pieces. Subsequently, it was processed with collagenase type I (0.5 mg/mL) in 37 °C for an hour. After homogenization of the tissue, the mesenchymal stem cell layer was isolated with centrifuge (2900 rpm, 20 min). Finally, the cell sediment was diluted in power buffer saline (PBS) to achieve a cellular solution of 5×10^6 cells/mL. The adipose-derived mesenchymal stromal cells were isolated according to the existing standardized protocol of the Laboratory of Biochemistry of our department. The AdMSCs were positive for CD44 and CD90 markers [45]. The primers used are mentioned in Appendix A Table A2.

2.4. Colitis Protocol

Dextran sodium sulfate (DSS) 5% 40 kPa was used for the induction of acute colitis in rats (Dextran Sulfate 40 Sodium Salt; AppliChem GmbH, Darmstadt, Germany) [46]. The chemical was added to the rats' water, and access to it was allowed ad libitum. The rats were observed clinically for 7 days. Loss of weight, diarrhea, bloody stool, general decline, anal inflammation, erected hair, and signs of self-neglect (soiled tails) were indicative of active colitis in the rats. The above findings were confirmed histologically in control animals that received DSS, as shown in Figures A1–A3.

2.5. Operative Procedure

The rats were anesthetized prior to the procedure, with an intraperitoneal administration of 50 mg/kg ketamine and 5 mg/kg xylazine. Hair removal was performed with a hair clipper and the abdomen was prepared with povidone iodine solution.

A midline 3 cm laparotomy was performed, and the large bowel was identified on the left of the abdominal cavity. A transection of the descending colon was performed, just above the pubic symphysis, taking care to preserve the vascularization. Following the transection, in group 1 an end-to-end primary anastomosis with a 5/0 polydioxanone (PDS) suture was performed, with interrupted stitches with the use of a microscope. In groups B and D, 5×10^6 AdMSCs in 70 µL PBS were injected in the bowel ends prior to anastomosis; in group C, 70 µL PBS was injected. After the anastomosis was completed, the bowel was returned to the abdominal cavity, and 10 mL of saline was used to wash the abdominal cavity. The surgical wound was closed with a 3/0 polyglactine suture, as shown in Figure A4.

After the operation, the rat was placed in an appropriately heated cage to recover and was allowed to consume water and food freely.

Seven days after the initial operation, all animals were sacrificed with use of a CO_2 cage according to local euthanasia protocols. A midline laparotomy was performed, and the abdomen was assessed macroscopically. After that, a 2.5 cm segment of the bowel containing the anastomosis was resected, and bursting strength was measured. Following the measurement of bursting strength, the specimen was frozen with the use of liquid CO_2 and was sent for biochemical measurements (hydroxyproline and real-time PCR).

2.6. Macroscopic Assessment

For the clinical assessment of the anastomosis, the anastomotic complication score was used, as proposed by Bosmans et al. [47], for the standardization of the clinical description of the experimental anastomosis outcomes (Table 1).

Table 1. Anastomotic complication score as endorsed by Bosmans et al. Reprinted from [47].

	Anastomotic Complication Score
0	No adhesions or abnormalities
1	Adhesion to fat pad, clean anastomosis underneath
2	Adhesion to intestinal loop, abdominal wall or other organ
3	Anastomotic defect found underneath adhesion, no other abnormalities
4	Signs of possible contamination (e.g., small abscesses)
5	Clear anastomotic complication; free pus, obstruction, signs of peritonitis
6	Fecal peritonitis/Death due to peritonitis

2.7. Bursting Pressure

The bursting pressure of the specimen was measured ex-situ, with the device depicted in Figure A5 of the Appendix A [48,49]. It consisted of a simple manometer, a tube connected to a three-way canula, and a syringe containing dyed water connected to the three-way. The specimen was fixed with a purse string to the tube and the free edge was clamped.

The dyed water was then infused slowly inside the specimen and the procedure was recorded with a camera to ensure an accurate recording. The pressure under which the anastomosis burst constituted the bursting pressure and was logged.

2.8. Hydroxyproline

Part of the resected bowel was sent for hydroxyproline measurement. All specimens were dried in cold air and homogenized before the procedure. A hydroxyproline concentration was estimated with the use of a spectrophotometry with a wavelength of 550 nm, after preparation with certain solutions (Table A1).

2.9. Real Time-Polymerase Chain Reaction

For the measurement of inflammatory cytokines (IL-6, TNFa, VEGF), a NucleoSpin RNA kit (Macherey-Nagel, Düren, Germany) was used according to the manufacturer's instructions. For the quantitative measurement of the cytokines, a One-Step qRT PCR kit (KAPABIOSYSTEMS, Wilmington, MA, USA) was used. The primers used can be found in Table A2.

2.10. Statistical Analysis

The measured variables were checked for the normality of their distribution by the Shapiro–Wilk test. Normally distributed continuous variables were expressed by the arithmetic mean ± standard deviation (mean ± SD), while continuous variables with a non-parametric distribution were expressed by the median and interquadrant range (median, IQR). Qualitative variables, categorical or ordinal, were presented as numbers and percentages per 100. The confidence interval was set at 95% which means that the differences between the groups were considered statistically significant when $p < 0.05$. To compare the independent variables in the two study groups, the Mann–Whitney U test was used. Non-parametric tests were preferred due to the small sample size. The statistical analysis of the results was performed using the statistical program Jamovi 1.6.18.0. All of the descriptive statistics can be found in Appendix B.

3. Results

3.1. AdMSCs Macroscopically Attenuate Intra-Abdominal Complications

Macroscopic evaluations of the abdominal cavities showed less intra-abdominal adhesions, colonic distention, and abscess formation. For groups A (operation only) and B (operation and AdMSCs), minimal complications were found, mainly adhesions to fat or other organs; group B, which received the AdMSCs, proved to have significantly less adhesions than group A ($p = 0.038$). As for the groups with acute inflammation, groups C and D, small abscesses, colonic dilatation, and other signs of intra-abdominal contamination were found, but again they were significantly more likely in group C, which did not receive AdMSCs. Group D had moderate complications compared to group C ($p = 0.02$); however, more significant morbidity was found in Group D compared to group B ($p = 0.008$). These results are illustrated in Figure 1 and Table A3.

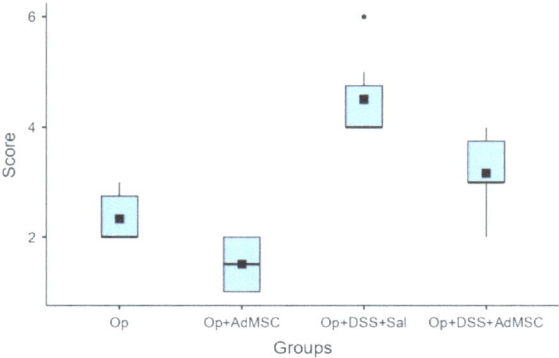

Figure 1. Macroscopic evaluation. Comparisons: A vs. B: $p = 0.038$, C vs. D: $p = 0.02$, B vs. D: $p = 0.008$.

3.2. Bursting Strength Is Significantly Higher in Groups with AdMSC

It seems that the groups that received AdMSCs (B and D) had a relatively higher bursting strength than their counterparts. The mean bursting pressures are lower in groups with inflammation, but the mean pressures are significantly higher in groups that received AdMSCs compared to those that did not. Also, it appears that the AdMSCs applied to the anastomosis which was subjected to a surgical strike had a significantly higher bursting pressure ($p = 0.037$) (Figure 2, Table A4).

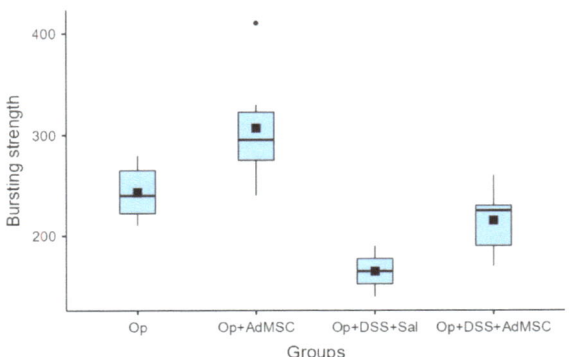

Figure 2. Bursting strength. Comparisons: A vs. B: $p = 0.037$, C vs. D: $p = 0.03$, B vs. D: $p = 0.008$.

3.3. Anastomoses with AdMSCs Had More Collagen Deposition

Enhanced anastomotic healing was found in anastomoses with AdMSCs, as indicated by higher mean hydroxyproline concentrations. The highest mean hydroxyproline concentration was found in Group B, which was significantly higher compared to Group A ($p = 0.041$). Inflammation reduced the collagen deposition in the anastomosis, and therefore hindered healing, but the AdMSCs reverse this effect, as shown from the comparison of groups C and D ($p = 0.004$) (Figure 3, Table A5).

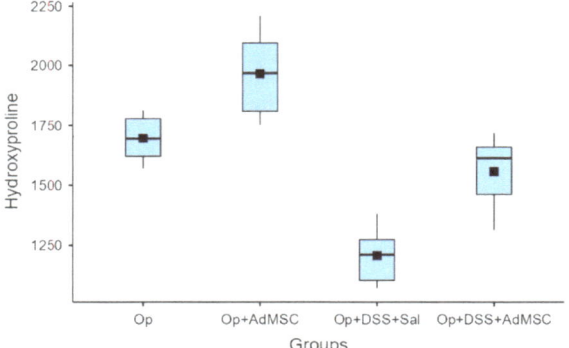

Figure 3. Hydroxyproline. Comparisons: A vs. B: $p = 0.041$, C vs. D: $p = 0.004$, B vs. D: $p = 0.002$.

3.4. Pro-Inflammatory Cytokine Expression Is Downregulated in Groups That Received AdMSC

The mRNAs of TNF-a and IL-6 were over-expressed in the groups that received DSS; it seems that the AdMSCs helped to downregulate the expression of these genes in the groups in which it was administered. Even in group B, the pro-inflammatory cytokines were significantly reduced compared to the control (Group A). These results are illustrated in Figures 4 and 5 and Tables A6 and A7.

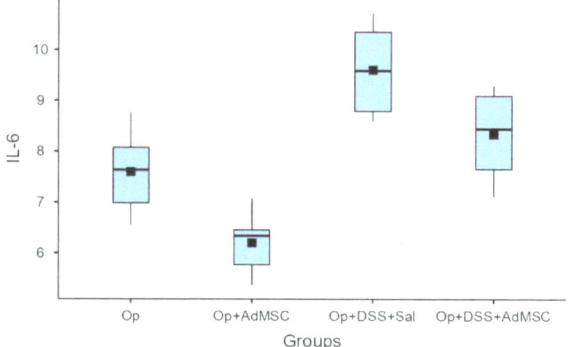

Figure 4. IL-6. Comparisons: A vs. B: $p = 0.009$, C vs. D: $p = 0.065$, B vs. D: $p = 0.002$.

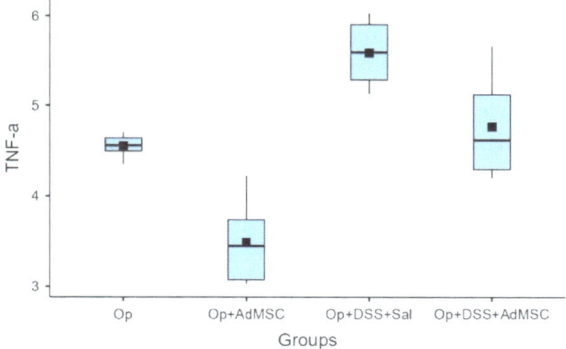

Figure 5. TNF-a. Comparisons: A vs. B: $p = 0.002$, C vs. D: $p = 0.026$, B vs. D: $p = 0.004$.

3.5. No Difference in Neo-Vascularization of the Anastomosis

With regards to neo-vascularization, we failed to see any significant differences between the groups. Although the mean values of VEGF were slightly higher in groups that received AdMSCs, there was no statistically significant difference between the respective groups. There was also a lower mean VEGF in group D compared to group B; therefore, the mean VEGF expression was lower in the group with acutely inflamed bowels, as shown in Figure 6 and Table A8.

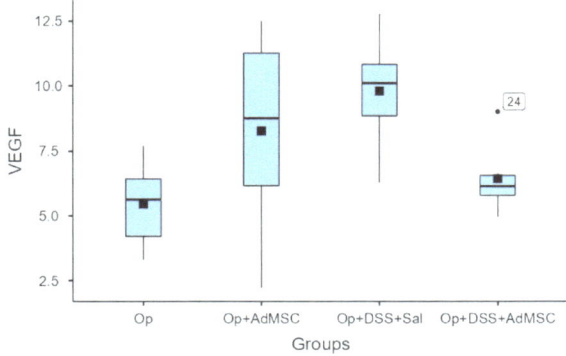

Figure 6. VEGF. Comparisons: A vs. B: $p = 0.18$, C vs. D: $p = 0.065$, B vs. D: $p = 0.31$.

4. Discussion

This study demonstrates that AdMSCs can be administered to colorectal anastomoses and attenuate inflammation. We showed that in the groups that received AdMSCs, bursting pressure was higher, local pro-inflammatory markers were not overexpressed, and anastomotic healing was enhanced, as shown by higher hydroxyproline levels.

The fact that inflammation impedes anastomotic healing is already a well-known fact in surgical practice, and is once again proved in our study, given that morbidity was higher in groups with acute inflammation. AdMSC administration reduced anastomotic-related morbidity, as shown by the macroscopic evaluation score, and by the lower rate of abscess formation, anastomotic dehiscence, and fecal peritonitis. There were no rat deaths in the groups that received AdMSCs, and there were fewer adhesions than the groups that did not receive AdMSCs. The low morbidity in groups that received AdMSCs has been found in similar research projects [39,40,50]. Yoo et al. reported significantly lower rates of infectious complications, strictures, and ulceration, but failed to show any significant difference in anastomotic leaks and adhesions in their ischemic anastomosis model [38].

Bursting strength was measured to be the highest in the groups that received AdMSCs in comparison to the groups that did not. Inflammation reduced the bursting strength of the anastomosis despite the administration of AdMSCs in group D, but bursting pressures were significantly higher compared to group C. Overall, the highest mean anastomotic pressure (mean, 307) was found in group B without the inflammation, with administration of AdMSCs [36–38]. In our study, the pressure measurements were measured ex-vivo so that inevitable local adhesions did not interfere with the bursting pressure and so we could gain a more objective appreciation of the anastomosis quality [35].

Hydroxyproline levels are a good marker of collagen accumulation in the anastomosis, but, in our view, its use as a marker of the quality of the anastomosis is oversimplified, because as far as we know, the anastomosis undergoes remodeling, which is mediated by cytokines like TGF-β, which induces the differentiation of fibroblasts to myofibroblasts [40,51,52]. In the remodeling phase, immature type III collagen is substituted by the more mature type I, which makes the anastomosis more durable [53]. Since our sampling takes place on the 8th post-operative day, we would argue that this period coincides with the proliferative phase of healing, during which we would expect an increased deposition of collagen in the anastomosis, which was demonstrated. Collagen was found to be higher in the groups that received AdMSCs [36–38].

Pro-inflammatory cytokines TNF-a and IL-6 were found to be significantly reduced in the groups that received AdMSCs and were following the same pattern as pro-inflammatory cytokines. We know that both these cytokines play an integral role in haemostasis/the inflammatory phase of anastomotic healing and are produced by M1 macrophages [54–57]. One of the mechanisms of action of AdMSCs is believed to be polarization of the M1 macrophage phenotype to the M2 type, which is believed to attenuate inflammation [34]. The M2 phenotype pro-inflammatory cytokines are downregulated and the cytokines involved in fibroblast proliferation and differentiation are increased. Gonzalez et al. administered AdMSCs to rats with colitis and sepsis. They have shown that AdMSCs had an anti-inflammatory effect by decreasing TNFa, IL6, and other proinflammatory cytokines, as well as increasing the expression of IL-10, thus downregulating the Th1 mediated inflammatory response, which is similar both in DSS colitis and Crohn's disease [58].

Another important component of granulomatous tissue formation in anastomoses is neo-vascularization, which plays a very important role in anastomosis viability. This is induced by the increased secretion of the vascular endothelial factor (VEGF). In studies with models of ischemic colitis, the VEGF was increased in groups that received bone marrow derived MSCs (BmMCSs) [36,37,59]. Similar results have been produced by Van de Putte et al. using their radiation-induced colitis protocol [34]. To our knowledge, our study is the first to investigate VEGF expression using an experimental colitis model. It is shown that VEGF expression tends to be increased in all groups compared to the control, but there is no significant difference between the groups. This could be a result of the sampling timing occurring early in the healing process.

Although mesenchymal cells have already been used in clinical trials with good results, we are still at a quite premature stage of understanding the complex mechanisms by which they work, react with other cells, and regulate inflammation. It is still too early to interpret these results in humans, as the standardization of experimental procedures, and more in-vivo and in-vitro experiments are needed. Most of the protocols are designed on the assumption of an ischemic rather than inflamed anastomosis; therefore, more experiments are needed with this type of high-risk anastomosis. There is still no universal agreement on the concentrations of cells that are sufficient to augment anastomotic healing; more experiments on this subject need to be performed in the future.

Our findings are in agreement with studies that have shown that administration on site can help the properties of AdMSCs work in a paracrine way on the organ target. Van de Putte et al. have shown that the local accumulation of MSCs was not significant at the side of the anastomosis weeks after the administration of therapy; therefore, it is speculated that the therapeutic properties in the indigenous cells are mediated by molecules excreted by MSCs [34]. Pascual et al. used sutures coated with MSCs and showed that the cells were homogenously distributed in the anastomoses and resulted in more durable anastomoses with fewer local adhesions [35]. Adas et al. conducted similar studies by administering MSC therapy both systemically and locally. They found that locally transplanted MSCs resulted in accelerated healing and attenuated inflammation for ischemic bowel anastomoses, whereas there was no improvement in inflammation when MSCs were administered systemically [36,37]. Alvarenga et al. and Castelo-Branco et al. have similarly shown that the systemic administration of MSCs failed to reach the organ target and attenuate inflammation, as compared to the intraperitoneal administration of MSCs. In their latest work, they instilled MSCs locally, which resulted in the attenuation of the inflammation by the downregulation of proinflammatory cytokines, the upregulation of anti-inflammatory cytokines, and a decrease in the expression of metalloproteases [40,60]. Lee et al. have reported that intravenously injected MSCs were found to be trapped in the lungs [61]. Also, Yu et al. have reported no therapeutic effect when they injected the secretome of MSCs intravenously, as compared to applying the therapy locally with the use of fibrin glue as a medium [62].

In terms of administration, we have found that directly administering MSCs on the anastomosis site worked in producing these results. This is in agreement with studies that have shown that the administration of AdMSCs on the site of the anastomosis can help the properties of the AdMSCs work in a paracrine way on the organ target [34–36,40,50]. Most of the related studies agree that by using a parenteral administration method, MSCs hardly ever reach the organ target [34,62]. Further studies are needed to reveal whether mesenchymal cell properties can be amplified by using a different medium of application. Yu et al. have proposed a novel cell free therapy by using fibrin glue as a medium. They have demonstrated that it is possible to deliver the healing properties of MSCs by administering their secretome with fibrin glue, enabling the slow release of healing and growth factors for up to 10 days in rats with ischemic anastomoses [62].

This study proves that AdMSC therapy is feasible and promising and could potentially be translated into human studies in the future; however, there is still more work to be done, as biological responses can vary between different species. There are still unanswered questions regarding the minimal dosage of MSCs that will have the optimal effect in the healing of anastomoses, as well as whether there are agents or mediums of application that could enhance the therapeutic properties of MSCs. One of the potential drawbacks of MSC therapy could be the hyperexcretion of growth factors that could theoretically lead to carcinogenesis. After proving that MSCs are effective at attenuating inflammation, the next step would be to prove their safety, before applying the treatment in human trials.

Key to the therapeutic properties of AdMSCs is the secretome by which they seem to regulate inflammation as well as enhance the healing properties of the cells; this might indicate future experimental directions. As indicated by the studies of Park et al. and Yu et al., using AdMSC secretome could be a way of using the properties of MSCs without using the actual cells [62,63]. More studies with secretome could potentially lead us to identify the molecule or the group of molecules produced by MSCs which have similar anti-inflammatory and regenerative properties as the cell culture of MSCs.

Nevertheless, regardless of the future findings and possible implementations in daily practice, MSC experiments help us to better understand and gain new insights into how anastomotic healing works.

5. Conclusions

In this study, we investigated the potential of adipose tissue-derived mesenchymal stromal cells (AdMSCs) for mitigating complications associated with high-risk anastomoses, particularly in the presence of acute intestinal inflammation. The results obtained reveal several significant outcomes. The administration of AdMSCs led to a notable reduction in intra-abdominal complications, including adhesions to fat and other organs, and significantly increased the bursting strength of anastomoses. Furthermore, AdMSCs promoted enhanced collagen deposition, which is indicative of enhanced healing in the early stages of the healing procedure, and downregulated the pro-inflammatory cytokines TNF-a and IL-6. Although AdMSCs had a potential positive effect on neo-vascularization, this difference was not statistically significant. These findings collectively support the clinical potential of AdMSCs in improving surgical outcomes and reducing inflammation in procedures with high-risk anastomoses, warranting further research and clinical investigation.

Author Contributions: Conceptualization, M.-G.P. and G.N.; methodology, G.N., M.-G.P., G.K., C.B., and A.C.; validation, S.S. and S.B.; formal analysis, G.N. and P.C.; investigation, G.N, S.B., S.S., M.K., C.B., A.T. and A.C.; resources, G.N.; data curation, G.N.; writing—original draft preparation, G.N.; writing—review and editing, M.-G.P. and O.I.; visualization, P.C.; supervision, M.P, G.K., and S.A.; project administration, S.A. All authors have read and agreed to the published version of the manuscript.

Funding: This research received no external funding.

Institutional Review Board Statement: The animal study protocol was approved by the Institutional Review Board (or Ethics Committee) of Aristotle University of Thessaloniki (protocol code #810556(3269) 07/02/2020).

Informed Consent Statement: Not applicable.

Data Availability Statement: Data are available to any qualified researchers upon request to gntampak@auth.gr.

Conflicts of Interest: The authors declare no conflict of interest.

Appendix A

Table A1. Solutions used for Hydroxyproline measurements.

#	Solution
1	Citric acid buffer pH = 6.5
2	50% k-propanol
3	Chloramine-T, 0.056 M
4	NaOH 10.125 N
5	Ehrlich 1 M reagent
6	Acetic acid 0.5N
7	Collagen standard solution 1 mg/mL

Table A2. Primers for RT-PCR.

	Ascending Primer (5′–3′)	Descending Primer (5′–3′)
TNF-a	TACTGAACTTCGG GGTGATCGGTCC	CAGCCTTGTCCCT TGAAGAGAACC
IL-6	CAAGAGACTT CCAGCCAGTTG	TTGCCGAGTAGAC CTCATAGTGACC
VEGF	CGCCTTGGCT TGTCACATC	GTCGGAGAGC AACGTCACTA
GAPDH	ACCACAGTC CATGCCATCAC	TCCACCACC CTGTTGCTGTA

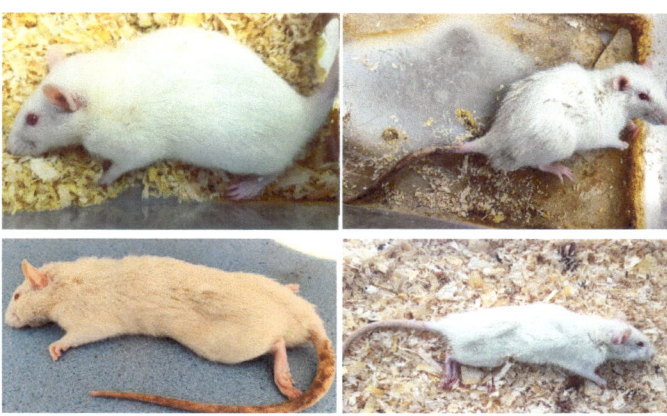

Figure A1. The first figure depicts the rat prior to DSS administration. The rest show their state after induction of colitis. Weight loss, hair erection, decreased mobility, and signs of neglected self-hygiene are noted.

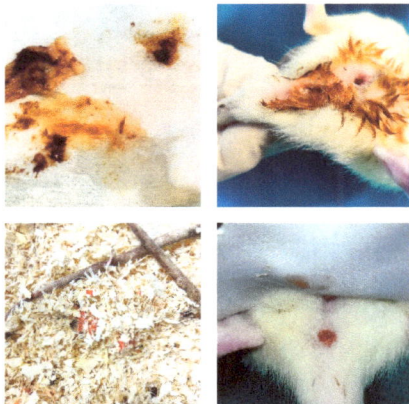

Figure A2. Mucous diarrhea, edematous anal mucosa, and blood in the stool after DSS administration.

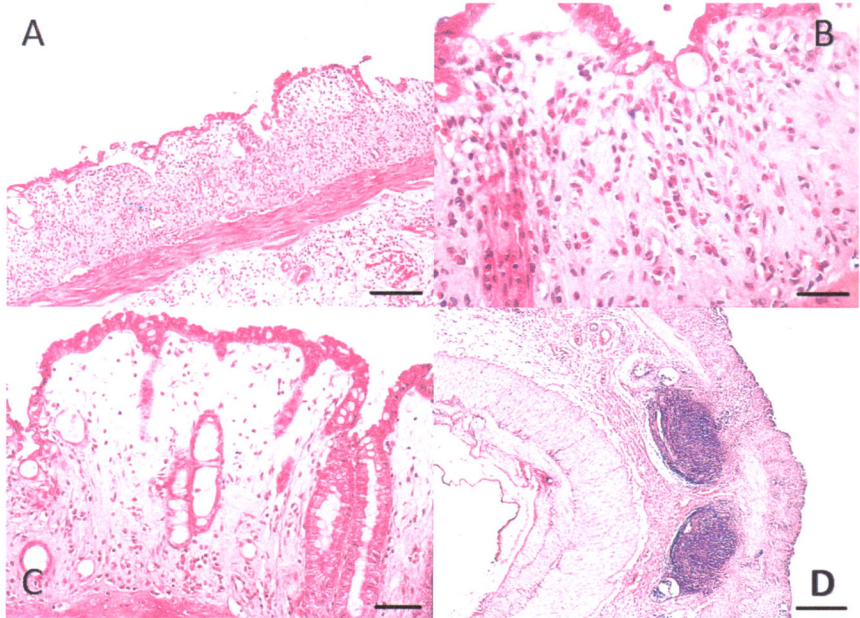

Figure A3. Histological confirmation of DSS colitis. H&E colon sections. ((**A**): ×100/scale bar 100 µm, (**B**): ×400/scale bar 20 µm, (**C**): ×200/scale bar 50 µm, (**D**): ×100/scale bar 100 µm). Figure A3 (**A–C**): Ulceration of the mucosa, inflammatory infiltration of mucosa, and submucosa from neutrophils. Obliteration of crypts and cryptic glands, as well as goblet cells. Loss of villous height. (**D**): Enlarged submucosal lymph nodes.

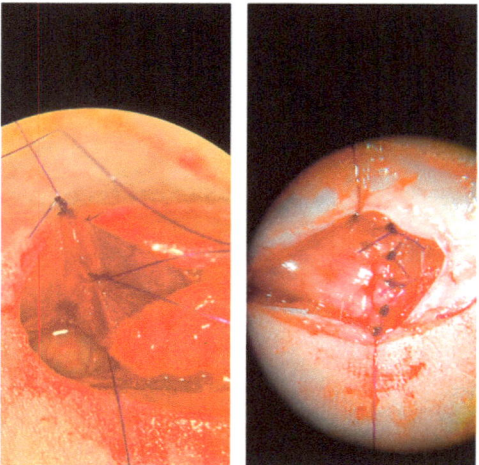

Figure A4. Anastomosis creation under the microscope.

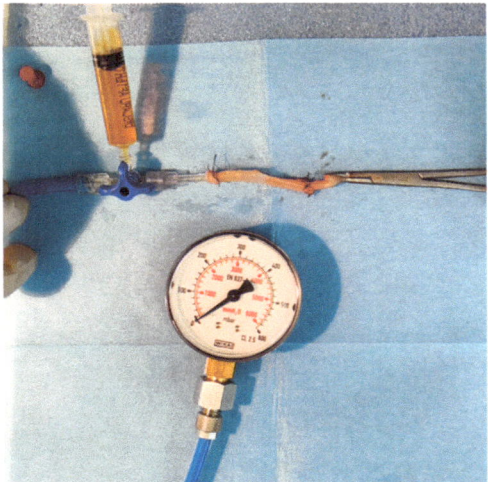

Figure A5. Device for measuring anastomotic bursting strength.

Appendix B

Table A3. Macroscopic evaluation.

Groups	Mean	Median	SD	Min	Max
A Op	2.33	2	0.516	2	3
B Op + AdMSC	1.50	1.5	0.548	1	2
C Op + DSS + Sal	4.50	4	0.837	4	6
D Op + DSS + AdMSC	3.17	3	0.753	2	4

Table A4. Bursting strength.

Groups	Mean	Median	SD	Min	Max
A Op	243	240	28.0	210	280
B Op + AdMSC	307	295	58.9	240	410
C Op + DSS + Sal	165	165	18.7	140	190
D Op + DSS + AdMSC	215	225	33.9	170	260

Table A5. Hydroxyproline.

Groups	Mean	Median	SD	Min	Max
A Op	1694	1692	103	1568	1813
B Op + AdMSC	1964	1967	186	1751	2210
C Op + DSS + Sal	1208	1212	120	1074	1383
D Op + DSS + AdMSC	1555	1609	155	1313	1715

Table A6. IL-6.

Groups	Mean	Median	SD	Min	Max
A Op	7.60	7.63	0.831	6.55	8.77
B Op + AdMSC	6.20	6.34	0.626	5.36	7.08
C Op + DSS + Sal	9.61	9.59	0.925	8.59	10.73
D Op + DSS + AdMSC	8.33	8.45	0.919	7.11	9.30

Table A7. TNF-a.

Groups	Mean	Median	SD	Min	Max
A Op	4.56	4.56	0.126	4.36	4.71
B Op + AdMSC	3.49	3.45	0.485	3.03	4.23
C Op + DSS + Sal	5.59	5.60	0.381	5.13	6.03
D Op + DSS + AdMSC	4.77	4.63	0.584	4.21	5.67

Table A8. VEGF.

Groups	Mean	Median	SD	Min	Max
A Op	5.45	5.63	1.67	3.30	7.72
B Op + AdMSC	8.28	8.76	3.91	2.22	12.52
C Op + DSS + Sal	8.94	8.89	2.62	5.30	12.79
D Op + DSS + AdMSC	6.10	6.14	2.03	3.84	9.54

References

1. Ananthakrishnan, A.N. Epidemiology and Risk Factors for IBD. *Nat. Rev. Gastroenterol. Hepatol.* **2015**, *12*, 205. [CrossRef] [PubMed]
2. Burisch, J.; Munkholm, P. The Epidemiology of Inflammatory Bowel Disease. *Scand. J. Gastroenterol.* **2015**, *50*, 942–951. [CrossRef] [PubMed]
3. Kamat, N.; Ganesh Pai, C.; Surulivel Rajan, M.; Kamath, A. Cost of Illness in Inflammatory Bowel Disease. *Dig. Dis. Sci.* **2017**, *62*, 2318–2326. [CrossRef]
4. Malik, T.A. Inflammatory Bowel Disease. *Surg. Clin. N. Am.* **2015**, *95*, 1105–1122. [CrossRef] [PubMed]
5. Tekkis, P.P.; Purkayastha, S.; Lanitis, S.; Athanasiou, T.; Heriot, A.G.; Orchard, T.R.; Nicholls, R.J.; Darzi, A.W. A Comparison of Segmental vs Subtotal/Total Colectomy for Colonic Crohn's Disease: A Meta-Analysis. *Color. Dis.* **2006**, *8*, 82–90. [CrossRef]
6. Gallo, G.; Kotze, P.G.; Spinelli, A. Surgery in Ulcerative Colitis: When? How? *Best Pract. Res. Clin. Gastroenterol.* **2018**, *32–33*, 71–78. [CrossRef]
7. Forbes, G.M. Mesenchymal Stromal Cell Therapy in Crohn's Disease. *Dig. Dis.* **2017**, *35*, 115–122. [CrossRef]
8. Yuan, Y.; Ni, S.; Zhuge, A.; Li, L.; Li, B. Adipose-Derived Mesenchymal Stem Cells Reprogram M1 Macrophage Metabolism via PHD2/HIF-1α Pathway in Colitis Mice. *Front. Immunol.* **2022**, *13*, 859806. [CrossRef]
9. Ko, J.Z.-H.; Johnson, S.; Dave, M. Efficacy and Safety of Mesenchymal Stem/Stromal Cell Therapy for Inflammatory Bowel Diseases: An Up-to-Date Systematic Review. *Biomolecules* **2021**, *11*, 82. [CrossRef]
10. Hu, Q.; Lyon, C.J.; Fletcher, J.K.; Tang, W.; Wan, M.; Hu, T.Y. Extracellular Vesicle Activities Regulating Macrophage- and Tissue-Mediated Injury and Repair Responses. *Acta Pharm. Sin. B* **2021**, *11*, 1493–1512. [CrossRef]
11. Gómez-Ferrer, M.; Amaro-Prellezo, E.; Dorronsoro, A.; Sánchez-Sánchez, R.; Vicente, Á.; Cosín-Roger, J.; Barrachina, M.D.; Baquero, M.C.; Valencia, J.; Sepúlveda, P. HIF-Overexpression and Pro-Inflammatory Priming in Human Mesenchymal Stromal Cells Improves the Healing Properties of Extracellular Vesicles in Experimental Crohn's Disease. *Int. J. Mol. Sci.* **2021**, *22*, 11269. [CrossRef]
12. Arabpour, M.; Saghazadeh, A.; Rezaei, N. Anti-Inflammatory and M2 Macrophage Polarization-Promoting Effect of Mesenchymal Stem Cell-Derived Exosomes. *Int. Immunopharmacol.* **2021**, *97*, 107823. [CrossRef]
13. Song, W.-J.; Li, Q.; Ryu, M.-O.; Ahn, J.-O.; Bhang, D.H.; Jung, Y.C.; Youn, H.-Y. TSG-6 Released from Intraperitoneally Injected Canine Adipose Tissue-Derived Mesenchymal Stem Cells Ameliorate Inflammatory Bowel Disease by Inducing M2 Macrophage Switch in Mice. *Stem Cell Res. Ther.* **2018**, *9*, 91. [CrossRef] [PubMed]
14. Park, H.J.; Kim, J.; Saima, F.T.; Rhee, K.-J.; Hwang, S.; Kim, M.Y.; Baik, S.K.; Eom, Y.W.; Kim, H.-S. Adipose-Derived Stem Cells Ameliorate Colitis by Suppression of Inflammasome Formation and Regulation of M1-Macrophage Population through Prostaglandin E2. *Biochem. Biophys. Res. Commun.* **2018**, *498*, 988–995. [CrossRef]
15. Luz-Crawford, P.; Djouad, F.; Toupet, K.; Bony, C.; Franquesa, M.; Hoogduijn, M.J.; Jorgensen, C.; Noël, D. Mesenchymal Stem Cell-Derived Interleukin 1 Receptor Antagonist Promotes Macrophage Polarization and Inhibits B Cell Differentiation. *Stem Cells* **2016**, *34*, 483–492. [CrossRef]
16. Abumaree, M.H.; Al Jumah, M.A.; Kalionis, B.; Jawdat, D.; Al Khaldi, A.; Abomaray, F.M.; Fatani, A.S.; Chamley, L.W.; Knawy, B.A. Human Placental Mesenchymal Stem Cells (pMSCs) Play a Role as Immune Suppressive Cells by Shifting Macrophage Differentiation from Inflammatory M1 to Anti-Inflammatory M2 Macrophages. *Stem Cell Rev. Rep.* **2013**, *9*, 620–641. [CrossRef]
17. Wang, S.; Lei, B.; Zhang, E.; Gong, P.; Gu, J.; He, L.; Han, L.; Yuan, Z. Targeted Therapy for Inflammatory Diseases with Mesenchymal Stem Cells and Their Derived Exosomes: From Basic to Clinics. *Int. J. Nanomed.* **2022**, *17*, 1757–1781. [CrossRef] [PubMed]

18. Wang, D.; Xue, H.; Tan, J.; Liu, P.; Qiao, C.; Pang, C.; Zhang, L. Bone Marrow Mesenchymal Stem Cells-Derived Exosomes Containing miR-539-5p Inhibit Pyroptosis through NLRP3/Caspase-1 Signalling to Alleviate Inflammatory Bowel Disease. *Inflamm. Res.* **2022**, *71*, 833–846. [CrossRef] [PubMed]
19. Yu, X.; Odenthal, M.; Fries, J.W.U. Exosomes as miRNA Carriers: Formation-Function-Future. *Int. J. Mol. Sci.* **2016**, *17*, 2028. [CrossRef]
20. Yang, S.; Liang, X.; Song, J.; Li, C.; Liu, A.; Luo, Y.; Ma, H.; Tan, Y.; Zhang, X. A Novel Therapeutic Approach for Inflammatory Bowel Disease by Exosomes Derived from Human Umbilical Cord Mesenchymal Stem Cells to Repair Intestinal Barrier via TSG-6. *Stem Cell Res. Ther.* **2021**, *12*, 315. [CrossRef]
21. Shen, Z.; Huang, W.; Liu, J.; Tian, J.; Wang, S.; Rui, K. Effects of Mesenchymal Stem Cell-Derived Exosomes on Autoimmune Diseases. *Front. Immunol.* **2021**, *12*, 749192. [CrossRef] [PubMed]
22. Liu, H.; Liang, Z.; Wang, F.; Zhou, C.; Zheng, X.; Hu, T.; He, X.; Wu, X.; Lan, P. Exosomes from Mesenchymal Stromal Cells Reduce Murine Colonic Inflammation via a Macrophage-Dependent Mechanism. *JCI Insight* **2019**, *4*, e131273. [CrossRef]
23. Wang, G.; Yuan, J.; Cai, X.; Xu, Z.; Wang, J.; Ocansey, D.K.W.; Yan, Y.; Qian, H.; Zhang, X.; Xu, W.; et al. HucMSC-exosomes Carrying miR-326 Inhibit Neddylation to Relieve Inflammatory Bowel Disease in Mice. *Clin. Transl. Med.* **2020**, *10*, e113. [CrossRef]
24. Sun, Z.; Shi, K.; Yang, S.; Liu, J.; Zhou, Q.; Wang, G.; Song, J.; Li, Z.; Zhang, Z.; Yuan, W. Effect of Exosomal miRNA on Cancer Biology and Clinical Applications. *Mol. Cancer* **2018**, *17*, 147. [CrossRef] [PubMed]
25. Heidari, M.; Pouya, S.; Baghaei, K.; Aghdaei, H.A.; Namaki, S.; Zali, M.R.; Hashemi, S.M. The Immunomodulatory Effects of Adipose-derived Mesenchymal Stem Cells and Mesenchymal Stem Cells-conditioned Medium in Chronic Colitis. *J. Cell. Physiol.* **2018**, *233*, 8754–8766. [CrossRef] [PubMed]
26. Cai, X.; Zhang, Z.; Yuan, J.; Ocansey, D.K.W.; Tu, Q.; Zhang, X.; Qian, H.; Xu, W.; Qiu, W.; Mao, F. hucMSC-Derived Exosomes Attenuate Colitis by Regulating Macrophage Pyroptosis via the miR-378a-5p/NLRP3 Axis. *Stem Cell Res. Ther.* **2021**, *12*, 416. [CrossRef]
27. Cao, Y.; Ding, Z.; Han, C.; Shi, H.; Cui, L.; Lin, R. Efficacy of Mesenchymal Stromal Cells for Fistula Treatment of Crohn's Disease: A Systematic Review and Meta-Analysis. *Dig. Dis. Sci.* **2017**, *62*, 851–860. [CrossRef]
28. Garcia-Olmo, D.; Garcia-Arranz, M.; Herreros, D. Expanded Adipose-Derived Stem Cells for the Treatment of Complex Perianal Fistula Including Crohn's Disease. *Expert Opin. Biol. Ther.* **2008**, *8*, 1417–1423. [CrossRef]
29. Ciccocioppo, R.; Gallia, A.; Sgarella, A.; Kruzliak, P.; Gobbi, P.G.; Corazza, G.R. Long-Term Follow-Up of Crohn Disease Fistulas After Local Injections of Bone Marrow-Derived Mesenchymal Stem Cells. *Mayo Clin. Proc.* **2015**, *90*, 747–755. [CrossRef]
30. Molendijk, I.; Bonsing, B.A.; Roelofs, H.; Peeters, K.C.M.J.; Wasser, M.N.J.M.; Dijkstra, G.; van der Woude, C.J.; Duijvestein, M.; Veenendaal, R.A.; Zwaginga, J.-J.; et al. Allogeneic Bone Marrow-Derived Mesenchymal Stromal Cells Promote Healing of Refractory Perianal Fistulas in Patients With Crohn's Disease. *Gastroenterology* **2015**, *149*, 918–927.e6. [CrossRef]
31. Duijvestein, M.; Vos, A.C.W.; Roelofs, H.; Wildenberg, M.E.; Wendrich, B.B.; Verspaget, H.W.; Kooy-Winkelaar, E.M.C.; Koning, F.; Zwaginga, J.J.; Fidder, H.H.; et al. Autologous Bone Marrow-Derived Mesenchymal Stromal Cell Treatment for Refractory Luminal Crohn's Disease: Results of a Phase I Study. *Gut* **2010**, *59*, 1662–1669. [CrossRef] [PubMed]
32. García-Olmo, D.; García-Arranz, M.; Herreros, D.; Pascual, I.; Peiro, C.; Rodríguez-Montes, J.A. A Phase I Clinical Trial of the Treatment of Crohn's Fistula by Adipose Mesenchymal Stem Cell Transplantation. *Dis. Colon Rectum* **2005**, *48*, 1416–1423. [CrossRef]
33. Dave, M.; Mehta, K.; Luther, J.; Baruah, A.; Dietz, A.B.; Faubion, W.A. Mesenchymal Stem Cell Therapy for Inflammatory Bowel Disease: A Systematic Review and Meta-Analysis. *Inflamm. Bowel Dis.* **2015**, *21*, 2696–2707. [CrossRef]
34. Van de Putte, D.; Demarquay, C.; Van Daele, E.; Moussa, L.; Vanhove, C.; Benderitter, M.; Ceelen, W.; Pattyn, P.; Mathieu, N. Adipose-Derived Mesenchymal Stromal Cells Improve the Healing of Colonic Anastomoses Following High Dose of Irradiation Through Anti-Inflammatory and Angiogenic Processes. *Cell Transplant.* **2017**, *26*, 1919–1930. [CrossRef] [PubMed]
35. Pascual, I.; Fernández de Miguel, G.; García Arranz, M.; García-Olmo, D. Biosutures Improve Healing of Experimental Weak Colonic Anastomoses. *Int. J. Color. Dis.* **2010**, *25*, 1447–1451. [CrossRef] [PubMed]
36. Adas, G.; Kemik, O.; Eryasar, B.; Okcu, A.; Adas, M.; Arikan, S.; Erman, G.; Kemik, A.S.; Kamali, G.; Dogan, Y.; et al. Treatment of Ischemic Colonic Anastomoses with Systemic Transplanted Bone Marrow Derived Mesenchymal Stem Cells. *Eur. Rev. Med. Pharmacol. Sci.* **2013**, *17*, 2275–2285.
37. Adas, G.; Arikan, S.; Karatepe, O.; Kemik, O.; Ayhan, S.; Karaoz, E.; Kamali, G.; Eryasar, B.; Ustek, D. Mesenchymal Stem Cells Improve the Healing of Ischemic Colonic Anastomoses (Experimental Study). *Langenbeck's Arch. Surg.* **2011**, *396*, 115–126. [CrossRef]
38. Yoo, J.H.; Shin, J.H.; An, M.S.; Ha, T.K.; Kim, K.H.; Bae, K.B.; Kim, T.H.; Choi, C.S.; Hong, K.H.; Kim, J.; et al. Adipose-Tissue-Derived Stem Cells Enhance the Healing of Ischemic Colonic Anastomoses: An Experimental Study in Rats. *J. Korean Soc. Coloproctol.* **2012**, *28*, 132. [CrossRef]
39. Morgan, A.; Zheng, A.; Linden, K.M.; Zhang, P.; Brown, S.A.; Carpenter, J.P.; Spitz, F.R.; Kwiatt, M.E. Locally Transplanted Adipose Stem Cells Reduce Anastomotic Leaks in Ischemic Colorectal Anastomoses: A Rat Model. *Dis. Colon Rectum* **2020**, *63*, 955–964. [CrossRef]

40. Alvarenga, V.; da Silva, P.T.; Bonfá, N.D.; Pêgo, B.; Nanini, H.; Bernardazzi, C.; Madi, K.; Baetas da Cruz, W.; Castelo-Branco, M.T.; de Souza, H.S.P.; et al. Protective Effect of Adipose Tissue–Derived Mesenchymal Stromal Cells in an Experimental Model of High-Risk Colonic Anastomosis. *Surgery* **2019**, *166*, 914–925. [CrossRef]
41. The ARRIVE Guidelines 2.0. Available online: https://arriveguidelines.org/arrive-guidelines (accessed on 23 July 2022).
42. Perše, M.; Cerar, A. Dextran Sodium Sulphate Colitis Mouse Model: Traps and Tricks. *J. Biomed. Biotechnol.* **2012**, *2012*, 718617. [CrossRef] [PubMed]
43. Perry, T.; Laffin, M.; Fedorak, R.N.; Thiesen, A.; Dicken, B.; Madsen, K.L. Ileocolic Resection Is Associated with Increased Susceptibility to Injury in a Murine Model of Colitis. *PLoS ONE* **2017**, *12*, e0184660. [CrossRef] [PubMed]
44. Perry, T.; Borowiec, A.; Dicken, B.; Fedorak, R.; Madsen, K. Murine Ileocolic Bowel Resection with Primary Anastomosis. *J. Vis. Exp.* **2014**, *92*, e52106. [CrossRef]
45. Karagergou, E.; Dionyssopoulos, A.; Karayannopoulou, M.; Psalla, D.; Theodoridis, A.; Demiri, E.; Koliakos, G. Adipose-Derived Stromal Vascular Fraction Aids Epithelialisation and Angiogenesis in an Animal Model. *J. Wound Care* **2018**, *27*, 637–644. [CrossRef] [PubMed]
46. Eichele, D.D.; Kharbanda, K.K. Dextran Sodium Sulfate Colitis Murine Model: An Indispensable Tool for Advancing Our Understanding of Inflammatory Bowel Diseases Pathogenesis. *World J. Gastroenterol.* **2017**, *23*, 6016–6029. [CrossRef]
47. Bosmans, J.W.A.M.; Moossdorff, M.; Al-Taher, M.; van Beek, L.; Derikx, J.P.M.; Bouvy, N.D. International Consensus Statement Regarding the Use of Animal Models for Research on Anastomoses in the Lower Gastrointestinal Tract. *Int. J. Color. Dis.* **2016**, *31*, 1021–1030. [CrossRef]
48. Pramateftakis, M.G.; Kanellos, D.; Mantzoros, I.; Despoudi, K.; Raptis, D.; Angelopoulos, S.; Koliakos, G.; Zaraboukas, T.; Lazaridis, C. Intraperitoneally Administered Irinotecan with 5-Fluorouracil Impair Wound Healing of Colonic Anastomoses in a Rat Model: An Experimental Study. *Tech. Coloproctol.* **2011**, *15*, 121–125. [CrossRef]
49. Cihan, A.; Armutcu, F.; Uçan, B.H.; Acun, Z.; Numanoglu, V.K.; Gürel, A.; Ulukent, S.C. Comparison of the Measurement Methods of Bursting Pressure of Intestinal Anastomoses. *Hepatogastroenterology* **2003**, *50* (Suppl. S2), ccxxxii–ccxxxiv.
50. Sukho, P.; Boersema, G.S.A.; Kops, N.; Lange, J.F.; Kirpensteijn, J.; Hesselink, J.W.; Bastiaansen-Jenniskens, Y.M.; Verseijden, F. Transplantation of Adipose Tissue-Derived Stem Cell Sheet to Reduce Leakage After Partial Colectomy in A Rat Model. *J. Vis. Exp.* **2018**, *138*, e57213. [CrossRef]
51. Lourenssen, S.R.; Blennerhassett, M.G. M2 Macrophages and Phenotypic Modulation of Intestinal Smooth Muscle Cells Characterize Inflammatory Stricture Formation in Rats. *Am. J. Pathol.* **2020**, *190*, 1843–1858. [CrossRef]
52. Duffield, J.S.; Lupher, M.; Thannickal, V.J.; Wynn, T.A. Host Responses in Tissue Repair and Fibrosis. *Annu. Rev. Pathol. Mech. Dis.* **2013**, *8*, 241–276. [CrossRef] [PubMed]
53. Wang, P.-H.; Huang, B.-S.; Horng, H.-C.; Yeh, C.-C.; Chen, Y.-J. Wound Healing. *J. Chin. Med. Assoc.* **2018**, *81*, 94–101. [CrossRef] [PubMed]
54. Mantovani, A.; Biswas, S.K.; Galdiero, M.R.; Sica, A.; Locati, M. Macrophage Plasticity and Polarization in Tissue Repair and Remodelling. *J. Pathol.* **2013**, *229*, 176–185. [CrossRef]
55. Mantovani, A.; Sica, A.; Locati, M. Macrophage Polarization Comes of Age. *Immunity* **2005**, *23*, 344–346. [CrossRef] [PubMed]
56. Davies, L.C.; Jenkins, S.J.; Allen, J.E.; Taylor, P.R. Tissue-Resident Macrophages. *Nat. Immunol.* **2013**, *14*, 986–995. [CrossRef]
57. Hidalgo-Garcia, L.; Galvez, J.; Rodriguez-Cabezas, M.E.; Anderson, P.O. Can a Conversation Between Mesenchymal Stromal Cells and Macrophages Solve the Crisis in the Inflamed Intestine? *Front. Pharmacol.* **2018**, *9*, 179. [CrossRef]
58. Gonzalez-Rey, E.; Anderson, P.; Gonzalez, M.A.; Rico, L.; Buscher, D.; Delgado, M. Human Adult Stem Cells Derived from Adipose Tissue Protect against Experimental Colitis and Sepsis. *Gut* **2009**, *58*, 929–939. [CrossRef]
59. Tadauchi, A.; Narita, Y.; Kagami, H.; Niwa, Y.; Ueda, M.; Goto, H. Novel Cell-Based Therapeutic Strategy for Ischemic Colitis with Use of Bone Marrow-Derived Mononuclear Cells in Rats. *Dis. Colon Rectum* **2009**, *52*, 1443–1451. [CrossRef]
60. Castelo-Branco, M.T.L.; Soares, I.D.P.; Lopes, D.V.; Buongusto, F.; Martinusso, C.A.; do Rosario, A.; Souza, S.A.L.; Gutfilen, B.; Fonseca, L.M.B.; Elia, C.; et al. Intraperitoneal but Not Intravenous Cryopreserved Mesenchymal Stromal Cells Home to the Inflamed Colon and Ameliorate Experimental Colitis. *PLoS ONE* **2012**, *7*, e33360. [CrossRef]
61. Lee, R.H.; Pulin, A.A.; Seo, M.J.; Kota, D.J.; Ylostalo, J.; Larson, B.L.; Semprun-Prieto, L.; Delafontaine, P.; Prockop, D.J. Intravenous hMSCs Improve Myocardial Infarction in Mice Because Cells Embolized in Lung Are Activated to Secrete the Anti-Inflammatory Protein TSG-6. *Cell Stem Cell* **2009**, *5*, 54–63. [CrossRef]
62. Yu, W.; Zhou, H.; Feng, X.; Liang, X.; Wei, D.; Xia, T.; Yang, B.; Yan, L.; Zhao, X.; Liu, H. Mesenchymal Stem Cell Secretome-Loaded Fibrin Glue Improves the Healing of Intestinal Anastomosis. *Front. Bioeng. Biotechnol.* **2023**, *11*, 1103709. [CrossRef] [PubMed]
63. Park, S.-R.; Kim, J.-W.; Jun, H.-S.; Roh, J.Y.; Lee, H.-Y.; Hong, I.-S. Stem Cell Secretome and Its Effect on Cellular Mechanisms Relevant to Wound Healing. *Mol. Ther.* **2018**, *26*, 606–617. [CrossRef] [PubMed]

Disclaimer/Publisher's Note: The statements, opinions and data contained in all publications are solely those of the individual author(s) and contributor(s) and not of MDPI and/or the editor(s). MDPI and/or the editor(s) disclaim responsibility for any injury to people or property resulting from any ideas, methods, instructions or products referred to in the content.

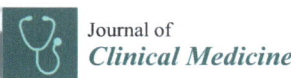 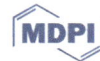

Article

The Significance of Preoperative Neutrophil-to-Lymphocyte Ratio (NLR), Platelet-to-Lymphocyte Ratio (PLR), and Systemic Inflammatory Index (SII) in Predicting Severity and Adverse Outcomes in Acute Calculous Cholecystitis

Dragos Serban [1,2,†], Paul Lorin Stoica [1,*], Ana Maria Dascalu [1,*], Dan Georgian Bratu [3,4,†], Bogdan Mihai Cristea [1,†], Catalin Alius [1,2,†], Ion Motofei [1,5], Corneliu Tudor [1,2], Laura Carina Tribus [6,7], Crenguta Serboiu [1], Mihail Silviu Tudosie [1], Denisa Tanasescu [8], Geta Vancea [1,9] and Daniel Ovidiu Costea [10,11]

1. Faculty of Medicine, Carol Davila University of Medicine and Pharmacy Bucharest, 020021 Bucharest, Romania; dragos.serban@umfcd.ro (D.S.); bogdan.cristea@umfcd.ro (B.M.C.); catalin.alius@umfcd.ro (C.A.); ion.motofei@umfcd.ro (I.M.); crenguta.serboiu@umfcd.ro (C.S.); geta.vancea@umfcd.ro (G.V.)
2. Fourth General Surgery Department, Emergency University Hospital Bucharest, 050098 Bucharest, Romania
3. Faculty of Medicine, University Lucian Blaga Sibiu, 550169 Sibiu, Romania; dan.bratu@ulbsibiu.ro
4. Department of Surgery, Emergency County Hospital Sibiu, 550245 Sibiu, Romania
5. Department of General Surgery, Emergency Clinic Hospital "Sf. Pantelimon" Bucharest, 021659 Bucharest, Romania
6. Faculty of Dental Medicine, Carol Davila University of Medicine and Pharmacy Bucharest, 020021 Bucharest, Romania
7. Department of Internal Medicine, Ilfov Emergency Clinic Hospital Bucharest, 022104 Bucharest, Romania
8. Department of Nursing and Dentistry, Faculty of General Medicine, University Lucian Blaga Sibiu, 550169 Sibiu, Romania; denisa.tanasescu@ulbsibiu.ro
9. Clinical Hospital of Infectious and Tropical Diseases "Dr. Victor Babes", 030303 Bucharest, Romania
10. Faculty of Medicine, Ovidius University Constanta, 900470 Constanta, Romania; daniel.costea@365.univ-ovidius.ro
11. General Surgery Department, Emergency County Hospital Constanta, 900591 Constanta, Romania
* Correspondence: paul.stoica@drd.umfcd.ro (P.L.S.); ana.dascalu@umfcd.ro (A.M.D.)
† These authors contributed equally to this work.

Abstract: The prediction of severity in acute calculous cholecystitis (AC) is important in therapeutic management to ensure an early recovery and prevent adverse postoperative events. We analyzed the value of the neutrophil-to-lymphocyte ratio (NLR), platelet-to-lymphocyte ratio (PLR), and systemic inflammatory index (SII) to predict advanced inflammation, the risk for conversion, and postoperative complications in AC. Advanced AC was considered the cases with empyema, gangrene, perforation of the gallbladder, abscesses, or difficulties in achieving the critical view of safety. A 3-year retrospective was performed on 235 patients admitted in emergency care for AC. The NLR was superior to the PLR and SII in predicting advanced inflammation and risk for conversion. The best predictive value was found to be at an NLR "cut-off" value of >4.19, with a sensitivity of 85.5% and a specificity of 66.9% (AUC = 0.824). The NLR, SII, and TG 13/18 correlate well with postoperative complications of Clavien–Dindo grade IV ($p < 0.001$ for all variables) and sepsis. For predicting early postoperative sepsis, TG 13/18 grading >2 and NLR > 8.54 show the best predicting power (AUC = 0.931; AUC = 0.888, respectively), although not significantly higher than that of the PLR and SII. The NLR is a useful biomarker in assessing the severity of inflammation in AC. The SII and PLR may be useful in the prediction of systemic inflammatory response.

Keywords: acute cholecystitis; systemic inflammatory biomarkers; NLR; PLR; SII; postoperative outcome

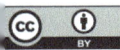

1. Introduction

Acute calculous cholecystitis (ACC) is a common cause of abdominal pain in emergencies. In a multicentric study designed by the World Society of Emergency Surgery in 2015,

ACC ranked as the second cause of complicated intra-abdominal infections, accounting for 18.5% of the total number of cases [1,2]. Early laparoscopic cholecystectomy (LC) is the gold standard in the current therapeutical approach, with favorable outcomes in most cases. However, recent studies found a 0.1–1% mortality risk and a 6–9% risk of major complications [3], such as main common bile duct lesions, myocardial infarction, and pulmonary complications, and this risk is highly increased in emergency LC performed in cases with severe inflammation. A recent study by Lucocq et al. [4] found that 36.7% of LCs performed in emergency had a non-standard outcome, including conversion, subtotal cholecystectomy, bile leak, and prolonged postoperative stay [4]. Most of these cases were related to the severity of local inflammation, intraoperative findings showing gangrenous cholecystitis, empyema, perforation of the gallbladder, and difficult dissection of the Calot Triangle, all these conditions being generally referred to as advanced acute cholecystitis [5] or severe cholecystitis [6,7] by different authors. Preoperative identification of these cases is important to optimize the therapeutic approach and improve the clinical outcome [5].

Currently, the role of different biomarkers with predictive value in acute cholecystitis is still a subject of research. TG13/18 guidelines propose a grading scale for evaluating local inflammation and its systemic involvement based on clinical evaluation, leukocytes, and CRP as well as the presence or not of the alterations of the vital functions related to the septic process [8,9].

However, a systematic review of Tufo et al. [3] found that while grade III TG 13/18 may be associated with higher mortality when compared with grade I, there is no consensus regarding the preoperatory predictive risk evaluation in patients with acute calculous cholecystitis.

Several studies found CRP to be a good predictive factor for conversion; however, the cut-off values varied widely from 76 mg/L to 220 mg/L [5,10–13]. Together with the valuable findings provided by ultrasound and CT exam, specific biomarkers were analyzed for the possible predictive role for the severity of local inflammation, such as the YKL-40 protein level [14], serum level of visfatin [15], procalcitonin [16], human neutrophil lipocalin [17], chitotriosidase, and neopterin [18]. However, their availability in emergencies is limited in many surgical departments.

Recently, the systemic inflammatory biomarkers, neutrophil-to-lymphocyte ratio (NLR) and platelet-to-lymphocyte ratio (PLR), were investigated for their predictive value in many inflammatory and septic conditions [18–22], such as septic shock, diabetic foot ulcer, acute appendicitis, and spontaneous bacterial peritonitis. They are cheap and inexpensive biomarkers, easy to calculate based on the complete blood count (CBC). Several studies found a good correlation between the NLR and PLR and the severity of inflammation in acute calculous cholecystitis as well as the length of postoperative stay. However, there is still conflicting evidence regarding the clinical significance of these biomarkers and their cut-off value that could be used in therapeutic management.

In the present study, we aimed to analyze the value of the NLR, PLR, and SII in predicting severe forms of acute cholecystitis, conversion to open surgery, and adverse postoperative outcomes.

2. Materials and Methods

2.1. Patient Selection

A 3-year retrospective study was carried out between January 2020 and December 2022 on the patients admitted for acute cholecystitis in the 4th Department of Surgery, Emergency University Hospital Bucharest. Data were collected from electronic patient records and operatory protocols. All patients admitted in emergency care, aged over 18 years, for whom the diagnosis of acute cholecystitis could be confirmed based on intraoperative findings were included in the statistical analysis. Along with local and systemic inflammatory signs, ultrasonography and/or abdominal CT were used to document the presence of calculi, the thickness of the gallbladder walls, common biliary duct (CBD) diameter, and the potential signs of pericholecystitis. For all patients, age, associated comorbidities, time elapsed from the onset of symptoms to presentation, and clinical signs were assessed at admission. Biological tests at admission included a complete blood count with differentials of fibrinogen, bilirubin, hepatic transaminases, INR, urea, and creatinine. Systemic inflammatory biomarkers were calculated based on the counts for neutrophils, platelets, and neutrophils measured from the same sample and expressed as their value in cells/L. SII was calculated using the formula SII = P × N/L, where P, N, and L are the counts of platelets, neutrophils, and lymphocytes, respectively [23].

C-reactive protein (CRP) was not available in an emergency in our hospital but was determined the next day, in cases in which surgical intervention was postponed due to local or general conditions. For this reason, CRP was not included in the statistical analysis.

Patients with associated malignancies as well as hematological and autoimmune diseases were excluded due to their previously documented impact on the blood cells and derivate systemic inflammatory indices.

2.2. Study Design

The patients included in the study were classified according to the intraoperative findings into mild and advanced acute cholecystitis, according to the intensity of local inflammation. Advanced forms were considered the cases with empyema, gangrene, perforation of the gallbladder, abscesses, adhesions, or difficulty in dissecting Calot's triangle, likely to be associated with increased operative difficulty [9,24].

The patients were classified according to TG 13/TG18 Tokyo guidelines for acute cholecystitis as grade I (mild) acute cholecystitis, grade II (moderate), and grade III (severe) if associated with organ dysfunction [9]. Systemic inflammatory biomarkers NLR, PLR, and SII were calculated based on the complete blood cell count at admission. The prediction values of TG 13/TG 18 severity grading, NLR, PLR, and SII were analyzed for advanced AC, postoperative complications, and hospital stay.

2.3. Statistical Analysis

Microsoft Excel and Med Calc® Statistical Software (version 22.006 Med Calc Software Ltd., Ostend, Belgium; https://www.medcalc.org; accessed on 10 August 2023) were used for data analysis. Pearson's Chi-squared test was used to evaluate the association between discrete variables, while ANOVA was used for continuous variables. For the statistically significant results, a post hoc analysis was performed to establish the differences within groups by using the Scheffe test for all pairwise comparisons.

The specificity and sensitivity of NLR, PLR, and SII in predicting the severity of inflammation, and local and systemic complications were analyzed by ROC curves. According to the widely accepted classification scale described by Safari et al. [25], the AUC values were categorized as 90–100 = excellent; 80–90 = good; 70–80 = fair; 60–70 = poor; and 50–60 = fail.

3. Results

3.1. General Data of the Patients Included in the Study Group

A total of 235 patients with acute cholecystitis were included in the study, with a mean age of 54.6 ± 16.3. Most of the cases were mild (70.6%) and of female patients (71.4%). In the advanced AC group, the mean age was significantly higher (61 ± 15.6 vs. 52 ± 15.9, <0.001), and there were significantly more male patients ($p = 0.008$) when compared to mild cases (Table 1).

Most patients included in the study group presented with two or more comorbidities. The subjects included in the advanced AC group had significantly more comorbidities than those admitted with mild AC ($p < 0.001$). Older age ($p < 0.001$), obesity ($p = 0.047$), diabetes ($p = 0.001$), ischemic cardiac disease ($p = 0.01$), chronic hepatic diseases ($p = 0.02$), and cardiac failure/shock at admission ($p = 0.01$) were correlated with advanced AC in the study group. According to the ASA risk scale, most patients were graded as grade II or III in both groups. However, there was an upward trend of distribution towards higher grades in the advanced AC group, confirmed by the linear-by-linear association test ($p = 0.0003$).

A similar upward trend was observed for the TG 13/18 severity scale, with more grade II and III cases in the advanced AC group (<0.0001).

Table 1. General data of the patients included in the study group.

Parameter	Total	Mild AC	Advanced AC	p Value
No. of patients	235	166 (70.6%)	69 (29.4%)	
Females	168 (71.4%)	127 (76.5%)	41 (59.4%)	0.008 [1]
Age	54.6 ± 16.3	52 ± 15.9	61 ± 15.6	<0.001 [1]
Comorbidities (No.):	2 ± 1.4	1.8 ± 1.3	2.6 ± 1.6	<0.001 [2]
Obesity	116 (49.4%)	75 (45.1%)	41 (59.4%)	0.047 [2]
Arterial hypertension	107 (45.5%)	57 (53.3%)	50 (46.7%)	0.093 [2]
Cardiac ischemic disease	28 (11.9%)	14 (8.4%)	14 (20.2%)	0.01 [2]
Chronic hepatic diseases	67 (28.5%)	40 (24%)	27 (39.1%)	0.02 [2]
Chronic respiratory diseases	31 (13.2%)	18 (10.8%)	13 (18.8%)	0.099 [2]
Chronic renal diseases	39 (16.6%)	25 (15%)	14 (20.2%)	0.327 [2]
Cardiac failure/shock	11 (4.7%)	4 (2.4%)	7 (10.1%)	0.01 [2]
Diabetes	32 (13.6%)	15 (9%)	17 (24.6%)	0.001 [2]
Others	84 (35.7%)	62 (37.3%)	22 (31.8%)	0.426 [2]
ASA PS risk scale				
I	16 (6.8%)	14 (8.4%)	2 (2.8%)	
II	124 (52.8%)	96 (57.8%)	28 (40.5%)	0.008 [2]
III	78 (33.2%)	48 (28.9%)	30 (43.4%)	(0.0003 [3] for trend)
IV	16 (6.8%)	8 (4.8%)	8 (11.5%)	
V	1 (0.4%)	0	1 (1.4%)	
TG 13/18 severity grading				
I	145 (61.7%)	121 (72.9%)	24 (37.4%)	<0.0001 [2] (<0.0001 [3] for trend)
II	73 (31.1%)	40 (24%)	33 (47.8%)	
III	17 (7.2%)	5 (3%)	12 (17.4%)	
Angiocholitis/CBD stones	18 (7.6%)	7 (4.2%)	11 (15.9%)	0.013 [2]
Leukocytes (/μL)	10,441 ± 4895.3	9187.6 ± 3787.4	13,456.2 ± 5882	<0.0001 [1]
Neutrophils (/μL)	7796 ± 4867.5	6413.4 ± 3728.6	11,124.9 ± 5646.6	0.001 [1]
Platelets (/μL)	239,767.1 ± 82,016.7	245,341.4 ± 77,532.9	226,356.5 ± 91,122	0.053 [1]
Fibrinogen (mg/dL)	450.1 ± 186.2	389.1 ± 119.1	596.8 ± 232.3	<0.001 [1]
INR	1.3 ± 1.1	1.2 ± 0.9	1.3 ± 1.2	0.327 [1]
Bilirubin	1.3 ± 2.0	0.95 ± 1.1	2.3 ± 3.1	<0.001 [1]
AST	68.9 ± 116	63.2 ± 116.2	125 ± 297.1	0.063 [1]
ALT	107.4 ± 165.9	85.8 ± 136.9	120 ± 179	0.056 [1]
Creatinine	1.3 ± 0.5	1.2 ± 0.3	1.5 ± 1.4	0.341 [1]
NLR	7.29 ± 12.2	4.3 ± 5.2	14.3 ± 19.4	<0.001 [1]
PLR	181.2 ± 229.4	143.8 ± 68.7	273.5 ± 397	<0.001 [1]
SII	1701.6 ± 3416.4	1009.5 ± 993.8	3366.8 ± 5812.4	<0.001 [1]

Footnote: [1] ANOVA; [2] Chi-squared test; [3] test of linear-by-linear association; ASA PS: American Society of Anesthesiologists Physical Status Classification; TG13/18: Tokyo Guidelines classification risk; AST: aspartate aminotransferase; ALT: Alanyl aminotransferase; NLR: neutrophil-to-lymphocyte ratio; PLR: platelet-to-lymphocyte ratio; SII: systemic inflammatory index.

Statistical analysis showed significantly higher values for leukocytes ($p < 0.0001$), neutrophils ($p = 0.001$), the NLR ($p < 0.001$), the PLR ($p < 0.001$), the SII ($p < 0.001$), fibrinogen ($p < 0.001$), and bilirubin ($p < 0.001$) with no significant difference for platelets, INR, transaminases, and creatinine levels.

3.2. Comparative Analysis of NLR, PLR, and SII Values with TG 13/18 Grading in the Study Group

Furthermore, we investigated how the TG13/18 severity grading scale for AC correlates with the values of NLR, PLR, and SII by using the Chi-squared test and Scheffe test for pairwise comparison. The statistical analysis found a significant positive correlation in all cases, with the mean values of the investigated systemic inflammatory biomarkers rising from the grade I to grade III groups. However, there are differences in the Scheffe test results, which may suggest that each of the biomarkers characterizes specific changes in the inflammation process (Table 2).

Table 2. Correlations between NLR, PLR, and SII with TG 13/18 grading in the study group.

	TG13/18 Grade I (1)	TG13/18 Grade II (2)	TG13/18 Grade III (3)	p Value (Chi-Squared Test)	Scheffe Test for Pairwise Comparison
NLR	3.6 ± 3	11.7 ± 14.6	18.8 ± 28	<0.001	(1) differs from (2) and (3)
PLR	147.8 ± 80.3	191.2 ± 123.6	432.1 ± 752	<0.001	(1) and (2) differ from (3)
SII	879.9 ± 726.5	2393.6 ± 2477	$5738.6 \pm 10{,}617$	<0.001	Each group differs significantly from the others.

While the NLR is an early inflammatory biomarker, which significantly raises between mild and moderate forms, the PLR seems to be significantly elevated in advanced stages, when local inflammation of the gallbladder and surrounding tissues reaches systemic involvement. SII values, combining in their formula both the number of neutrophils and platelets, discriminate best among the three stages defined by the TG 13/18 scale.

3.3. Prediction Value of NLR, PLR, SII, and TG 13/18 Grading Scale for Advanced Acute Cholecystitis

The sensitivity and specificity of the NLR, PLR, SII, total leukocytes, and TG 13/18 grading scale for predicting advanced forms of AC were analyzed by the ROC curves (Figure 1).

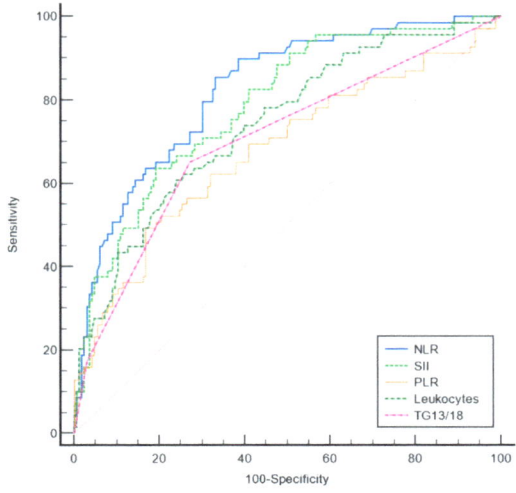

Figure 1. Comparative ROC curves for NLR, PLR, SII, TG13/18, and total leukocytes in predicting advanced AC.

Only the NLR showed a good predictive value (AUC = 0.824). The pairwise comparison of ROC curves for predicting advanced AC found that the predictive value of the NLR was significantly superior to that of the SII ($p = 0.0065$), PLR ($p < 0.0001$), total leukocytes ($p = 0.0103$), and TG 13/18 grading ($p = 0.0006$). The best predictive value was found to be at a cut-off value of >4.19, with a sensitivity of 85.5% and a specificity of 66.9% (Table 3).

Table 3. Sensitivity and specificity at the "cut-off" value predicting advanced forms.

	Sensitivity	Specificity	Cut-Off Value	AUC	p
NLR	85.5	66.9	>4.19	0.824	<0.001
PLR	49.3	83.1	>189.3	0.679	<0.001
SII	63.8	80.7	>1442.4	0.787	<0.001
TG13/18	65.22	72.8	>1(mild)	0.704	<0.001
Leukocytes	60.87	75.9	>11,300	0.741	<0.001

3.4. Surgical Approach and Postoperative Outcomes

Laparoscopic cholecystectomy was the most common procedure in both groups. However, the number of cases that required conversion, open surgical procedures, Kehr drainage, or perioperative ERCP was significantly higher in the advanced AC group (Table 4).

Table 4. Surgical treatment and outcomes.

	Total (n = 235)	Mild AC (n = 166)	Advanced AC (n = 69)	p Value
Types of surgery:				
LC	208 (88.6%)	162 (97.6%)	46 (66.6%)	<0.0001 [1] (<0.0001 [2] for trend)
LC-conversion	16 (6.8%)	1 (0.6%)	15 (21.7%)	
CC	10 (4.2%)	3 (1.8%)	7 (10.2%)	
Cholecystostomy	1 (0.4%)	0	1 (1.5%)	
Kehr drainage	5 (2.1%)	1 (0.6%)	4 (5.8%)	0.012 [1]
ERCP + calculi removal (pre or postop)	17 (7.2%)	7 (4.2%)	10 (14.5%)	0.005 [1]
Postoperative hospital stay (days)	3.6 ± 3.4	2.9 ± 2.8	5.1 ± 4	<0.001 [3]
Length of stay (days)	7.1 ± 4.5	6.1 ± 3.9	9.3 ± 5.2	<0.001 [3]

Footnote: LC = laparoscopic cholecystectomy; CC = classic (open) cholecystectomy; ERCP = endoscopic retrograde cholecysto-pancreatography; [1]—Chi-squared test; [2]—Scheffe test for pairwise comparison; [3]—ANOVA.

The reason for conversion to open surgery in the mild AC group was the unclear anatomy of the Calot triangle due to extensive fibrosis. In the advanced AC group, most cases were converted due to a friable hemorrhagic gangrenous gallbladder wall (five cases) and the impossibility of achieving the critical view of safety (CVS) due to inflammation and adherences (six cases). Other causes of conversion included biliary fistula (one case), Mirizzi Syndrome (one case), biliary peritonitis due to a perforated gallbladder abscess (one case), and a pericholecystic abscess (one case).

Open surgery as the first choice was mainly dictated by the general status and associated comorbidities in patients graded as ASA IV or V (seven cases, including the three cases in the mild AC group), for whom the laparoscopic approach was not considered safe to be performed by the intensive care team. In three cases, the decision was made based on the clinical and imagistic data: pseudo-tumoral pericholecystic mass (one case) and gallbladder abscess (two cases). There was one case treated by cholecystostoma, an 85-year-old patient with piocholecystitis and septic shock at admission, who died 3 days after surgery in the intensive care unit due to sepsis and acute limb ischemia.

In the study group, there were 16 patients who were COVID-19-positive at the moment of admission. Out of these, 14 were treated safely by laparoscopic cholecystectomy, after all the required safety measures were taken to prevent the contamination of the operatory team. In the remaining cases, open surgery was performed due to associated septic shock (one case) and COVID-19 severe pneumonia (one case).

Furthermore, we analyzed the postoperative complications encountered in the study group, registered after Clavien–Dindo classification (Table 5).

Table 5. Postoperative complications according to Clavien–Dindo Classification.

	Total (n = 235)	Mild AC (n = 166)	Advanced AC (n = 69)	p-Value *
I (surgical site infections)	4 (1.7%)	1 (0.6%)	3 (4.3%)	0.043
II (requiring pharmacological treatment) surgical-related complications, treated conservatory	11 (4.6%)	5 (3%)	6 (8.6%)	0.064
Nosocomial infections	15 (6.4%)	6 (3.6%)	9 (13%)	0.007
III (surgical-related complications requiring endoscopic/surgical/ Rx approach)	2 (0.8%)	1 (0.6%)	1 (1.4%)	1.00
IV (general complications requiring intensive care)	16 (6.8%)	4 (2.4%)	12 (17.3%)	0.002
Malign hypertension	4 (1.7%)	1 (0.6%)	3 (4.3%)	0.043
Hemodynamic instability	1 (0.4%)	0	1 (1.4%)	0.12
Sepsis	8 (3.4%)	2 (1.2%)	6 (8.6%)	0.004
Pulmonary edema/pleurisy	3 (1.3%)	1 (0.6%)	2 (2.8%)	0.15
V (deceased)	5 (2.1%)	2 (1.2%)	3 (4.3%)	0.129

Footnote: * p-value was calculated by Chi-squared test.

Statistically significant differences observed between the mild and advanced AC groups for surgical site infections ($p = 0.043$) and nosocomial infections ($p = 0.007$) could be correlated with higher numbers of open surgeries and conversions, as well as with increased hospital stays in the advanced AC group. General complications requiring intensive care were more frequent in the advanced AC group ($p = 0.002$), including sepsis ($p = 0.004$) and postoperative malign hypertension ($p = 0.043$).

3.5. Correlations between Inflammatory Parameters and Types of Surgery in the Study Group

NLR and TG13/18 grading correlated well with the type of surgery performed ($p = 0.001$; and $p < 0.0001$, respectively), while the PLR and SII mean values were higher in the conversion and open surgery groups but not statistically significant (Table 6).

Table 6. Correlations between the types of surgery and NLR, PLR, SII, and TG13/18 in the study group.

	LC (1)	LC-Conversion (2)	CC/Cholecystostomy (3)	p-Value	Scheffe Test for Pairwise Comparison
NLR	6.2 ± 11.8	12.1 ± 7	20.2 ± 17.3	0.001 [1]	(1) differs from (3)
PLR	178.5 ± 241.9	182 ± 82.7	248.1 ± 73.4	0.823 [1]	NS
SII	1583.8 ± 3572.4	2323.2 ± 1474.2	3014.5 ± 1779.5	0.49 [1]	NS
TG 13/18 grading				<0.0001 [2]	Each group differs significantly from the others
I	139 (66.9%)	4 (25%)	2 (18.2%)		
II	58 (27.9%)	10 (62.5%)	5 (45.4%)		
III	11 (5.2%)	2 (12.5%)	4 (36.4%)		

[1] ANOVA; [2] Chi-squared test; NS: not significant.

The predictive value for conversion for the NLR, PLR, SII, TG 13/18, and total leukocytes was analyzed by ROC curves (Figure 2).

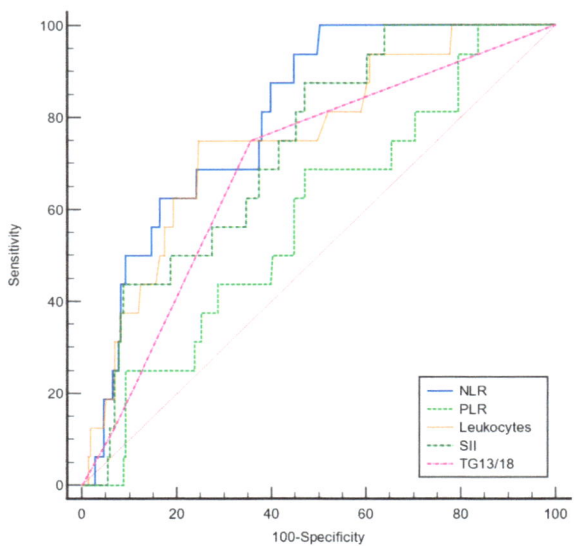

Figure 2. Comparative ROC curves for NLR, PLR, SII, TG13/18, and total leukocytes in predicting conversion to open cholecystectomy.

Out of the studied parameters, only the NLR showed a good predictive value for conversion, with a cut-off value of 4.24 (AUC = 0.802, $p < 0.001$), significantly higher compared to that of leukocytes (AUC = 0.755), SII (AUC = 0.734), and TG13/18 (AUC = 0.690) (Table 7).

Table 7. Prediction value of NLR, PLR, SII, and TG 13/18 for conversion to open surgery.

	PDR Sensitivity	PDR Specificity	Cut-Off Value	AUC	p
NLR	93.7	55.2	>4.24	0.802	<0.001
PLR	68.7	53	>141.8	0.582	0.246
SII	87.5	53	>949.6	0.734	<0.001
TG13/18	75	64.3	>1	0.690	0.001
Leukocytes	75	75.3	>12,200	0.755	<0.001

3.6. Correlations between Inflammatory Parameters and Postoperative Outcomes in the Study Group

ANOVA showed a good correlation between the NLR, PLR, SII, and TG 13/18 grading scale and the postoperative hospital stay ($p < 0.001$; $p < 0.001$; $p < 0.001$; and $p = 0.008$, respectively) and total hospital stay ($p = 0.002$; $p < 0.001$; $p < 0.001$; and $p = 0.001$, respectively).

In the present study, the NLR, PLR, SII, and TG 13/18 grading scales had a poor prognostic value for predicting local postoperative complications, almost equal to a coin toss (Table 8, Figure 3), and did not correlate well with the postoperative complications related to surgery, Clavien–Dindo grades II and III ($p = 0.83$; $p = 0.843$; and $p = 0.898$, respectively).

Table 8. Prediction value of NLR, PLR, SII, and TG 13/18 for surgical-related postoperative complications.

	PDR Sensitivity	PDR Specificity	Cut-Off Value	AUC	p
NLR	45.45	80.8	>8.88	0.595	0.33
PLR	45.45	75.45	>194.6	0.528	0.776
SII	45.45	70.54	>1525.9	0.530	0.3
TG13/18	54.5	62.5	>1	0.583	0.31
Leukocytes	72.73	5	<17,800	0.510	0.935

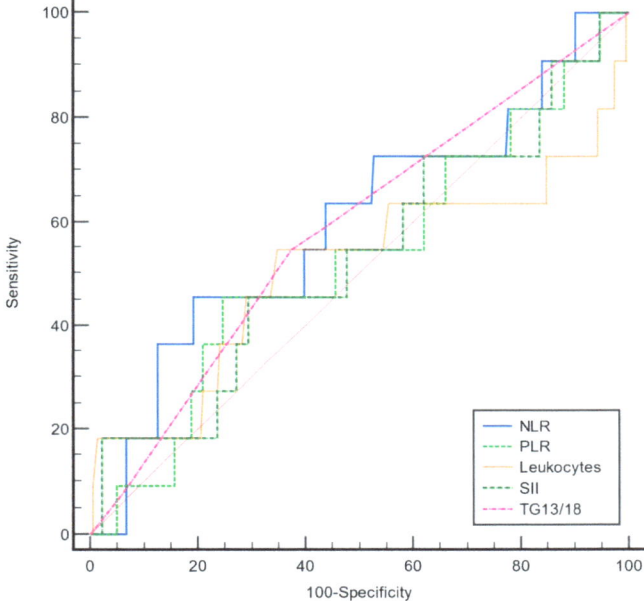

Figure 3. Comparative ROC curves for NLR, PLR, SII, TG13/18, and total leukocytes in predicting postoperative local complications.

However, the NLR, SII, and TG 13/18 correlated well with postoperative complications of Clavien–Dindo grade IV ($p < 0.001$ for all variables), while the values were not statistically significant for the PLR ($p = 0.113$). However, their predictive power evaluated by ROC curves varied from poor (PLR and SII) to fair (TG 13/18 grading and NLR), as shown in Table 9, Figure 4.

Table 9. Prediction value of NLR, PLR, SII, and TG 13/18 for general postoperative complications requiring intensive care (Clavien–Dindo IV).

	Sensitivity	Specificity	Cut-Off Value	AUC	p
NLR	66.7	80.6	>7.67	0.758	<0.001
PLR	45.8	83.9	>221.3	0.640	0.02
SII	83.3	51.7	>858.3	0.697	0.001
TG13/18	70.83	65.4	>1	0.715	<0.001
Leukocytes	79.2	54.4	>9100	0.668	0.006

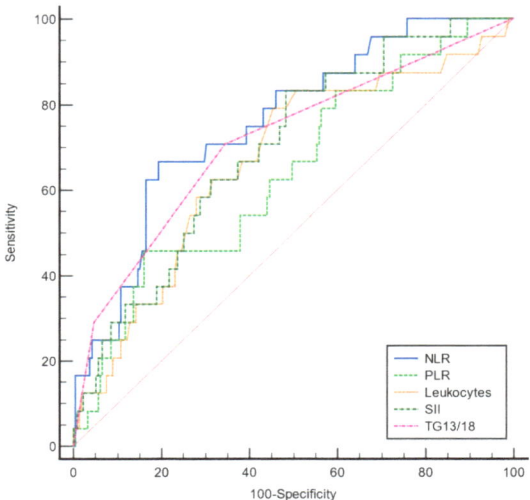

Figure 4. Comparative ROC curves for NLR, PLR, SII, TG13/18, and total leukocytes in predicting general complications requiring intensive care support (Clavien–Dindo grade IV).

For predicting early postoperative sepsis, a TG 13/18 grading > 2 and NLR > 8.54 showed the best predicting power (AUC = 0.931; AUC = 0.888, respectively), though not significantly higher than that of the PLR and SII (Table 10, Figure 5).

Table 10. Prediction value of NLR, PLR, SII, and TG 13/18 for postoperative sepsis.

	PDR Sensitivity	PDR Specificity	Cut-Off Value	AUC	p
NLR	87.5	81	>8.54	0.888	<0.001
PLR	75	83.2	>222.46	0.807	<0.001
SII	87.5	70.04	>1447.68	0.845	<0.001
TG13/18	75	92.1	>2	0.931	<0.0001
Leukocytes	87.5	66.9	>11,300	0.753	0.025

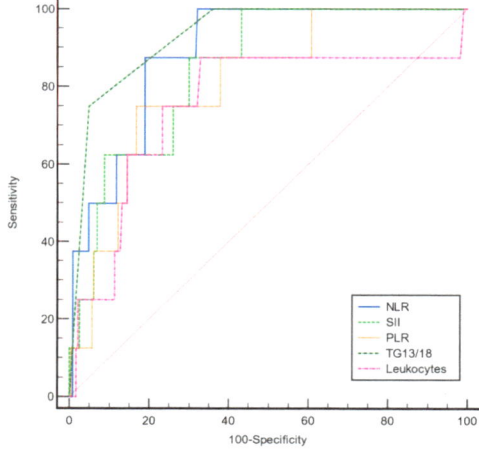

Figure 5. Comparison of ROC curve for NLR, SII, PLR, TG13/18, and total leukocytes in predicting sepsis in the early postoperative period.

4. Discussion

Predicting the severity of acute cholecystitis is important to achieve the best therapeutic outcomes and prevent adverse postoperative events [2,26–29]. Local inflammation and surgical trauma induce metabolic and systemic inflammatory responses, which may lead to systemic complications [30]. Understanding and addressing inflammation and the possible systemic imbalances that it may cause is important to prevent adverse outcomes and unnecessarily prolonged hospital stays in cases with AC.

Commonly used for diagnosis, CT and ultrasound examination may not accurately predict advanced AC [30,31]. In a study on 1115 patients who underwent surgery for acute calculous cholecystitis, Goiayev et al. [31] found that even in cases with a gallbladder wall of ≤ 4.85 mm, if the NLR > 5.65 and the total leukocytes exceed $8100/mm^3$, there is a 92% probability of complicated AC, including gangrenous, perforated, emphysematous, or necrotizing AC. NLR is a cheap, easy-to-calculate inflammatory biomarker that combines the relative ratio of neutrophils—the first line of cellular defense in acute inflammation—and the lymphocytes, with an immunomodulatory role [30].

Although several studies have found a significant correlation between the NLR and the severity of inflammation in AC [30,32–34], there is limited evidence regarding the specific cut-off value, with possible clinical use.

In the present study, we comparatively examined NLR, PLR, SII, total leukocytes, and TG13/18 grading scale for predicting severe inflammation in acute cholecystitis, risk for conversion, and adverse outcomes. We found that the NLR performed best for predicting advanced AC, with an AUC of 0.824 at a cut-off value >4.19. The NLR also has a good predictive value for conversion (AUC = 0.804, cut-off value of 4.24), with high sensitivity (93.7%) but low sensitivity (55.7%).

A previous study by Micic et al. [24] on 136 patients who underwent LC for acute cholecystitis found a similar cut-off value of 4.18 for predicting advanced AC with a 78.3% sensitivity and 74.3% specificity [24], while another recent study found a cut-off value of 4.17 for moderate to severe AC [35], with a predictive value similar to that of CRP.

A higher "cut-off" value of 5.5 for the NLR was found by Turhan et al. [36] with a good predictive value, 80.8% sensitivity, and 80.1% specificity. This may be explained, however, by the selection criteria the authors defined for the complicated AC group in their study, which included very advanced changes of the gallbladder wall, such as perforation, gangrenous cholecystitis, and emphysematous cholecystitis. The definition of "difficult cholecystectomy" is still a challenging subject, with no international consensus being reached. In the present study, we followed the recommendations of Manuel Velasques et al. [37], so we also included severe local inflammation which led to the impossibility of achieving the critical view of safety. On the other hand, Turhan et al. [37] also found that the PLR correlated with inflammation, but with a lower predictive value when compared to that of the NLR for complicated AC (AUC = 0.704 vs. 0.873, respectively), which is consistent with our findings. Diez Ares et al., in a study on 130 patients operated on for AC, found that an NLR value of >5 and a CRP value of >100 mg/dL were independent risk factors for gangrenous cholecystitis, with good predictive value estimated by ROC curves (AUC = 0.75 vs. AUC = 0.80, respectively), and should be taken into account in the therapeutic decision, considering that early laparoscopic cholecystectomy provides the best outcomes in gangrenous AC [38].

A different approach was used by Unal et al. [34], who analyzed the correlation between the NLR and the TG 13/18 grading scale. He found that an NLR cut-off value of 5.2 may discriminate well between TG13/18 grade 1 vs. grades 2 and 3 with a sensitivity of 76.76% and specificity of 76.17% (AUC of 0.817), while a NRL > 8.5 is a good predictor for TG 13/18 grade 3, which associates with systemic imbalance due to inflammation [34]. In our study, we also found a cut-off value of >8.54 to be a good predictor for early postoperative sepsis.

Kartal and Kalayci [38] found no correlation between the NLR and postoperative overall morbidity in the elderly with AC [38]. In the present study, we found no correlation between the systemic inflammatory biomarkers and Clavien–Dindo complications grades II and III. This finding may support the current recommendation that early cholecystectomy may be performed safely in all cases of acute cholecystitis, even those with severe inflammation. However, inflammatory biomarkers were well-correlated with the grade IV Clavien–Dindo complications, requiring intensive care. In the present study, we found that an NLR value of >8.54 has 87.5% sensitivity and 81% specificity for early postoperative sepsis. Although postoperative complications are more frequent in the severe cholecystitis group, there is no correlation between postoperative surgical complications and the values of the NLR, SII, PLR, or TG 13/18 grading scale. This supports, on the one hand, the idea that choosing the appropriate technique for each case allows for a successful solution regardless of the severity of the local inflammation [1,39–41]. On the other hand, repeated inflammatory relapses that lead to local fibrous rearrangements, but also the involvement of the human factor (perception errors of the struts during dissection), can generate vascular-biliary lesions [42,43].

In our study, we found that the PLR is an important biomarker in predicting sepsis in patients with AC admitted in emergency care. Part of the complicated underlying pathophysiology of sepsis syndrome is clot formation and bleeding diathesis associated with platelet disfunction, endothelial activation, and disseminated intravascular coagulation [44]. Prompt identification of these patients is essential for improving the survival rate in these patients [44–46].

Mitigation of perioperative inflammation and pain is important for enhanced recovery after surgery (ERAS) and preventing postoperative complications [47–49]. Postoperative analgesia is a very important part of perioperative management in patients with AC. The pain pattern after LC seems to be different from that after other laparoscopic surgeries [48], and good pain management should be based on an individualized approach. The intensity of preoperative inflammation may sensibilize the peritoneal nociceptors, so a multimodal analgesia could be the best option to control the pain with minimal adverse effects [48]. Several studies found that choosing non-opioid combinations, such as paracetamol and parecoxib 40 mg IV or lornoxicam quick-release 8 mg PO every 12 h, results in the same anti-algic effect as opioids, but limits the risk of pulmonary complications and allows a quick recovery [50,51].

Our study has some limitations: it is a monocentric retrospective study on a limited number of patients. The analyzed values are those from admission, not those from the operative moment. Also, the dynamics of biomarkers regarding the development of postoperative complications were not analyzed. We also could not differentiate between the cases that needed conversion due to sclerosis after multiple previous episodes of mild AC and the impossibility of achieving the critical view of safety due to active inflammation. This might be an explanation for the lower cut-off value found for the NLR when compared to other studies that focus on the gangrenous gallbladder only. However, our study brings valuable information regarding the correlations between the NLR, PLR, and SII and the severity of AC, risk for conversion, and postoperative morbidity.

5. Conclusions

The NLR, PLR, and SII are useful in the preoperative assessment of the AC. The NLR is an early biomarker of inflammation, with higher predictive value when compared to that of PLR, SII, and total leukocytes, and is more versatile than the TG 13/18 scale, being a continuous variable. An NLR value of >4.19 is suggestive of advanced inflammation, while a value of >8.54 is a good predictor for early postoperative sepsis. The PLR and SII correlate significantly with the severity of the inflammation and may be useful in the prediction of the systemic inflammatory response, but they have fair predictive value for advanced AC and risk for conversion in LC.

Author Contributions: Conceptualization, D.S., P.L.S., A.M.D., D.G.B. and C.A.; methodology: P.L.S., B.M.C. and I.M.; software, A.M.D., L.C.T. and G.V.; validation, D.S., C.T, C.S. and D.O.C.; formal analysis, I.M., C.T., M.S.T. and L.C.T.; investigation, D.O.C., C.A., B.M.C. and. D.G.B.; resources, D.S.; data curation, C.A. writing—original draft preparation, D.S., P.L.S., A.M.D., D.G.B., B.M.C., I.M., L.C.T. and C.A.; writing—review and editing, C.S., D.T., G.V., D.O.C. and M.S.T.; visualization, D.S., D.O.C. and C.A.; supervision, D.S.; project administration, P.L.S.; funding acquisition, D.S. Dan Georgian Bratu (D.G.B.), Bogdan Mihai Cristea (B.M.C.) and Catalin Alius (C.A.) contributed equally as the first author at the manuscript. All authors have read and agreed to the published version of the manuscript.

Funding: This research received no external funding.

Institutional Review Board Statement: Ethical review and approval were waived for this study due to the retrospective nature of the study.

Informed Consent Statement: Not applicable.

Data Availability Statement: The data presented in this study are available on request from the corresponding author. The data are not publicly available due to privacy.

Conflicts of Interest: The authors declare no conflict of interest.

References

1. Sartelli, M.; Abu-Zidan, F.M.; Catena, F.; Griffiths, E.A.; Di Saverio, S.; Coimbra, R.; Ordoñez, C.A.; Leppaniemi, A.; Fraga, G.P.; Coccolini, F. Global validation of the WSES Sepsis Severity Score for patients with complicated intra-abdominal infections: A prospective multicentre study (WISS Study). *World J. Emerg. Surg.* **2015**, *10*, 61. [CrossRef] [PubMed]
2. Gomes, C.; Junior, C.S.; Di Saverio, S.; Sartelli, M.; Kelly, M.D.; Gomes, C.C.; Gomes, F.C.; Corrêa, L.D.; Alves, C.B.; Guimarãesm, S.F. Acute calculous cholecystitis: Review of current best practices. *World J. Gastrointest. Surg.* **2017**, *9*, 118–126, Erratum in *World J. Gastrointest. Surg.* **2017**, *9*, 214. [CrossRef]
3. Tufo, A.; Pisano, M.; Ansaloni, L.; de Reuver, P.; van Laarhoven, K.; Davidson, B.; Gurusamy, K.S. Risk Prediction in Acute Calculous Cholecystitis: A Systematic Review and Meta-Analysis of Prognostic Factors and Predictive Models. *J. Laparoendosc. Adv. Surg. Technol. A* **2021**, *31*, 41–53. [CrossRef]
4. Lucocq, J.; Patil, P.; Scollay, J. Acute cholecystitis: Delayed cholecystectomy has lesser perioperative morbidity compared to emergency cholecystectomy. *Surgery* **2022**, *172*, 16–22. [CrossRef]
5. Bouassida, M.; Zribi, S.; Krimi, B.; Laamiri, G.; Mroua, B.; Slama, H.; Mighri, M.M.; M'saddak Azzouz, M.; Hamzaoui, L.; Touinsi, H. C-reactive Protein Is the Best Biomarker to Predict Advanced Acute Cholecystitis and Conversion to Open Surgery. A Prospective Cohort Study of 556 Cases. *J. Gastrointest. Surg.* **2020**, *24*, 2766–2772. [CrossRef]
6. Turhan, V.B.; Gök, H.F.; Ünsal, A.; Akpınar, M.; Güler Şimşek, G.; Buluş, H. Pre-operative neutrophil/lymphocyte and platelet/lymphocyte ratios are effective in predicting complicated acute cholecystitis. *Ulus. Travma Acil Cerrahi Derg.* **2022**, *28*, 471–476. [CrossRef] [PubMed]
7. Díez Ares, J.Á.; Martínez García, R.; Estellés Vidagany, N.; Peris Tomás, N.; Planells Roig, M.; Valenzuela Gras, M.; Ripollés González, T. Can inflammatory biomarkers help in the diagnosis and prognosis of gangrenous acute cholecystitis? A prospective study. *Rev. Esp. Enfermedades Dig.* **2021**, *113*, 41–44. [CrossRef]
8. Yokoe, M.; Takada, T.; Strasberg, S.M.; Solomkin, J.S.; Mayumi, T.; Gomi, H.; Pitt, H.A.; Garden, O.J.; Kiriyama, S.; Hata, J.; et al. TG13 diagnostic criteria and severity grading of acute cholecystitis (with videos). *J. Hepato-Biliary-Pancreat. Sci.* **2013**, *20*, 35–46. [CrossRef]
9. Yokoe, M.; Hata, J.; Takada, T.; Strasberg, S.M.; Asbun, H.J.; Wakabayashi, G.; Kozaka, K.; Endo, I.; Deziel, D.J.; Miura, F.; et al. Tokyo Guidelines 2018: Diagnostic criteria and severity grading of acute cholecystitis (with videos). *J. Hepato-Biliary-Pancreat. Sci.* **2018**, *25*, 41–54. [CrossRef] [PubMed]
10. Jessica Mok, K.W.; Goh, Y.L.; Howell, L.E.; Date, R.S. Is C-reactive protein the single most useful predictor of difficult laparoscopic cholecystectomy or its conversion? A pilot study. *J. Minimal Access Surg.* **2016**, *12*, 26–32. [CrossRef]
11. Wevers, K.P.; van Westreenen, H.L.; Patijn, G.A. Laparoscopic cholecystectomy in acute cholecystitis: C-reactive protein level combined with age predicts conversion. *Surg. Laparosc. Endosc. Percutan. Technol.* **2013**, *23*, 163–166. [CrossRef]
12. Díaz-Flores, A.; Cárdenas-Lailson, E.; Cuendis-Velázquez, A.; Rodríguez-Parra, A.; Trejo-Ávila, M.E. C-Reactive Protein as a Predictor of Difficult Laparoscopic Cholecystectomy in Patients with Acute Calculous Cholecystitis: A Multivariate Analysis. *J. Laparoendosc. Adv. Surg. Technol. Part A* **2017**, *27*, 1263–1268. [CrossRef]
13. Vural, S.; Aydin, I.; Kesicioglu, T. Association of Serum C-Reactive Protein Level and Treatment Duration in Acute Cholecystitis Patients Treated Conservatively. *Cureus* **2022**, *14*, e22146. [CrossRef]
14. Çeliktürk, E.; Salt, Ö.; Sayhan, M.B.; Dıbırdık, İ. A novel biomarker in acute cholecystitis: YKL-40. *Asian J. Surg.* **2023**, *46*, 1564–1570. [CrossRef] [PubMed]

15. Park, J.W.; Kim, O.H.; Lee, S.C.; Kim, K.H.; Hong, H.E.; Seo, H.; Choi, H.J.; Kim, S.J. Serum level of visfatin can reflect the severity of inflammation in patients with acute cholecystitis. *Ann. Surg. Treat. Res.* **2020**, *99*, 26–36. [CrossRef]
16. Yaow, C.Y.L.; Chong, R.I.H.; Chan, K.S.; Chia, C.T.W.; Shelat, V.G. Should Procalcitonin Be Included in Acute Cholecystitis Guidelines? A Systematic Review. *Medicina* **2023**, *59*, 805. [CrossRef] [PubMed]
17. Li, D.; Yue, Z.; Weng, Y.; Zhen, G. Diagnostic value of ROC curve evaluation of serum markers in acute cholecystitis with bacterial infection. *J. Pak. Med. Assoc.* **2022**, *72*, 1133–1136. [CrossRef]
18. Nechita, V.I.; Hajjar, N.A.; Drugan, C.; Cătană, C.-S.; Moiș, E.; Nechita, M.-A.; Graur, F. Chitotriosidase and Neopterin as Potential Biomarkers for the Evaluation of Complicated Cholecystitis—A Pilot Study. *J. Clin. Med.* **2023**, *12*, 1641. [CrossRef]
19. Modica, R.; Minotta, R.; Liccardi, A.; Cannavale, G.; Benevento, E.; Colao, A. Evaluation of Neutrophil-to-Lymphocyte Ratio (NLR), Platelet-to-Lymphocyte Ratio (PLR) and Systemic Immune–Inflammation Index (SII) as Potential Biomarkers in Patients with Sporadic Medullary Thyroid Cancer (MTC). *J. Pers. Med.* **2023**, *13*, 953. [CrossRef]
20. Xia, W.; Tan, Y.; Hu, S.; Li, C.; Jiang, T. Predictive Value of Systemic Immune-Inflammation index and Neutrophil-to-Lymphocyte Ratio in Patients with Severe COVID-19. *Clin. Appl. Thromb. Hemost.* **2022**, *28*, 10760296221111391. [CrossRef]
21. Serban, D.; Papanas, N.; Dascalu, A.M.; Kempler, P.; Raz, I.; Rizvi, A.A.; Rizzo, M.; Tudor, C.; Silviu Tudosie, M.; Tanasescu, D.; et al. Significance of Neutrophil to Lymphocyte Ratio (NLR) and Platelet Lymphocyte Ratio (PLR) in Diabetic Foot Ulcer and Potential New Therapeutic Targets. *Int. J. Low Extrem. Wounds* **2021**, 15347346211057742. [CrossRef] [PubMed]
22. Seyedi, S.A.; Nabipoorashrafi, S.A.; Hernandez, J.; Nguyen, A.; Lucke-Wold, B.; Nourigheimasi, S.; Khanzadeh, S. Neutrophil to Lymphocyte Ratio and Spontaneous Bacterial Peritonitis among Cirrhotic Patients: A Systematic Review and Meta-analysis. *Can. J. Gastroenterol. Hepatol.* **2022**, *2022*, 8604060. [CrossRef] [PubMed]
23. Hajibandeh, S.; Hajibandeh, S.; Hobbs, N.; Mansour, M. Neutrophil-to-lymphocyte ratio predicts acute appendicitis and distinguishes between complicated and uncomplicated appendicitis: A systematic review and meta-analysis. *Am. J. Surg.* **2020**, *219*, 154–163. [CrossRef] [PubMed]
24. Yan, Q.; Ertao, Z.; Zhimei, Z.; Weigang, D.; Jianjun, P.; Jianhui, C.; Chuangqi, C. Systemic immune-inflammation index (SII): A More Promising Inflammation-Based Prognostic Marker for Patients with synchronic colorectal peritoneal carcinomatosis. *J. Cancer* **2020**, *11*, 5264–5272. [CrossRef] [PubMed]
25. Mićić, D.; Stanković, S.; Lalić, N.; Đukić, V.; Polovina, S. Prognostic Value of Preoperative Neutrophil-to-lymphocyte Ratio for Prediction of Severe Cholecystitis. *J. Med. Biochem.* **2018**, *37*, 121–127. [CrossRef] [PubMed]
26. Safari, S.; Baratloo, A.; Elfil, M.; Negida, A. Evidence Based Emergency Medicine; Part 5 Receiver Operating Curve and Area under the Curve. *Emergency* **2016**, *4*, 111–113.
27. Er, S.; Ozden, S.; Celik, C.; Yuksel, B.C. Can we predict severity of acute cholecystitis at admission? *Pak. J. Med. Sci.* **2018**, *34*, 1293–1296. [CrossRef] [PubMed]
28. Yilmaz, S.; Aykota, M.R.; Ozgen, U.; Birsen, O.; Simsek, S.; Kabay, B. Might simple peripheral blood parameters be an early indicator in the prediction of severity and morbidity of cholecystitis? *Ann. Surg. Treat. Res.* **2023**, *104*, 332–338. [CrossRef] [PubMed]
29. Kao, C.H.; Liu, Y.H.; Chen, W.K.; Huang, F.W.; Hsu, T.Y.; Cheng, H.T.; Hsueh, P.R.; Hsiao, C.T.; Wu, S.Y.; Shih, H.M. Value of monocyte distribution width for predicting severe cholecystitis: A retrospective cohort study. *Clin. Chem. Lab. Med.* **2023**, *61*, 1850–1857. [CrossRef] [PubMed]
30. Paul, S.; Khataniar, H.; Ck, A.; Rao, H.K. Preoperative scoring system validation and analysis of associated risk factors in predicting difficult laparoscopic cholecystectomy in patients with acute calculous cholecystitis: A prospective observational study. *Turk. J. Surg.* **2022**, *38*, 375–381. [CrossRef]
31. Önder, A.; Kapan, M.; Ülger, B.V.; Oğuz, A.; Türkoğlu, A.; Uslukaya, Ö. Gangrenous cholecystitis: Mortality and risk factors. *Int. Surg.* **2015**, *100*, 254–260. [CrossRef] [PubMed]
32. Prakash, G.; Hasan, M. The Accuracy of Neutrophil-to-Lymphocyte Ratio and Abdominal Computed Tomography to Predict the Severity of Acute Cholecystitis. *Cureus* **2022**, *14*, e32243. [CrossRef]
33. Gojayev, A.; Karakaya, E.; Erkent, M.; Yücebaş, S.C.; Aydin, H.O.; Kavasoğlu, L.; Aydoğan, C.; Yildirim, S. A novel approach to distinguish complicated and non-complicated acute cholecystitis: Decision tree method. *Medicine* **2023**, *102*, e33749. [CrossRef] [PubMed]
34. Ünal, Y.; Tuncal, S.; Küçük, B.; Barlas, A.M.; Altıner, S.; Balık, R.; Aydın, S.M.; Senlikci, A.; Pekcici, M.R. An effective and reliable marker in grading the severity of acute cholecystitis: Increased immature granulocyte percentage. Akut kolesistitin şiddetini derecelendirmede etkili ve güvenilir bir belirteç: Artmış immatür granülosit yüzdesi. *Ulus. Travma Acil Cerrahi Derg.* **2022**, *28*, 1716–1722. [CrossRef]
35. Sato, N.; Kinoshita, A.; Imai, N.; Akasu, T.; Yokota, T.; Iwaku, A.; Koike, K.; Saruta, M. Inflammation-based prognostic scores predict disease severity in patients with acute cholecystitis. *Eur. J. Gastroenterol. Hepatol.* **2018**, *30*, 484–489. [CrossRef]
36. Cakcak, İ.E.; Kula, O. Predictive evaluation of SIRI, SII, PNI, and GPS in cholecystostomy application in patients with acute cholecystitis. *Ulus. Travma Acil Cerrahi Derg.* **2022**, *28*, 940–946. [CrossRef]
37. Beliaev, A.M.; Angelo, N.; Booth, M.; Bergin, C. Evaluation of neutrophil-to-lymphocyte ratio as a potential biomarker for acute cholecystitis. *J. Surg. Res.* **2017**, *209*, 93–101. [CrossRef]
38. Kartal, M.; Kalaycı, T. Can neutrophil-lymphocyte ratio, platelet-lymphocyte ratio, prognostic nutrition index, and albumin be used to predict cholecystectomy morbidity in super-elderly patients? *Ulus. Travma Acil Cerrahi Derg.* **2023**, *29*, 890–896. [CrossRef]

39. Manuel-Vázquez, A.; Latorre-Fragua, R.; Alcázar, C.; Requena, P.M.; de la Plaza, R.; Blanco Fernández, G.; Serradilla-Martín, M.; Ramia, J.M.; SCORELAP Group. Reaching a consensus on the definition of "difficult" cholecystectomy among Spanish experts. A Delphi project. A qualitative study. *Int. J. Surg.* **2022**, *102*, 106649. [CrossRef]
40. Dumitrescu, D.; Savlovschi, C.; Borcan, R.; Pantu, H.; Serban, D.; Gradinaru, S.; Smarandache, G.; Trotea, T.; Branescu, C.; Musat, L.; et al. Clinical case—voluminous diaphragmatic hernia—surgically acute abdomen: Diagnostic and therapeutical challenges. *Chirurgia* **2011**, *106*, 657–660. [PubMed]
41. Savlovschi, C.; Serban, D.; Trotea, T.; Borcan, R.; Dumitrescu, D. Post-surgery morbidity and mortality in colorectal cancer in elderly subjects. *Chirurgia* **2013**, *108*, 177–179. [PubMed]
42. Serban, D.; Badiu, D.C.; Davitoiu, D.; Tanasescu, C.; Tudosie, M.S.; Sabau, A.D.; Dascalu, A.M.; Tudor, C.; Balasescu, S.A.; Socea, B.; et al. Systematic review of the role of indocyanine green near-infrared fluorescence in safe laparoscopic cholecystectomy (Review). *Exp. Ther. Med.* **2022**, *23*, 187. [CrossRef]
43. Pisano, M.; Allievi, N.; Gurusamy, K.; Borzellino, G.; Cimbanassi, S.; Boerna, D.; Coccolini, F.; Tufo, A.; Di Martino, M.; Leung, J.; et al. 2020 World Society of Emergency Surgery updated guidelines for the diagnosis and treatment of acute calculus cholecystitis. *World J. Emerg. Surg.* **2020**, *15*, 61. [CrossRef]
44. Karamouzos, V.; Paraskevas, T.; Mulita, F.; Karteri, S.; Oikonomou, E.; Ntoulias, N.; Pantzaris, N.D.; Bourganou, V.; Velissaris, D. Neutrophil to Lymphocyte Ratio and Platelet to Lymphocyte Percentage Ratio as Predictors of In-hospital Mortality in Sepsis. An Observational Cohort Study. *Mater. Socio-Medica* **2022**, *34*, 33–36. [CrossRef]
45. Boicean, A.; Neamtu, B.; Birsan, S.; Batar, F.; Tanasescu, C.; Dura, H.; Roman, M.D.; Hașegan, A.; Bratu, D.; Mihetiu, A.; et al. Fecal Microbiota Transplantation in Patients Co-Infected with SARS-CoV2 and *Clostridioides difficile*. *Biomedicines* **2023**, *11*, 7. [CrossRef] [PubMed]
46. Shen, Y.; Huang, X.; Zhang, W. Platelet-to-lymphocyte ratio as a prognostic predictor of mortality for sepsis: Interaction effect with disease severity-a retrospective study. *BMJ Open* **2019**, *9*, e022896. [CrossRef]
47. Mansour, N.O.; Boraii, S.; Elnaem, M.H.; Elrggal, M.E.; Omar, T.; Abdelraouf, A.; Abdelaziz, D.H. Evaluation of preoperative duloxetine use for postoperative analgesia following laparoscopic cholecystectomy: A randomized controlled trial. *Front. Pharmacol.* **2022**, *13*, 944392. [CrossRef]
48. Chicea, R.; Bratu, D.; Chicea, A.L.; Mihetiu, A.; Preluca, V.; Tantar, C.; Sava, M. A comparative Histologic and Immunohistochemistry Evaluation Between Normal Aponeurotic Tissue, Fibrotic Aponeurotic Scars and Polypropylene Embedded Aponeurotic Scars. *Mater. Plast.* **2017**, *54*, 510–512. [CrossRef]
49. Yu, T.; Zhao, L.; Zhao, H.; Fu, H.; Li, J.; Yu, A. The enhanced recovery after surgery (ERAS) protocol in elderly patients with acute cholecystitis: A retrospective study. *Medicine* **2023**, *102*, e32942. [CrossRef]
50. Mulita, F.; Karpetas, G.; Liolis, E.; Vailas, M.; Tchabashvili, L.; Maroulis, I. Comparison of analgesic efficacy of acetaminophen monotherapy versus acetaminophen combinations with either pethidine or parecoxib in patients undergoing laparoscopic cholecystectomy: A randomized prospective study. *Med. Glas.* **2021**, *18*, 27–32. [CrossRef]
51. Kouroukli, I.; Zompolas, V.; Tsekoura, V.; Papazoglou, I.; Louizos, A.; Panaretou, V. Comparison between lornoxicam quick-release and parecoxib for post-operative analgesia after laparoscopic cholecystectomy: A prospective randomized, placebo-controlled trial. *J. Anaesthesiol. Clin. Pharmacol.* **2013**, *29*, 485–490. [CrossRef]

Disclaimer/Publisher's Note: The statements, opinions and data contained in all publications are solely those of the individual author(s) and contributor(s) and not of MDPI and/or the editor(s). MDPI and/or the editor(s) disclaim responsibility for any injury to people or property resulting from any ideas, methods, instructions or products referred to in the content.

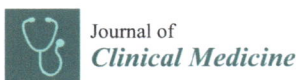 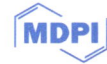

Article

Systemic Inflammatory Response and the Noble and Underwood (NUn) Score as Early Predictors of Anastomotic Leakage after Esophageal Reconstructive Surgery

Elke Van Daele [1,*], Hanne Vanommeslaeghe [1], Flo Decostere [2], Louise Beckers Perletti [2], Esther Beel [2], Yves Van Nieuwenhove [1,2], Wim Ceelen [1,2] and Piet Pattyn [1,2]

[1] Department of Gastrointestinal Surgery, Ghent University Hospital, C. Heymanslaan 10, B-9000 Ghent, Belgium; wim.ceelen@ugent.be (W.C.)
[2] Faculty of Medicine, Ghent University, C. Heymanslaan 10, B-9000 Ghent, Belgium; flo.decostere@ugent.be (F.D.); louise.beckers@ugent.be (L.B.P.); esther.beel@ugent.be (E.B.)
* Correspondence: elke.vandaele@uzgent.be

Abstract: Anastomotic leakage (AL) remains the main cause of post-esophagectomy morbidity and mortality. Early detection can avoid sepsis and reduce morbidity and mortality. This study evaluates the diagnostic accuracy of the Nun score and its components as early detectors of AL. This single-center observational cohort study included all esophagectomies from 2010 to 2020. C-reactive protein (CRP), albumin (Alb), and white cell count (WCC) were analyzed and NUn scores were calculated. The area under the curve statistic (AUC) was used to assess their predictive accuracy. A total of 74 of the 668 patients (11%) developed an AL. CRP and the NUn-score proved to be good diagnostic accuracy tests on postoperative day (POD) 2 (CRP AUC: 0.859; NUn score AUC: 0.869) and POD 4 (CRP AUC: 0.924; NUn score AUC: 0.948). A 182 mg/L CRP cut-off on POD 4 yielded a 87% sensitivity, 88% specificity, a negative predictive value (NPV) of 98%, and a positive predictive value (PPV) of 47.7%. A NUn score cut-off > 10 resulted in 92% sensitivity, 95% specificity, 99% NPV, and 68% PPV. Albumin and WCC have limited value in the detection of post-esophagectomy AL. Elevated CRP and a high NUn score on POD 4 provide high accuracy in predicting AL after esophageal cancer surgery. Their high negative predictive value allows to select patients who can safely proceed with enhanced recovery protocols.

Keywords: NUn score; esophagectomy; anastomotic leakage; risk score; esophageal cancer; inflammatory biomarkers

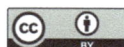

1. Introduction

The incidence of esophageal cancer (EC) is increasing, making it the sixth leading cause of cancer-related mortality worldwide [1]. The prognosis remains poor with 5-year overall survival rates varying from 90% for stage I cancer to <10% for stage IV cancer patients. For locally advanced cancer, multimodality therapy followed by surgery has convincingly improved both local control and overall survival [2–5]. Surgical resection and lymphadenectomy remain crucial in the treatment of non-metastatic esophageal cancer patients [5,6]. However, the procedure is known for its potentially complicated postoperative course. Large benchmarking series report postoperative complications in more than 50% of cases, even in high-volume centers. Pulmonary complications (15–25%), cardiac events (14–15%), and the failure of the esophagogastric anastomosis (12–16%) remain the most important sources of both morbidity and mortality after esophagectomy [7–9]. Considerable improvements in surgical technique and perioperative care have resulted in 90-day mortality rates after esophagectomy of less than 5% in experienced centers [7–9]. However, the mortality of AL remains high, ranging from 7 to 17% [10,11]. The severity of AL depends on the location of the anastomosis, the estimated surface and circumference of the defect, the extent of contamination, the degree of sepsis, and the time from occurrence to diagnosis and therapy [12]. The early detection and management of an AL can prevent the development of mediastinitis-related sepsis and is critical to improving its outcome [13].

Inflammatory biomarkers have been previously proposed as easy and cheap tests for the early diagnosis of postoperative infectious complications after major surgery. C-reactive protein (CRP) is an acute-phase protein produced in response to infection, tissue damage, and ischemia. A low CRP on postoperative day (POD) 3 and 5 may rule out AL after esophagectomy [13]. However, it can be difficult to distinguish the normal systemic inflammatory response to surgical stress from AL-associated sepsis. Identifying a clinically relevant, easy-to-use scoring system may be helpful in the early diagnosis of AL, selecting patients for imaging, and tailoring AL management. Noble and Underwood introduced the NUn score, using the acute-phase markers white cell count (WCC), CRP, and albumin (Alb) as a predictor of AL and major postoperative complications [14]. The attempts to validate the score are limited and conflicting [15–18]. We aimed to determine the diagnostic accuracy of these inflammatory response biomarkers and the combined NUn score as early predictors of post-esophagectomy AL.

2. Materials and Methods

The study protocol was approved by the institutional review board of the Ghent University Hospital (reference: B670201111232).

2.1. Surgery and Postoperative Care

Transthoracic (sub)total esophagectomy with 2- or 3-field lymphadenectomy and a right intrathoracic (Ivor Lewis, IL or Transhiatal, THE) or cervical esophagogastric anastomosis (McKeown, McK) were performed. All procedures were performed by 2 surgeons (PP and EVD). The surgical approach included open as well as hybrid minimally invasive procedures (introduced in 2013). Fully minimal invasive esophagectomy (MIE) was introduced in 2014. All patients received an intrathoracic end-to-side or end-to-end circular esophagogastric anastomosis using a Premium Plus EEA™ (Medtronic, Dublin, Ireland) stapler (25 or 28 mm), or a standardized cervical end-to-side hand-sewn anastomosis. Patients recovered at the intensive care unit for 12–24 h and were then discharged to a dedicated gastrointestinal surgery ward. A nasogastric tube was kept in place during a period of 2–3 days. A water-soluble contrast swallow was obtained on the third postoperative day as a routine screening before initiating oral intake. Patients suspected of AL received an emergency CT scan with oral contrast and/or upper endoscopy. Anastomotic leakage was treated conservatively, endoscopically, or surgically, according to clinical presentation. Nutritional support was provided by a feeding jejunostomy. Since 2018, patients have been treated according to an Enhanced Recovery After Surgery (ERAS) protocol.

2.2. Patient Selection

This cohort study was based on data gathered from a prospective institutional database supplemented with data from the electronic patient records. Consecutive patients undergoing esophagectomy for cancer between January 2010 and December 2020, and fitting the criteria were included. Patients in whom the esophagus was replaced with a small bowel or colon, or who underwent concurrent laryngectomy, were excluded.

2.3. Outcomes

Individual collected data included demographics, American Society of Anesthesiologists (ASA) score, tumor characteristics, the type of neoadjuvant therapy, surgical details, pathology reports, laboratory results, and postoperative morbidity and mortality until 90 days postoperatively. Pathological staging was based on the 7th AJCC TNM classification manual. Postoperative morbidity and mortality were classified using the European Complication Consensus Group (ECCG) platform [19] and graded according to the Clavien Dindo classification [20]. Anastomotic leakage was defined as a full thickness gastrointestinal defect involving the esophagus, anastomosis, staple line, or conduit, irrespective of presentation or method of identification, according to the ECCG classification. Results are reported according to the "Strengthening the Reporting of Observational Studies in Epidemiology" (STROBE) guidelines [21].

2.4. Inflammatory Biomarkers and the NUn Score

Acute-phase markers were retrieved from the daily blood samples postoperatively. WCC was measured in cells $\times 10^3/\mu L$ (reference range 3.6–9.3 $10^3/\mu L$) and converted to $10^9/L$ for the NUn score calculation. Serum concentrations of albumin were expressed in g/L (normal range 35–52 g/L) and CRP in mg/L (normal range < 0.5 mg/L). The NUn score was calculated according the original Noble formula: $11.3894 + (0.005 \times CRP$ in mg/L$) + (0.186 \times WCC$ in $10^9/L) - (0.174 \times$ albumin in g/L$)$. Missing data were replaced using the last observation carried forward approach.

2.5. Statistical Analysis

All analyses were performed using IBM SPSS® version 28 for Windows® and Sigmaplot® version 13 for Windows®. Continuous data are summarized as means with standard deviations (SD), or as medians with interquartile ranges (IQR). Categorical data are reported using frequencies and percentages. Independent samples t test, Pearson chi square, Fisher's exact, and Mann–Whitney U tests were used to compare means and proportions. The significance of the different covariates in the prediction of AL was assessed using univariate analysis. The predictive accuracy of the biomarkers and the NUn score was assessed using receiver operating curve (ROC) analyses and the area under the curve (AUC). Sensitivity, specificity, and positive and negative predictive value were calculated for the determined cut-off values of the biomarkers and the NUn score.

3. Results

3.1. Demographics of the Study Cohort

Between January 2010 and December 2020, 668 esophagectomy patients were identified matching the inclusion criteria. Demographic data and their univariable association with AL are detailed in Table 1. The mean age was 64.0 ± 12.2 years (78.9% male). Overall, 74 patients (11.1%) experienced an AL. The majority of patients were treated for an adenocarcinoma (67.5%). Univariable analysis could not identify statistically significant differences in demographics, comorbidities, neoadjuvant treatment regimens, histology, or clinical staging between the patients with and without leakage, except for a higher percent of ASA 3 patients in the AL group. The surgical procedure, approach, and conditions did, however, significantly influence the AL rate, with a significantly higher AL rate in patients with a cervical anastomosis (McK 28% vs. IL 10.9% vs. THE 5.2%, $p = 0.010$), after total minimally invasive surgery (16.8% vs. 8.6% after both open and hybrid procedures, $p = 0.008$), and when an emergency procedure was performed. AL was defined according to the ECCG guidelines, diagnosed on CT-scan and/or upper GI endoscopy, and graded according to both the CD (17.6% gr 2; 1.4% gr 3a; 43.2% gr 3b; 27% gr 4a; 8.1% gr 4b; and 2.7% gr 5) and ECCG grading system (18.9% type 1; 12.2% type 2; and 68.9% type 3).

Table 1. Baseline characteristics.

			All Patients (n = 668)	No AL (n = 594)	AL (n = 74)	p Value
Age, (y)		Mean ± SD	64.0 ± 12.2	64.8 ± 10.2	65.6 ± 8.9	0.508
BMI (kg/m^2)		Mean ± SD	25.3 ± 4.6	25.2 ± 4.5	25.9 ± 4.9	0.252
ASA score, n (%)		1	27 (4.0%)	24 (4.1%)	3 (4.1%)	**0.036**
		2	286 (42.8%)	261 (43.9%)	25 (33.7%)	
		3	335 (50.1%)	292 (49.2%)	43 (58.1%)	
		4	4 (0.6%)	2 (0.3%)	2 (2.7%)	

Table 1. Cont.

		All Patients (*n* = 668)	No AL (*n* = 594)	AL (*n* = 74)	*p* Value
Gender, *n* (%)	Male	527 (78.9%)	468 (78.8%)	59 (79.7%)	0.851
	Female	141 (21.1%)	126 (21.2%)	15 (20.3%)	
Comorbidities, *n* (%)	Kidney disease	21 (3.1%)	19 (3.2%)	2 (2.7%)	0.818
	Cardiovascular disease	257 (38.5%)	226 (38.0%)	31 (41.9%)	0.522
	Pulmonary disease	161 (24.1%)	140 (23.6%)	21 (28.4%)	0.362
	Diabetes	88 (13.2%)	75 (12.6%)	13 (17.6%)	0.236
	Smoking	230 (34.4%)	200 (33.7%)	30 (40.5%)	0.241
	Corticosteroids	20 (3.0%)	16 (2.7%)	4 (5.4%)	0.197
Tumor Location, *n* (%)	Proximal	17 (2.5%)	12 (2.0%)	5 (6.8%)	0.094
	Mid	121 (18.1%)	110 (18.5%)	11 (14.9%)	
	Distal	402 (60.2%)	357 (60.1%)	45 (60.8%)	
	GEJ	128 (19.2%)	115 (19.4%)	13 (17.6%)	
Neoadjuvant therapy, *n* (%)	None	179 (26.8%)	158 (26.6%)	21 (28.4%)	0.932
	Chemotherapy	97 (14.5%)	87 (14.6%)	10 (13.5%)	
	Radiochemotherapy	392 (58.7%)	349 (58.8%)	43 (58.1%)	
Histology, *n* (%)	Adeno Ca	451 (67.5%)	402 (67.7%)	49 (66.2%)	0.719
	Squamous cell Ca	200 (29.9%)	176 (29.6%)	24 (32.4%)	
	Other	17 (2.5%)	16 (2.7%)	1 (1.4%)	
cT-stage, *n* (%) *	Tx	8 (1.2%)	7 (1.2%)	1 (1.4%)	0.641
	T1	56 (8.4%)	49 (8.2%)	7 (9.5%)	
	T2	136 (20.4%)	118 (19.9%)	18 (24.3%)	
	T3	455 (68.1%)	407 (68.5%)	48 (64.9%)	
	T4	13 (1.9%)	13 (2.2%)	0 (0.0%)	
cN-stage, *n* (%) *	N0	227 (34.0%)	203 (34.2%)	24 (32.4%)	0.898
	N1	308 (46.1%)	276 (46.5%)	32 (43.2%)	
	N2	112 (16.8%)	97 (16.3%)	15 (20.3%)	
	N3	13 (1.9%)	11 (1.9%)	2 (2.7%)	
cM-stage, *n* (%) *	M0	625 (93.6%)	556 (93.6%)	69 (93.2%)	0.989
	M1	35 (5.2%)	31 (5.2%)	4 (5.4%)	
Procedure, *n* (%)	IL	586 (87.7%)	522 (87.9%)	64 (86.5%)	**0.010**
	McK	25 (3.7%)	18 (3.0%)	7 (9.5%)	
	THE	57 (8.5%)	54 (9.1%)	3 (4.1%)	
Approach, *n* (%)	Open	327 (49.0%)	299 (50.3%)	28 (37.8%)	**0.008**
	Hybride	139 (20.8%)	127 (21.4%)	12 (16.2%)	
	MIE	202 (30.2%)	168 (28.3%)	34 (45.9%)	
Type of surgery, *n* (%)	Elective	608 (91.0%)	545 (91.8%)	63 (85.1%)	**<0.001**
	Emergency	5 (0.7%)	1 (0.2%)	4 (5.4%)	
	Salvage	55 (8.2%)	48 (8.1%)	7 (9.5%)	

SD, standard deviation; BMI, body mass index; ASA, American Society of Anesthesiologists; GEJ, gastro esophageal junction; IL, Ivor Lewis; McK, McKeown; THE, transhiatal esophagectomy; * cTNM staging according to the AJCC 8th edition. Bold values state statistical significance.

3.2. Mean Levels of Inflammatory Biomarkers and Severity of the AL

CRP was available in 642 patients on POD 2 and 613 patients on POD 4. WCC was measured in 645 patients on POD 2 and 662 patients on POD 4. Albumin was available for 596 patients on POD 2 and 615 on POD 4. Missing data were replaced using the last observation carried forward approach. NUn scores were calculated for all but five patients on POD 2 and four patients on POD 4. Mean CRP, WCC, and combined NUn scores were significantly higher in AL patients compared to the non-AL patients, and this significance was confirmed for all ECCG AL types. Mean Alb was significantly lower in the AL group. Mean CRP and WCC levels were higher in patients with a more sever ECCG AL grade, specifically when type 1 leaks were compared to type 2 and type 3 leaks. The significance was present for the evaluated biomarkers both on POD 2 and POD 4 (Figure 1). All biomarkers were identified as significant markers for AL on univariate analysis (Table 2).

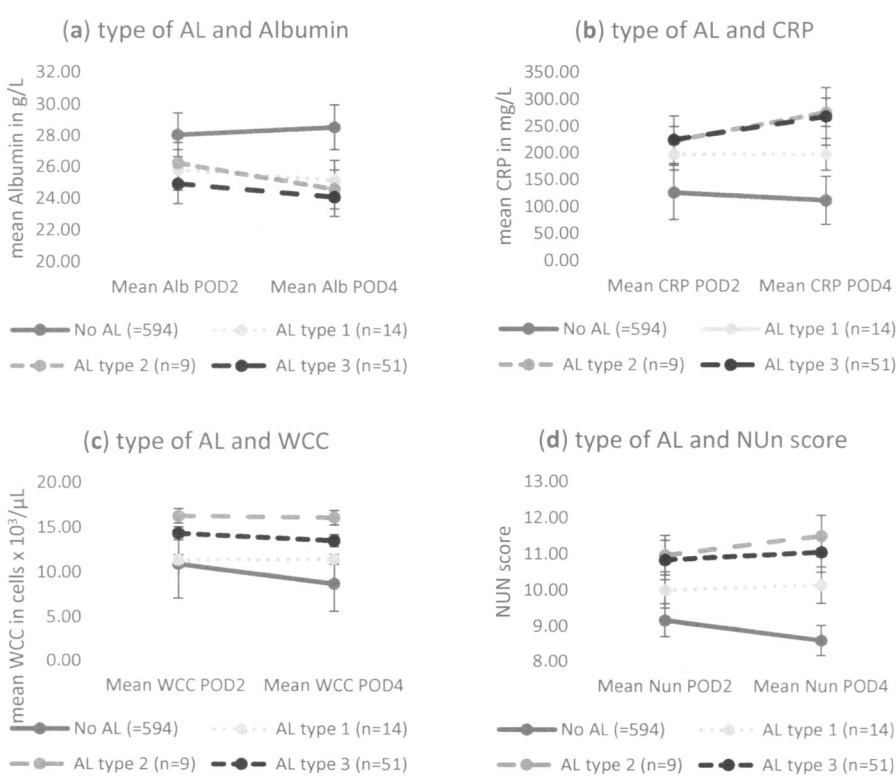

Figure 1. Mean levels of albumin, CRP, WCC, and NUn score on postoperative day 2 and 4 in patients with and without AL, stratified by ECCG type of AL (data displayed as means with standard deviation). (**a**) Correlation between mean Alb and type of AL, (**b**) correlation between mean CRP and type of AL, (**c**) correlation between mean WCC and type of AL, and (**d**) correlation between mean NUn and type of AL.

Table 2. Univariate analysis of the mean biomarkers and NUn score on POD 2 and 4 according to the ECCG type of AL.

	No AL (=594)	AL Type 1 (n = 14)	AL Type 2 (n = 9)	AL Type 3 (n = 51)	p Value
Alb POD 2 (mean ± SD)	28.0 (±3.7)	25.8 (±2.6)	26.2 (±4.4)	24.9 (±4.1)	<0.001
Alb POD 4 (mean ± SD)	28.5 (±3.9)	25.1 (±3.4)	24.6 (±4.0)	24.1 (±3.2)	<0.001
CRP POD 2 (mean ± SD)	125.9 (±55.4)	197.0 (±89.8)	222.3 (±73.2)	224.4 (±67.9)	<0.001
CRP POD 4 (mean ± SD)	111.1 (±62.8)	196.8 (±84.9)	275.4 (±86.4)	267.6 (±74.0)	<0.001
WCC POD 2 (mean ± SD)	10.9 (±5.2)	11.4 (±3.6)	16.3 (±6.5)	14.3 (±4.2)	<0.001
WCC POD 4 (mean ± SD)	8.7 (±2.9)	11.46 (±3.7)	16.1 (±5.7)	13.5 (±4.5)	<0.001
NUn POD 2 (mean ± SD)	9.2 (±1.2)	10.0 (±0.8)	10.9 (±1.4)	10.8 (±1.0)	<0.001
NUn POD 4 (mean ± SD)	8.6 (±1.0)	10.1 (±1.2)	11.5 (±0.8)	11.1 (±0.9)	<0.001

3.3. Optimal Cut-Off and Predictive Accuracy of Albumin

Mean albumin levels for patients with and without AL were 25.2 versus 28.0 g/L on POD 2 (p < 0.001) and 24.3 versus 28.5 g/L on POD 4 (p < 0.001). Figure 2 shows the ROC curve analyses of albumin, with a fair performance on POD 2 (AUC 0.710, 95% CI: 0.646–0.774) and POD 4 (AUC 0.799, 95% CI: 0.746–0.853). A POD 4 albumin threshold of

26.5 g/L had the highest, but still limited diagnostic accuracy, with a sensitivity of 80% and a specificity of 68%.

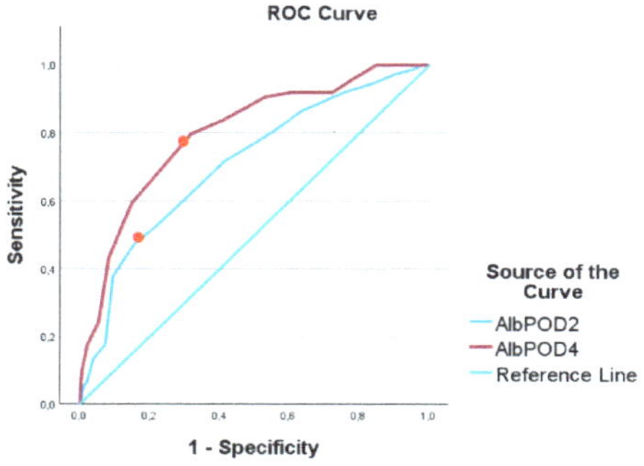

(a) ALB	AUC	95% CI	Cut-off	sens	spec
POD2	0.710	0.646–0.774	24.5	47.30%	84.40%
POD4	0.799	0.746–0.853	26.5	79.70%	68.20%

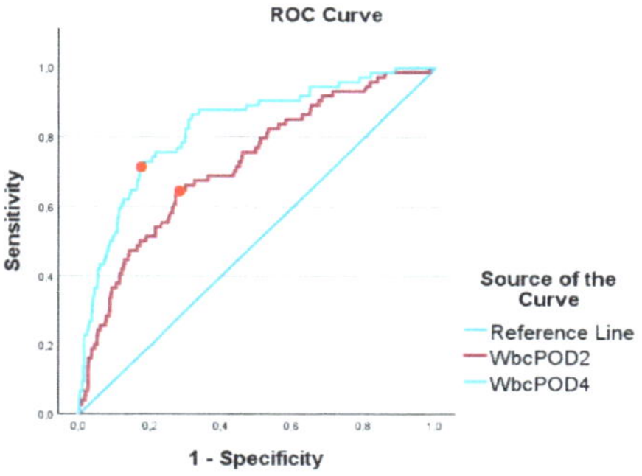

(b) WBC	AUC	95% CI	Cut-off	sens	spec
POD2	0.724	0.662–0.786	12.255	64.90%	72.30%
POD4	0.829	0.777–0.880	10.885	73.00%	82.00%

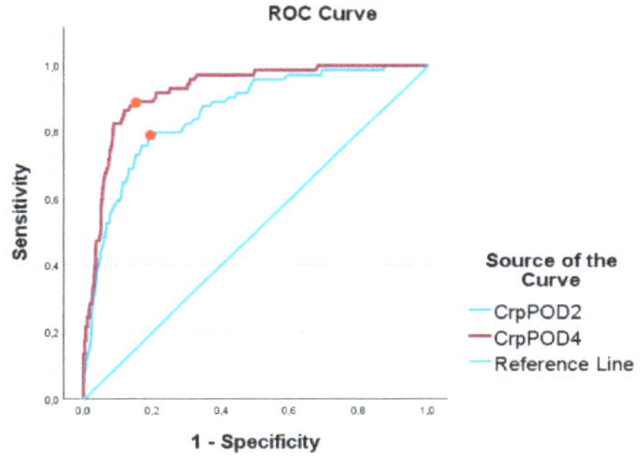

(c) CRP	AUC	95% CI	Cut-Off	sens	spec
POD2	0.859	0.816–0.903	165.5	79.70%	79.30%
POD4	0.924	0.896–0.953	181.5	86.50%	88.20%

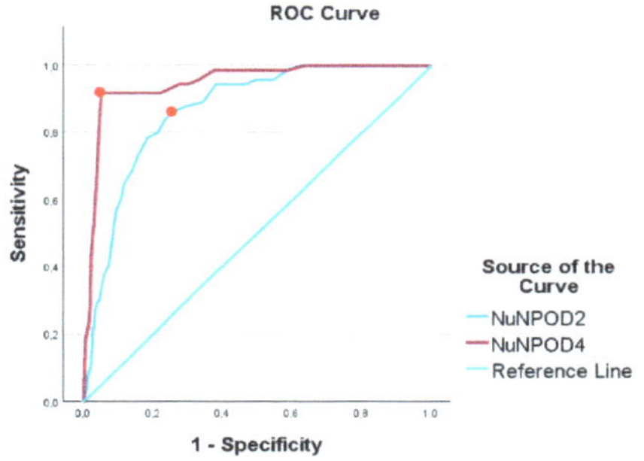

(d) NUn	AUC	95% CI	Cut-off	sens	spec
POD2	0.869	0.833–0.905	9.75	83.80%	76.80%
POD4	0.948	0.923–0.972	10.05	91.90%	94.70%

Figure 2. Receiver operating curve (ROC) for albumin, C-reactive protein, white cell count, and the NUn score on POD 2 (light blue) and POD 4 (dark red) and their diagnostic accuracy in detecting AL. (**a**) ROC curve for Alb, (**b**) ROC curve for WCC, (**c**) ROC curve for CRP, and (**d**) ROC curve for the NUn score. The X axis resembles the true positive rate (=sensitivity) and the Y axis resembles the false positive rate (=1-specificity). The red dot is the cut-off value, and Youden's J statistic is used to select the optimal predicted probability cut-off. It is the maximum vertical distance between the ROC curve and the diagonal line.

3.4. Optimal Cut-Off and Predictive Accuracy of CRP

The mean CRP levels for patients with and without AL were 218.9 versus 125.9 mg/L, respectively, on POD 2 ($p < 0.001$) and 255.2 mg/L versus 111.1 on POD 4 ($p < 0.001$). Figure 2 shows the ROC curve analyses of CRP, with a good performance on POD 2 (AUC 0.859, 95% CI: 0.816–0.903) and an excellent performance on POD 4 (AUC 0.924, 95% CI: 0.896–0.953). A POD 4 CRP threshold of 181.5 mg/L had the highest diagnostic accuracy compared to all the other individual markers. This resulted in a sensitivity of 87%, a specificity of 88%, a negative predictive value of 98%, and a positive predictive value of 48%.

3.5. Optimal Cut-Off and Predictive Accuracy of WCC

Mean WCC levels were significantly higher for patients with AL (14.0 and 13.4 $\times 10^3/\mu L$ on POD 2 and 4) compared to the those for patients without an AL (10.9 and 8.7 $\times 10^3/\mu L$ on POD 2 and 4) ($p < 0.001$). Figure 2 shows the ROC curve analyses of WCC, with a fair performance on POD 2 (AUC 0.724 95% CI: 0.662–0.786) but a good performance on POD 4 (AUC 0.829, 95% CI: 0.777–0.880). A POD 4 WCC cut-off of 10.9 $\times 10^3/\mu L$ resulted in a sensitivity of 73%, a specificity of 82%, a negative predictive value of 96%, and a positive predictive value of 33%.

3.6. Optimal Cut-Off and Predictive Accuracy of the NUn Score

Patients with AL presented a mean NUn score of 10.7 on POD 2 and 10.9 on POD 4, compared to a 9.2 score on POD 2 and 8.6 score on POD 4 in the non-AL group ($p < 0.001$). The presence of a NUn score > 10 on POD4, as presented by Noble and Underwood, was identified as a significant risk factor for AL both in the univariate and multivariate analysis in this study group. Figure 2 shows the ROC curve analyses of the NUn score, with a good performance on POD 2 (AUC 0.869, 95% CI: 0.833–0.905) and an excellent performance on POD 4 (AUC 0.948, 95% CI: 0.923–0.972). A POD 4 NUn score of >10 had the highest diagnostic accuracy compared to all the other individual markers, with a sensitivity of 92%, a specificity of 95%, a negative predictive value of 99%, and a positive predictive value of 68% (Table 3).

Table 3. Threshold values for Alb, CRP, WCC, and the NUn score and their diagnostic accuracy for AL.

Variable		AUC	95% CI	p Value	Cut-Off	Sens	Spec	PPV	NPV	PLR	NLR
Alb	POD2	0.710	0.646–0.774	<0.001	24.5	47.30%	84.40%	27.42%	92.78%	3.032	0.624
	POD4	0.799	0.746–0.853	<0.001	26.5	79.70%	68.20%	23.79%	96.42%	2.506	0.298
CRP	POD2	0.859	0.816–0.903	<0.001	165.5	79.70%	79.30%	32.42%	96.90%	3.850	0.256
	POD4	0.924	0.896–0.953	<0.001	181.5	86.50%	88.20%	47.73%	98.13%	7.330	0.153
WCC	POD2	0.724	0.662–0.786	<0.001	12.255	64.90%	72.30%	22.59%	94.30%	2.343	0.486
	POD4	0.829	0.777–0.880	<0.001	10.885	73.00%	82.00%	33.57%	96.06%	4.056	0.329
NUn	POD2	0.869	0.833–0.905	<0.001	9.75	83.80%	76.80%	31.03%	97.44%	3.612	0.211
	POD4	0.948	0.923–0.972	<0.001	10.05	91.90%	94.70%	68.36%	98.95%	17.340	0.086

AUC, area under the curve; CI, confidence interval; Sens, sensitivity; Spec, specificity; PPV, positive predictive value; NPV, negative predictive value; PLR, positive likelihood ratio; NLR, negative likelihood ratio.

4. Discussion

The failure of the esophagogastric anastomosis (12–16%) remains the most important source of prolonged hospital stay, increased risk for reoperation, stenosis, short-term reduced quality of live, increased costs, and increased perioperative death [12,22]. The effect of post-esophagectomy AL on long term oncological and functional outcome is still under debate [23–26]. The clinical presentation of AL is diverse and its severity ranges widely, mainly determined by the location and extent of the defect, the presence of contamination and sepsis, and the time from onset to treatment [12]. Early diagnosis and treatment helps to prevent subsequent sepsis and improves AL-related outcomes. This observational study demonstrates the clinical utility of both CRP and the NUn score in postoperative AL monitoring in esophagectomy patients. The high NPV and the rather low PPV, however, suggest that their main value is not the early detection, but rather the exclusion of an AL.

A postoperative drop in **Albumin** (Alb) is thought to be a marker for surgical stress. The low concentrations of Alb and prealbumin on POD 4–6 are identified as potential risk factors for AL. Five studies evaluated postoperative Alb in relation to AL but only Noble reported a significant association with a POD 5 cut-off < 22.5 g/L with fair performance (AUC 0.742) [14–16,27–30]. Our analyses identified an equally fair performance for Alb with threshold values of <24.5 on POD 2 (AUC 0.710) and <26.5 g/L on POD 4 (AUC

0.799). Given its limited accuracy, the authors do not advocate Alb alone as a predictive marker of AL. However, pre albumin, Alb in combined scores (e.g., Alb/CRP ratio, CART algorithm), and a perioperative Alb decrease of 11 g/L seem more promising as predictive markers [28,30,31].

Elevated **CRP** levels are the most commonly identified markers for post-esophagectomy complications [14–18,28–47]. CRP is an acute-phase protein synthesized in the liver in response to endotoxins, and its levels commonly increase within 6 h after the onset of the inflammation. It is a marker for acute inflammation with a high sensitivity but often low specificity for its inflammatory origin. CRP values have been studied from POD 1 to 10, with most studies focusing on POD 3–5. However, the earlier the AL is suspected, the better. We therefore focused on POD 2–4, as POD1 CRP showed low diagnostic performance in previous studies. In this study, the mean CRP levels on POD 2–4 were significantly higher in the AL group and proportionally correlated to the ECCG type of the AL, a finding consistent with Hagens et al.'s observations; however, due to the small sample size in that cohort, they could not prove statistical significance [47]. ROC curves were plotted to identify a CRP cut-off level of 165 mg/L on POD 2 with good diagnostic performance (AUC 0.859) and a cut-off level of 181 mg/L on POD 4 with excellent performance (AUC 0.924). Six other studies evaluated POD 2 CRP with varying thresholds from 177 to 300 mg/L [14,34,36,40–42]. All studies identified higher thresholds than ours on POD 2, and with lower AUCs, except Ji who identified a cut-off of 177 mg/L on POD 2 with a good performance (AUC 0.994, sens 90%, and spec 95%) similar to this study. Our POD 4 cut-off of 181 mg/L was significantly higher than the cut-off level of 111 mg/L reported by Miki [44] and 106 mg/L by Stuart [45], probably because they only included MIE patients. But it was in line with the threshold value of 177 mg/L published in a meta-analysis by Aiolfi who included all types of esophagectomy [13]. Based on the high AUC, the relevant sensitivity, specificity, low PPV, but high NPV, we could identify POD 2–4 CRP levels only to be useful in the exclusion and not in the diagnosis of an AL. This is consistent with most other studies that identify CRP as a negative predictor for AL.

Mean **WCC** levels were significantly different between the AL and the non-AL patients. However, our study identified WCC on POD 2 to have only a fair diagnostic accuracy (AUC 0.724) while in POD 4 it had a good diagnostic performance (AUC 0.829). The high NPV and low PPV again suggest clinical use as negative predictor instead of a diagnostic tool. Multiple studies evaluated WCC but only three reported cut-off values; however, they did so only on POD 3 and 5 and with poor diagnostic accuracy, eliminating the possibility for comparison [14–16,18,27,32–34,44,48].

Noble combined CRP, Alb, and white cell count in the **NUn score**, in an attempt to increase their accuracy as a AL predictor [14]. Findlay and Paireder failed to validate the score, potentially because they included all AL types, both symptomatic and asymptomatic, compared to Noble who included only "leaks sufficient to cause symptoms" [15,17]. Bundred, however, successfully validated the score's cut-off value of 10 on POD 4, with a fair diagnostic accuracy (AUC 0.77) and including only symptomatic leaks, confirmed by radiology or endoscopy consistent to Noble's definition [16]. Liesenfeld identified a sign difference between the mean NUn score of AL negative and positive patients (8.6 vs. 9.1, $p = 0.006$), but the optimal cut-off value recommended by Noble could not be confirmed as an AL predictor [18]. In this study, the NUn score seemed to have the highest accuracy of all tested biomarkers, and not just for the symptomatic AL patients as initially proven by Noble and validated by Bundred, but in all ECCG types of AL (whereas Findlay and Paireder failed to validate the score in a similar cohort).The presence of a NUn score > 10 on POD 4 was identified as a significant risk factor for AL, and the ROC curve analysis showed good performance on POD 2 (AUC 0.869) and an excellent performance on POD 4 (AUC 0.948), validating the score in this cohort.

This study has multiple pitfalls, as it is retrospective in nature, but based on prospectively collected data. We analyzed a heterogenic esophagectomy population including different procedures, approaches, and types of surgery, all known to have an impact on the AL rate, potentially biasing the results. However, we wanted to evaluate cheap and easily available tests and standardize their clinical use in postoperative monitoring for all esophagectomy patients. EC cancer is a rare disease resulting in a limited amount of annual esophagectomies. Nevertheless, we present a large population for a single-center observational study. Moreover, this is the first study to validate the NUn-score for all ECCG types in AL.

5. Conclusions

CRP and the NUn score both show good diagnostic performance on POD 2 and excellent performance on POD 4. They are, however, only valuable for AL exclusion, which can be useful in algorithms for a safe and early discharge. There is no single non-invasive test that can rule out AL, but patients with a CRP < 165 mg/L on POD 2 can proceed with oral intake according to the local ERAS protocol, and patients with a CRP < 181 mg/L or a NUn score < 10 on POD 4 are unlikely to develop an AL and can safely be discharged when clinically possible.

While highly elevated CRP levels have been consistently associated with post-operative inflammation and inflammatory complications, it is essential to acknowledge that they should not be used in isolation. CRP and NUn score kinetics over time may provide additional insights into the severity and the progression of a post-esophagectomy complications. However, daily CRP monitoring in the postoperative follow-up of esophagectomy patients seems to be a valuable strategy for the early detection of AL. Its negative predictive value and dynamic response make it a useful tool. However, clinical assessment, imaging studies, and endoscopic evaluations should be considered in junction with CRP. Based on our results, we created a center-specific diagnostic algorithm including clinical signs, CRP, NUn score, drain amylase, chest CT scan, and upper GI endoscopy to facilitate early diagnostic and surgical decision making for patients suspected for AL.

Author Contributions: Conceptualization, E.V.D., H.V., and P.P.; data curation, E.V.D., H.V., F.D., L.B.P. and E.B.; formal analysis, E.V.D. and W.C.; investigation, F.D., L.B.P. and E.B.; methodology, E.V.D.; supervision, Y.V.N., W.C. and P.P.; writing—original draft, E.V.D.; writing—review and editing, H.V., Y.V.N., W.C. and P.P. All authors have read and agreed to the published version of the manuscript.

Funding: This research received no external funding.

Institutional Review Board Statement: Ethical approval for the creation and maintenance of an observational prospective database for patients after esophageal resections was granted by the institutional Ethical Committee of the Ghent University Hospital. Belgian registration number: B670201111232 (25 June 2020). Ethical approval for this retrospective data analysis was granted by the same Ethical Committee of the Ghent University Hospital, registration number: BC-07939.

Informed Consent Statement: Informed consent was obtained from all subjects involved in the study for inclusion in the institutional dataset. The authors received a statement from their ethical committee stating that no additional informed consent is required for this retrospective analysis.

Data Availability Statement: All relevant data are available within the paper. Additional data if needed can be obtained from the corresponding author after approval by the local ethical committee.

Acknowledgments: We thank our study and data nurses for their help in constructing and supporting our esophageal database.

Conflicts of Interest: The authors declare no conflicts of interest.

References

1. Sung, H.; Ferlay, J.; Siegel, R.L.; Laversanne, M.; Soerjomataram, I.; Jemal, A.; Bray, F. Global cancer statistics 2020: GLOBOCAN estimates of incidence and mortality worldwide for 36 cancers in 185 countries. *CA A Cancer J. Clin.* **2021**, *71*, 209–249. [CrossRef]
2. van Hagen, P.; Hulshof, M.C.C.M.; Van Lanschot, J.J.B.; Steyerberg, E.W.; van Berge Henegouwen, M.I.; Wijnhoven, B.P.L.; Richel, D.J.; Nieuwenhuijzen, G.A.P.; Hospers, G.A.P.; Bonenkamp, J.J.; et al. Preoperative chemo radiotherapy for esophageal or junctional cancer. *N. Engl. J. Med.* **2012**, *366*, 2074–2084. [CrossRef]

3. Shapiro, J.; van Lanschot, J.J.B.; Hulshof, M.C.C.M.; van Hagen, P.; van Berge Henegouwen, M.I.; Wijnhoven, B.P.L.; van Laarhoven, H.W.M.; Nieuwenhuijzen, G.A.P.; Hospers, G.A.P.; Bonenkamp, J.J.; et al. Neoadjuvant chemoradiotherapy plus surgery versus surgery alone for oesophageal or junctional cancer (CROSS): Long-term results of a randomised controlled trial. *Lancet Oncol.* **2015**, *16*, 1090–1098. [CrossRef] [PubMed]
4. van der Wilk, B.J.; Eyck, B.M.; Lagarde, S.M.; van der Gaast, A.; Nuyttens, J.J.M.E.; Wijnhoven, B.P.L.; van Lanschot, J.J.B. The optimal neoadjuvant treatment of locally advanced esophageal cancer. *J. Thorac. Dis.* **2019**, *11*, S621–S631. [CrossRef]
5. Obermannová, R.; Alsina, M.; Cervantes, A.; Leong, T.; Lordick, F.; Nilsson, M.; van Grieken, N.; Vogel, A.; Smyth, E.; ESMO Guidelines Committee. Oesophageal cancer: ESMO Clinical Practice Guideline for diagnosis, treatment and follow-up. *Ann. Oncol.* **2022**, *33*, 992–1004. [CrossRef] [PubMed]
6. Lordick, F.; Mariette, C.; Haustermans, K.; Obermannová, R.; Arnold, D.; ESMO Guidelines Committee. Oesophageal cancer: ESMO CLinical proactive guidelines for diagnosis, treatment and follow up. *Ann. Oncol.* **2016**, *27*, v50–v57. [CrossRef] [PubMed]
7. Low, D.E.; Kuppusamy, M.K.; Alderson, D.; Cecconello, I.; Chang, A.C.; Darling, G.; Davies, A.; D'journo, X.B.; Gisbertz, S.S.; Griffin, S.M.; et al. Benchmarking Complications Associated with Esophagectomy. *Ann. Surg.* **2019**, *269*, 291–298. [CrossRef] [PubMed]
8. Schmidt, H.M.; Gisbertz, S.S.; Moons, J.; Rouvelas, I.; Kauppi, J.; Brown, A.; Asti, E.; Luyer, M.; Lagarde, S.M.; Berlth, F.; et al. Defining Benchmarks for Transthoracic Esophagectomy: A Multicenter Analysis of Total Minimally Invasive Esophagectomy in Low Risk Patients. *Ann. Surg.* **2017**, *266*, 814–821. [CrossRef]
9. Oesophago-Gastric Anastomosis Study Group; Fergusson, J.; Beenen, E.; Mosse, C.; Salim, J.; Cheah, S.; Wright, T.; Cerdeira, M.; McQuillan, P.; Richardson, M.; et al. Comparison of short-term outcomes from the International Oesophago-Gastric Anastomosis Audit (OGAA), the Esophagectomy Complications Consensus Group (ECCG), and the Dutch Upper Gastrointestinal Cancer Audit (DUCA). *BJS Open* **2021**, *5*, zrab010. [CrossRef]
10. Turrentine, F.E.; Denlinger, C.E.; Simpson, V.B.; Garwood, R.A.; Guerlain, S.; Agrawal, A.; Friel, C.M.; LaPar, D.J.; Stukenborg, G.J.; Jones, S.R. Morbidity, mortality, cost, and survival estimates of gastrointestinal anastomotic leaks. *J. Am. Coll. Surg.* **2015**, *220*, 195–206. [CrossRef]
11. Kassis, E.S.; Kosinski, A.S.; Ross, P.; Koppes, K.E.; Donahue, J.M.; Daniel, V.C. Predictors of anastomotic leak after esophagectomy: An analysis of the society of thoracic surgeons general thoracic database. *Ann. Thorac. Surg.* **2013**, *96*, 1919–1926. [CrossRef] [PubMed]
12. Ubels, S.; Verstegen, M.; Klarenbeek, B.; Bouwense, S.; Henegouwen, M.v.B.; Daams, F.; van Det, M.J.; A Griffiths, E.; Haveman, J.W.; Heisterkamp, J.; et al. Severity of oEsophageal Anastomotic Leak in patients after oesophagectomy: The SEAL score. *Br. J. Surg.* **2022**, *109*, 864–871. [CrossRef] [PubMed]
13. Aiolfi, A.; Asti, E.; Rausa, E.; Bonavina, G.; Bonitta, G.; Bonavina, L. Use of C-reactive protein for the early prediction of anastomotic leak after esophagectomy: Systematic review and Bayesian meta-analysis. *PLoS ONE* **2018**, *13*, e0209272. [CrossRef] [PubMed]
14. Noble, F.; Curtis, N.; Harris, S.; Kelly, J.J.; Bailey, I.S.; Byrne, J.P.; Underwood, T.J.; South Coast Cancer Collaboration–Oesophago-Gastric (SC-OG). Risk assessment using a novel score to predict anastomotic leak and major complications after oesophageal resection. *J. Gastrointest. Surg.* **2012**, *16*, 1083–1095. [CrossRef] [PubMed]
15. Findlay, J.M.; Tilson, R.C.; Harikrishnan, A.; Sgromo, B.; Marshall, R.E.K.; Maynard, N.D.; Gillies, R.S.; Middleton, M.R. Attempted validation of the NUn score and inflammatory markers as predictors of esophageal anastomotic leak and major complications. *Dis. Esophagus* **2015**, *28*, 626–633. [CrossRef] [PubMed]
16. Bundred, J.; Hollis, A.C.; Hodson, J.; Hallissey, M.T.; Whiting, J.L.; A Griffiths, E. Validation of the NUn score as a predictor of anastomotic leak and major complications after Esophagectomy. *Dis. Esophagus* **2020**, *33*, doz041. [CrossRef]
17. Paireder, M.; Jomrich, G.; Asari, R.; Kristo, I.; Gleiss, A.; Preusser, M.; Schoppmann, S.F. External validation of the NUn score for predicting anastomotic leakage after oesophageal resection. *Sci. Rep.* **2017**, *7*, 9725. [CrossRef]
18. Liesenfeld, L.F.; Sauer, P.; Diener, M.K.; Hinz, U.; Schmidt, T.; Müller-Stich, B.P.; Hackert, T.; Büchler, M.W.; Schaible, A. Prognostic value of inflammatory markers for detecting anastomotic leakage after esophageal resection. *BMC Surg.* **2020**, *20*, 324. [CrossRef]
19. Low, D.E.; Alderson, D.; Cecconello, I.; Chang, A.C.; Darling, G.; D'journo, X.B.; Griffin, S.M.; Hölscher, A.H.; Hofstetter, W.L.; Jobe, B.A.; et al. International Consensus on Standardization of Data Collection for Complications Associated with Esophagectomy: Esophagectomy Complications Consensus Group (ECCG). *Ann. Surg.* **2015**, *262*, 286–294. [CrossRef]
20. Dindo, D.; Demartines, N.; Clavien, P.-A. Classification of Surgical Complications: A New Proposal with Evaluation in a Cohort of 6336 Patients and Re-sults of a Survey. *Ann. Surg.* **2004**, *240*, 205–213. [CrossRef]
21. von Elm, E.; Altman, D.G.; Egger, M.; Pocock, S.J.; Gøtzsche, P.C.; Vandenbroucke, J.P.; STROBE Initiative. The Strengthening the Reporting of Observational Studies in Epidemiology (STROBE) Statement: Guidelines for reporting observational studies. *Int. J. Surg.* **2014**, *12*, 1495–1499. [CrossRef] [PubMed]
22. Oesophago-Gastric Anastomosis Study Group on behalf of the West Midlands Research Collaborative. Rates of Anastomotic Complications and Their Management Following Esophagectomy: Results of the Oesophago-Gastric Anastomosis Audit (OGAA). *Ann. Surg.* **2022**, *275*, e382–e391. [CrossRef] [PubMed]
23. Aiolfi, A.; Griffiths, E.A.; Sozzi, A.; Manara, M.; Bonitta, G.; Bonavina, L.; Bona, D. Effect of Anastomotic Leak on Long-Term Survival After Esophagectomy: Multivariate Meta-analysis and Restricted Mean Survival Times Examination. *Ann. Surg. Oncol.* **2023**, *30*, 5564–5572. [CrossRef] [PubMed]

24. Markar, S.; Gronnier, C.; Duhamel, A.; Mabrut, J.-Y.; Bail, J.-P.; Carrere, N.; Lefevre, J.H.; Brigand, C.; Vaillant, J.-C.; Adham, M.; et al. The impact of severe anastomotic leak on long-term survival and cancer recurrence after surgical resection for esophageal malignancy. *Ann. Surg.* **2015**, *262*, 972–980. [CrossRef]
25. Fransen, L.F.C.; Berkelmans, G.H.K.; Asti, E.; van Berge Henegouwen, M.I.; Berlth, F.; Bonavina, L.; Brown, A.; Bruns, C.; van Daele, E.; Gisbertz, S.S.; et al. Eso-Benchmark Collaborative. The effect of postoperative complications after minimally invasive esophagectomy on long-term survival: An international multicenter cohort study. *Ann. Surg.* **2021**, *274*, e1129–e1137. [CrossRef]
26. Kamarajah, S.K.; Navidi, M.; Wahed, S.; Immanuel, A.; Hayes, N.; Griffin, S.M.; Phillips, A.W. Anastomotic Leak Does Not Impact on Long-Term Outcomes in Esophageal Cancer Patients. *Ann. Surg. Oncol.* **2020**, *27*, 2414–2424. [CrossRef]
27. Gao, C.; Xu, G.; Wang, C.; Wang, D. Evaluation of preoperative risk factors and postoperative indicators for anastomotic leak of minimally invasive McKeown esophagectomy: A single-center retrospective analysis. *J. Cardiothorac. Surg.* **2019**, *14*, 46. [CrossRef]
28. Shao, C.; Liu, K.; Li, C.; Cong, Z.; Hu, L.; Luo, J.; Diao, Y.; Xu, Y.; Ji, S.; Qiang, Y.; et al. C-reactive protein to albumin ratio is a key indicator in a predictive model for anastomosis leakage after esophagectomy: Application of classification and regression tree analysis. *Thorac. Cancer* **2019**, *10*, 728–737. [CrossRef] [PubMed]
29. Lindenmann, J.; Fink-Neuboeck, N.; Porubsky, C.; Fediuk, M.; Anegg, U.; Kornprat, P.; Smolle, M.; Maier, A.; Smolle, J.; Smolle-Juettner, F.M. A nomogram illustrating the probability of anastomotic leakage following cervical esophagogastrostomy. *Surg. Endosc.* **2020**, *35*, 6123–6131. [CrossRef] [PubMed]
30. Zhang, C.; Li, X.K.; Hu, L.W.; Zheng, C.; Cong, Z.Z.; Xu, Y.; Luo, J.; Wang, G.M.; Gu, W.F.; Xie, K.; et al. Predictive value of postoperative C-reactive protein-to-albumin ratio in anastomotic leakage after esophagectomy. *J. Cardiothorac. Surg.* **2021**, *16*, 133. [CrossRef]
31. Labgaa, I.; Mantziari, S.; Genety, M.; Elliott, J.A.; Kamiya, S.; Kalff, M.C.; Winiker, M.; Pasquier, J.; Allemann, P.; Messier, M.; et al. Early postoperative decrease of albumin is an independent predictor of major complications after oncological esophagectomy: A multicenter study. *J. Surg. Oncol.* **2021**, *123*, 462–469. [CrossRef]
32. Asti, E.; Bonitta, G.; Melloni, M.; Tornese, S.; Milito, P.; Sironi, A.; Costa, E.; Bonavina, L. Utility of C-reactive protein as predictive biomarker of anastomotic leak after minimally invasive esophagectomy. *Langenbeck's Arch. Surg.* **2018**, *403*, 235–244. [CrossRef]
33. Tsujimoto, H.; Ono, S.; Takahata, R.; Hiraki, S.; Yaguchi, Y.; Kumano, I.; Matsumoto, Y.; Yoshida, K.; Aiko, S.; Ichikura, T.; et al. Systemic inflammatory response syndrome as a predictor of anastomotic leakage after esophagectomy. *Surg. Today* **2012**, *42*, 141–146. [CrossRef]
34. Hoeboer, S.H.; Groeneveld, A.B.J.; Engels, N.; van Genderen, M.; Wijnhoven, B.P.L.; van Bommel, J. Rising C-reactive protein and procalcitonin levels precede early complications after esophagectomy. *J. Gastrointest. Surg.* **2015**, *19*, 613–624. [CrossRef]
35. Gordon, A.C.; Cross, A.J.; Foo, E.W.; Roberts, R.H. C-reactive protein is a useful negative predictor of anastomotic leak in oesophago-gastric resection. *ANZ J. Surg.* **2018**, *88*, 223–227. [CrossRef]
36. Kil Park, J.; Kim, J.J.; Moon, S.W. C-reactive protein for the early prediction of anastomotic leak after esophagectomy in both neoadjuvant and non-neoadjuvant therapy case: A propensity score matching analysis. *J. Thorac. Dis.* **2017**, *9*, 3693–3702. [CrossRef]
37. Giulini, L.; Dubecz, A.; Solymosi, N.; Tank, J.; Renz, M.; Thumfart, L.; Stein, H.J. Prognostic Value of Chest-Tube Amylase Versus C-Reactive Protein as Screening Tool for Detection of Early Anastomotic Leaks After Ivor Lewis Esophagectomy. *J. Laparoendosc. Adv. Surg. Tech.* **2019**, *29*, 192–197. [CrossRef]
38. McAnena, P.; Neary, C.; Doyle, C.; Kerin, M.J.; McAnena, O.J.; Collins, C. Serial CRP levels following oesophagectomy: A marker for anastomotic dehiscence. *Ir. J. Med. Sci.* **2020**, *189*, 277–282. [CrossRef] [PubMed]
39. Kunovsky, L.; Prochazka, V.; Marek, F.; Svaton, R.; Farkasova, M.; Potrusil, M.; Moravcik, P.; Kala, Z. C-reactive protein as predictor of anastomotic complications after minimally invasive oesophagectomy. *J. Minimal Access Surg.* **2019**, *15*, 46–50. [CrossRef] [PubMed]
40. Dutta, S.; Fullarton, G.M.; Forshaw, M.J.; Horgan, P.G.; McMillan, D.C. Persistent elevation of C-reactive protein following esophagogastric cancer resection as a predictor of postopera-tive surgical site infectious complications. *Mol. Med.* **2011**, *35*, 1017–1025. [CrossRef]
41. Ji, L.; Wang, T.; Tian, L.; Gao, M. The early diagnostic value of C-reactive protein for anastomotic leakage post radical gastrectomy for esophagogastric junction carcinoma: A retrospective study of 97 patients. *Int. J. Surg.* **2016**, *27*, 182–186. [CrossRef] [PubMed]
42. Babic, B.; Tagkalos, E.; Gockel, I.; Corvinus, F.; Hadzijusufovic, E.; Hoppe-Lotichius, M.; Lang, H.; van der Sluis, P.C.; Grimminger, P.P. C-reactive Protein Levels After Esophagectomy Are Associated with Increased Surgical Trauma and Complications. *Ann. Thorac. Surg.* **2020**, *109*, 1574–1583. [CrossRef]
43. Neary, C.; McAnena, P.; McAnena, O.; Kerin, M.; Collins, C. C-Reactive Protein-Lymphocyte Ratio Identifies Patients at Low Risk for Major Morbidity after Oesophagogastric Resection for Cancer. *Dig. Surg.* **2020**, *37*, 515–523. [CrossRef] [PubMed]
44. Miki, Y.; Toyokawa, T.; Kubo, N.; Tamura, T.; Sakurai, K.; Tanaka, H.; Muguruma, K.; Yashiro, M.; Hirakawa, K.; Ohira, M. C-Reactive Protein Indicates Early Stage of Postoperative Infectious Complications in Patients Following Minimally Invasive Esophagectomy. *World J. Surg.* **2016**, *41*, 796–803. [CrossRef] [PubMed]
45. Stuart, S.K.; Kuypers, T.J.L.; Martijnse, I.S.; Heisterkamp, J.; Matthijsen, R.A. C-reactive protein and drain amylase: Their utility in ruling out anastomotic leakage after minimally invasive Ivor-Lewis esophagectomy. *Scand. J. Gastroenterol.* **2022**, *58*, 448–452. [CrossRef] [PubMed]

46. Rat, P.; Piessen, G.; Vanderbeken, M.; Chebaro, A.; Facy, O.; Rat, P.; Boisson, C.; Ortega-Deballon, P. C-reactive protein identifies patients at low risk of anastomotic leak after esophagectomy. *Langenbeck's Arch. Surg.* **2022**, *407*, 3377–3386. [CrossRef]
47. Hagens, E.R.C.; Feenstra, M.L.; Lam, W.C.; Eshuis, W.J.; Lameris, W.; Henegouwen, M.I.v.B.; Gisbertz, S.S. C-Reactive Protein as a Negative Predictive Marker for Anastomotic Leakage After Minimally Invasive Esophageal Surgery. *Mol. Med.* **2023**, *47*, 1995–2002. [CrossRef]
48. Baker, E.H.; Hill, J.S.; Reames, M.K.; Symanowski, J.; Hurley, S.C.; Salo, J.C. Drain amylase aids detection of anastomotic leak after esophagectomy. *J. Gastrointest. Oncol.* **2016**, *7*, 181–188. [CrossRef]

Disclaimer/Publisher's Note: The statements, opinions and data contained in all publications are solely those of the individual author(s) and contributor(s) and not of MDPI and/or the editor(s). MDPI and/or the editor(s) disclaim responsibility for any injury to people or property resulting from any ideas, methods, instructions or products referred to in the content.

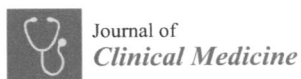 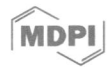

Review

Are Surgeons Going to Be Left Holding the Bag? Incisional Hernia Repair and Intra-Peritoneal Non-Absorbable Mesh Implant Complications

Andrew W. Kirkpatrick [1,2,*], Federico Coccolini [3], Matti Tolonen [4], Samual Minor [5], Fausto Catena [6], Andrea Celotti [7], Emanuel Gois, Jr. [8], Gennaro Perrone [9], Giuseppe Novelli [10], Gianluca Garulli [11], Orestis Ioannidis [12], Michael Sugrue [13], Belinda De Simone [14], Dario Tartaglia [15], Hanna Lampella [16], Fernando Ferreira [17], Luca Ansaloni [18], Neil G. Parry [19], Elif Colak [20], Mauro Podda [21], Luigi Noceroni [11], Carlo Vallicelli [6], Joao Rezende-Netos [22], Chad G. Ball [23], Jessica McKee [2], Ernest E. Moore [24] and Jack Mather [23]

1. Regional Trauma Services, Department of Surgery, Critical Care Medicine, University of Calgary, Calgary, AB T2N 2T9, Canada
2. TeleMentored Ultrasound Supported Medical Interventions (TMUSMI) Research Group, University of Calgary, Calgary, AB T3H 3W8, Canada; jessicamckee05@gmail.com
3. General, Emergency and Trauma Surgery Department, Pisa University Hospital, 56124 Pisa, Italy; federico.coccolini@gmail.com
4. Emergency Surgery Department, HUS Helsinki University Hospital, 00029 Helsinki, Finland; matti.tolonen@hus.fi
5. Department of Surgery and Critical Care Medicine, Dalhousie University, Halifax, NS B3H 4R2, Canada; sam.minor@nshealth.ca
6. Head Emergency and General Surgery Department, Bufalini Hospital, 47521 Cesena, Italy; faustocatena@gmail.com (F.C.); carlo.vallicelli@auslromagna.it (C.V.)
7. Surgery Department, ASST Cremona, 26100 Cremona, Italy; andrea.celotti@asst-cremona.it
8. Department of Surgery, Londrina State University, Londrina 86038-350, Brazil; emanuelgoisjr@me.com
9. Department of Emergency Surgery, Parma University Hospital, 43125 Parma, Italy; gennaro.perrone82@gmail.com
10. Chiurgia Generale e d'Urgenza, Osepedale Buffalini Hospital, 47521 Cesna, Italy; giuseppe.novelli@auslromagna.it
11. Hospital Infermi Rimini, 47923 Rimini, Italy; lucagarulli@gmail.com (G.G.); luigi.noceroni@auslromagna.it (L.N.)
12. 4th Department of Surgery, Medical School, Aristotle University of Thessaloniki, General Hospital "George Papanikolaou", 57010 Thessaloniki, Greece; telonakos@hotmail.com
13. Letterkenny University Hospital, F92 AE81 Donegal, Ireland; michaelesugrue@gmail.com
14. Unit of Emergency Minimally Invasive Surgery, Academic Hospital of Villeneuve-Saint-Georges, 91560 Villeneuve-Saint-Georges, France; desimone.belinda@gmail.com
15. Emergency and General Surgery Unit, New Santa Chiara Hospital, University of Pisa, 56126 Pisa, Italy; dario.tartaglia@unipi.it
16. Gastrointestinal Surgery Unit, Helsinki University Hospital, Helsinki University, 00100 Helsinki, Finland; hanna.lampela@hus.fi
17. GI Surgery and Complex Abdominal Wall Unit, Hospital CUF Porto, Faculty of Medicine of the Oporto University, 4200-319 Porto, Portugal; med1873@gmail.com
18. San Matteo Hospital of Pavia, University of Pavia, 27100 Pavia, Italy; aiace63@gmail.com
19. Department of Surgery and Medicine, Schulich School of Medicine and Dentistry, Western University, London, ON N6A 3K7, Canada; neil.parry@lhsc.on.ca
20. Samsun Training and Research Hospital, University of Samsun, 55000 Samsun, Turkey; elifmangancolak@hotmail.com
21. Department of Surgical Science, University of Cagliari, 09124 Cagliari, Italy; mauropodda@ymail.com
22. Trauma and Acute Care Surgery, General Surgery, St. Michael's Hospital, University of Toronto, Toronto, ON M5T 1P8, Canada; joao.rezende-neto@unityhealth.to
23. Acute Care, and Hepatobiliary Surgery and Regional Trauma Services, University of Calgary, Calgary, AB T2N 1N4, Canada; ball.chad@gmail.com (C.G.B.); jpmather@gmail.com (J.M.)
24. Ernest E Moore Shock Trauma Center at Denver Health, Denver, CO 80204, USA; ernest.moore@dhha.org
* Correspondence: andrew.kirkpatrick@ahs.ca or andrew.kirkpatrick@albertahealthservices.ca; Tel.: +403-944-4262; Fax: +403-944-8799

Citation: Kirkpatrick, A.W.; Coccolini, F.; Tolonen, M.; Minor, S.; Catena, F.; Celotti, A.; Gois, E., Jr.; Perrone, G.; Novelli, G.; Garulli, G.; et al. Are Surgeons Going to Be Left Holding the Bag? Incisional Hernia Repair and Intra-Peritoneal Non-Absorbable Mesh Implant Complications. *J. Clin. Med.* 2024, 13, 1005. https://doi.org/10.3390/jcm13041005

Academic Editor: Fabio Francesco Di Mola

Received: 3 January 2024
Revised: 29 January 2024
Accepted: 31 January 2024
Published: 9 February 2024

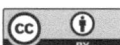

Copyright: © 2024 by the authors. Licensee MDPI, Basel, Switzerland. This article is an open access article distributed under the terms and conditions of the Creative Commons Attribution (CC BY) license (https://creativecommons.org/licenses/by/4.0/).

Abstract: Ventral incisional hernias are common indications for elective repair and frequently complicated by recurrence. Surgical meshes, which may be synthetic, bio-synthetic, or biological, decrease recurrence and, resultingly, their use has become standard. While most patients are greatly benefited, mesh represents a permanently implanted foreign body. Mesh may be implanted within the intra-peritoneal, preperitoneal, retrorectus, inlay, or onlay anatomic positions. Meshes may be associated with complications that may be early or late and range from minor to severe. Long-term complications with intra-peritoneal synthetic mesh (IPSM) in apposition to the viscera are particularly at risk for adhesions and potential enteric fistula formation. The overall rate of such complications is difficult to appreciate due to poor long-term follow-up data, although it behooves surgeons to understand these risks as they are the ones who implant these devices. All surgeons need to be aware that meshes are commercial devices that are delivered into their operating room without scientific evidence of efficacy or even safety due to the unique regulatory practices that distinguish medical devices from medications. Thus, surgeons must continue to advocate for more stringent oversight and improved scientific evaluation to serve our patients properly and protect the patient–surgeon relationship as the only rationale long-term strategy to avoid ongoing complications.

Keywords: incisional hernia; ventral hernia; mesh; complications; enteroprosthetic fistula; regulatory oversight

1. Introduction

Each year, more than 20 million hernia repairs are performed around the world. Moreover, the costs associated with these procedures are expected to reach almost USD 6.5 billion by 2027 [1]. While inguinal hernias occur most frequently, ventral incisional hernias are particularly common and uniquely problematic [2]. Indeed, in high-risk patients, this condition can be expected to occur after the index laparotomy more than 40% of the time [3–6]. Adding further complexity is that recurrence rates following repairs of these hernias can be almost 20% [7]. Thus, repair of ventral incisional hernias is frequently complicated by recurrence and, clearly, the perfect operation has yet to be found. While many patients opt not to have their hernia repaired, many others undergo different operations with varied success; indeed, many repairs often fail, leading to yet further operative interventions [8]. Ultimately, a small incisional hernia that has been the initial event can cascade into abdominal wall failure, with loss of domain of the viscera, and leaving the patient an "abdominal wall cripple."

Beginning in the late 20th century, there was increasing evidence that hernia mesh improved outcomes in management of groin hernias. As a result, more and more frequently mesh was also being used to manage ventral hernias, although this strong recommendation had very low evidence [8]. The remainder of this discussion will be specific to the use of mesh for ventral or incisional hernias. Surgical mesh is a medical device that supports the repair of a hernia as it heals. The use of mesh decreases hernia recurrences and has thus become standard practice [9–18], and has even be considered prophylactically when closing an incision at the first laparotomy [19,20]. The vast majority of patients are greatly benefited by the use of mesh, and it would be hard, if not impossible, to practice hernia surgery currently without mesh except at specialized centers or in low resource settings. Indeed, a number of different techniques have been described for the management of these hernias and for the placement of mesh. Thus, every incisional hernia repair now requires this dual choice, merging a surgical technique to a surgical implant choice.

Like almost anything in medicine, however, mesh hernia repair has a small but constant complication rate, with consequences ranging from inconvenient to devastating. Prompt and diligent attention of the surgeon can often mitigate the affects on the patient. Prompt and skillful post-operative care can rescue many mesh complications. Thus, all surgeons must be familiar with these complications and the strategies to address them. Realistically, contemporary hernia surgery is now practiced under the bright lights of medicolegal challenges and social media misinformation, and this is then combined with a bewildering array of mesh choices, providing for significant confusion amongst practitioners. Yet, despite this context, there is a distinct lack of regulatory oversight. Thus, any thorough discussion of managing complications in ventral incisional hernia must not only consider the operating room and the post-operative wards, but also the courtroom many years hence. We thus hope to comprehensively review the known complications and management options for incisional hernia repair, while highlighting areas in need of further research and understanding, specifically including the regulatory background for existing and potentially new mesh adjuncts.

2. Surgical Mesh

Historically, ventral hernia repair has been a challenging operation for the patient with a recurrence rate often exceeding 50% [21–24]. However, augmentation of the primary tissue repair with a reinforcing mesh may decrease these recurrence rates to between 2 and 36% [4]. Luijenijk's randomized trial comparing mesh repair to primary suture repair of ventral hernias demonstrated a nearly doubled recurrence rate with suture repair alone at a three-year follow-up [25]. In this study, the prosthetic mesh was sutured to the dorsal side of the fascia with either the peritoneum closed, the omentum sutured between, or an absorbable polyglactin mesh interposed between the prosthetic mesh and the viscera [25]. These authors subsequently followed their mesh-repaired patients for an average of 98 months and noted that, while the recurrence rate in the mesh group was half the suture repair rate, 17% of mesh-repaired patients had a repair related complication which consisted of small bowel obstructions (12%), fistula from mesh to skin (5%), infected mesh (2%), and enterocutaneous fistula (3%) [26]. Thus, even in this well-designed study, conclusions regarding the use of mesh, method of mesh of placement, and whether mesh is even appropriate remain complex. There thus remains a lack of objective data and much subjective opinion regarding the appropriate use of mesh in incisional hernia repair.

2.1. Mesh Classifications

In theory, surgical mesh is meant to achieve physical integrity of the components of the musculofascial layers of the abdominal wall equivalent to the native structures [22]. An ideal mesh should be non-toxic, have sufficient mechanical strength and stable physical and chemical properties, ease of handling without displacement, anti-adhesive and anti-infective properties, and it should be cost effective [17,22]. To date, the ideal mesh does not exist.

As the science continues to advance, there are now many different manufacturing processes for mesh. In addition, numerous attempts have been made to classify mesh types; from simple to complex [22]. At perhaps the most basic level, mesh can be classified into absorbable and non-absorbable. In evaluation of prosthetic meshes, they can also be classified by mesh weight, pore shape, and pore size [16,22]. Prosthetic meshes may also be differentiated as to whether they are reticular, laminar, or composite and whether they are knit or woven [1,16]. A common system is to classify synthetic mesh by porosity. Type I is considered to be "macroporous" with pore size > 10 microns; type II is "microporous" with pore size < 10 microns; and type III is a composite of both micro- and macroporous elements. Nearly all synthetic nondegradable meshes are made of polypropylene, polyvinylidene fluoride (PVDF), polyethylene terephthalate polyester, or expanded polytetrafluoroethylene (ePTFE) [16]. Composite meshes are made of two or more components and typically require a specific orientation with placement. They contain a traditional mesh component which will permit tissue ingrowth as well as a protected peritoneal side with a non-adherent mesh surface or surface coating [2,16,22,27–29]. Reticular meshes allow better ingrowth of cells between their fibers, while lamellar prostheses such as PTFE do not support cellular ingrowth within their substance [1]. Thus, PTFE meshes have been associated with poor resistance to infection as white blood cells are prevented from accessing mesh [30]. Alternatively, polypropylene has been developed with larger pore sizes and lower density. These two factors allow easier ingrowth of native tissue and vascularization which increases the resistance to infection [1]. Some macroporous prostheses contain pore sizes greater than 75 microns, which is large enough to allow ingress of cellular fibroplasia and angiogenesis. A totally microporous mesh has pores less than 10 microns in at least one dimension and can thus resist cellular ingrowth [31]. Polypropylene is the most common hernia mesh used globally but is known to cause dense adhesions to any bowel to which it is exposed [16,17,22,23]. Further, the heavy-weight mesh may be associated with chronic pain from a profound foreign body response and fibrosis in both ventral and inguinal hernias [16,32].

2.2. Biological Meshes

Biological prostheses (biological meshes or bioprosthetic materials) are classically used for complex or contaminated abdominal hernia repairs, as they may cause less inflammation and fibrosis than synthetic meshes, making them suitable for infected or potentially infected fields [33,34]. They are typically derived from human (allogenic) or animal tissues (xenogenic), such as porcine or bovine, and processed to remove cellular components, leaving behind a collagen scaffold [35]. In theory, biological meshes are designed to integrate with the patient's own tissue over time, potentially leading to a more natural and durable repair, which may result in fewer complications, especially in a contaminated field [34]. The use of biological mesh, however, comes at a high economic cost; these meshes can cost up to 200 times more than synthetic mesh. Indeed, there remain many questions regarding surgical technique, long-term outcomes, and health economics with respect to the use of biological mesh. A well-performed multi-centre randomized trial comparing synthetic versus biological mesh in contaminated ventral hernia fields (with a retromuscular placement) reported a recurrence rate nearly 4 times higher in the biological mesh group but no difference in risk of surgical site infectious complications between groups at 2-year follow-up. Moreover, the median cost of the biologic mesh was $21,539 vs. $105 for the synthetic mesh. [36]. However, intraperitoneal placement of biological meshes has not been associated with the same long-term complications as non-biological prosthetic intraperitoneal mesh placement, as we shall see below.

2.3. Anatomic Review of Mesh Placement

Surgical meshes may be implanted into a number of anatomic positions in the anterior abdominal wall (Table 1) (Figure 1). These positions constitute the intra-peritoneal, preperitoneal, retrorectus, inlay, and onlay positions [10,24,37]. These will be discussed below.

Table 1. Anatomic locations within the anterior abdominal wall utilized for permanent mesh implantation.

Location	Posterior Structures	Anterior Structures	Location-Pros	Location-Cons
Intraperitoneal	Peritoneal cavity	Peritoneum	Biomechanically strong	Adjacent to viscera Inaccessible if infected
Preperitoneal	Peritoneum	Transversalis fascia	Biomechanically strong	Potentially adjacent to viscera (peritoneal defect)
Retrorectus	Posterior Rectus Sheath	Rectus Abdominus Muscle	Biomechanically strong	Limited width of mesh (except TAR [1] uses very large mesh)
Inlay	Mesh inlaid between edges of hernia defect with no overlap	Subcutaneous tissue	None	Adjacent to Viscera Biochanically very weak
Onlay	Anterior rectus sheath and External oblique	Subcutaneous tissue	Accessible to local salvage therapies in case of infection Distant from viscera	Less biomechanically strong

[1] TAR = Transversus abdominus release.

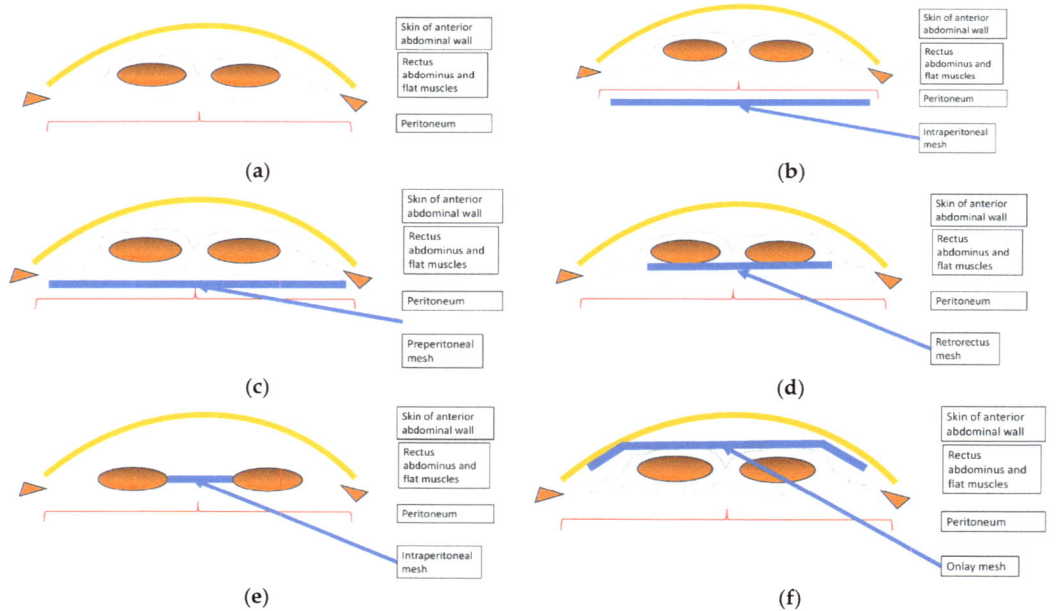

Figure 1. Schematic diagram of anatomic abdominal incisional hernia mesh placement locations. (**a**) Normal Abdominal Wall. (**b**) Intraperitoneal mesh. (**c**) Preperitoneal mesh. (**d**) Retrorectus mesh. (**e**) Inlay mesh. (**f**) Onlay mesh.

2.3.1. Intra-Peritoneal Placement of Mesh

These meshes are intended to be implanted within the peritoneal cavity proper and are, therefore, in direct contact with the intra-abdominal viscera. These devices may utilize anti-adherent physical barriers and can include prosthetic-coated, composite-coated, or biological [1]. There are also examples of intra-peritoneal non-coated synthetic meshes that are protected from visceral adhesions by interposing omentum with reportedly acceptable results in uncontrolled series [38].

2.3.2. Intra-Peritoneal Onlay Mesh (IPOM) Placement

Since the introduction of minimally invasive ventral hernia repair which consists of an intra-peritoneal onlay mesh (IPOM) technique, there has been uncertainty as to whether it benefits patients. The technique seems to confidently decrease local wound complications and may shorten hospital stay [23,24,39–41]. However, despite a moderate evidence base and numerous randomized controlled trials, there has been no conclusive determination of whether open or laparoscopic techniques, with mesh in an intra-peritoneal position, provides a benefit to patients [39,42,43]. Indeed, a pertinent comment made by the Cochrane review group is that there is a "rare but theoretically higher risk that intraabdominal organs are more likely to be injured during a laparoscopic procedure [39]". The Italian Laparoscopic Ventral Hernia Guideline group meta-analysis showed that the laparoscopic technique was associated with increased accidental full-thickness enterotomies [9]. Further, a nation-wide population-based review from France concluded that laparoscopic IPOM placement significantly increased the risk of bowel obstruction compared to patients with a previous laparotomy but no intra-peritoneal mesh [18]. The most recent Midline Incisional hernia guidelines from the European Hernia Society also state that any mesh in the abdominal cavity exposed to the abdominal viscera should be used with caution due to the risk of long-term complications at any subsequent abdominal surgery," and to "keep the mesh out of the peritoneal cavity where possible to limit contact with the viscera" [8].

2.4. Complications of Mesh Placement

Complications of intraperitoneal mesh have been generally classified as minor versus major [3]. Minor complications include seromas, hematomas, recurrent pain, and superficial surgical site infections. Major complications include hernia recurrence, complications of subsequent surgery, adhesive bowel obstruction, mesh contraction, deep prosthetic infection (i.e., mesh infection), enterocutaneous fistulae [17,18,22], and protracted medicolegal proceedings (Table 2).

Table 2. Mesh complications.

Minor
Seroma
Hematoma
Recurrent pain
Surgical site infection
Not-validated
Autoimmune reactions
Male infertility
Major
Hernia recurrence
Complication of subsequent surgery
Adhesive bowel obstruction
Mesh contraction
Mesh infection
Enteroprosthethic fistula
Enterocutaneous fistula

2.4.1. Management of Minor Complications of Incisional Hernia Repair with Mesh

Seromas frequently complicate hernia repairs when the surgical site must be dissected in order to create an anatomic space for mesh implantation. Surgeons have long been taught to liberally use wound drains to prevent post-operative fluid collections and their sequalae, such as wound dehiscence and infection. This practice, however, has not been particularly well studied in the hernia population. [44–48]. While one recent randomized study demonstrated no difference between the size of residual fluid collection between a drain vs. no-drain group, they also demonstrated a significantly lower complication rate in the drainage group, including less risk of dehiscence [46]. When a seroma does occur post-operatively, it can most frequently be managed conservatively and most resolve with time, especially if there are no features suggestive of superimposed infection. If the seroma is symptomatic and persistent, we offer repeat percutaneous aspiration or drainage. As part of the informed discussion with the patient, it is vital to reiterate that there is a small risk of introducing infection with every aspiration. If there are concerns for potential or actual infection, this can typically be confirmed with aspiration of the seroma, most easily done under ultrasound guidance. If a surgical site infection (SSI) is strongly suspected or confirmed, appropriate antibiotics should be administered early for an appropriate length of time according to the clinical response of the wound and ideally directed by culture results. The local microbiological characteristics of the hospital should be known, and infectious disease consultation may be appropriate both to treat the patient properly, but also to prevent overuse of antibiotics and development of antibiotic resistance [49]. If there is purulence or frank pus within a wound, it should be opened, and the wound packed with regular dressing changes. SSIs may or may not involve any contiguous mesh. Exposure or infection within the anatomic compartment containing the mesh intuitively increases the complexity of the problem, and a mesh infection whether acute or chronic constitutes a major complication.

Autoimmune Complications Have Not Been Validated

Fortunately, autoimmune reactions to mesh, while dramatized in the lay press after being suggested by a methodologically poor case series [50], have not been scientifically validated [51,52]. Neither has any valid evidence to support male infertility been published [53].

2.4.2. Major Complications of Incisional Hernia Repair with Mesh

Complications of Subsequent Surgery

When formulating a plan for repair of a ventral hernia, an important waypoint is to consider any ramifications of the repair on any future operative interventions. For example, mesh placement is associated with more peri-operative complications at a subsequent operation when that mesh is placed in an intra-peritoneal position [4]. Indeed, a review of such outcomes found that, after re-laparotomy, 76% of patients with previous intraperitoneal mesh placement had perioperative complications compared with only 29% in patients with pre-peritoneal mesh. Moreover, in the intraperitoneal mesh group, 21% of patients required a small bowel resection compared with none in the preperitoneal group [4].

Mesh Infection

Prosthetic mesh infection (PMI) is often a devastating complication for which there are sparingly few well-controlled scientific studies beyond biased opinion and previous experience [54]. The risk of mesh infection has been reported to be from 1% to as high as 25.6% depending on the technique, patient population, and type of mesh [16,23,28,41,55]. In particular, the incidence of infection depends heavily on mesh selection and surgical technique. Polypropylene meshes have been reported to have infection rates ranging from 2.0 to 4.2%, while ePTFE infection rates may vary from 0.0% to 9.2% [56]. Multifilament polyester meshes show the highest infection rates that may range from 7.0% to 16% [56,57]. Some authors do not consider incisional hernia repair as clean surgical cases owing to marked infection rates in some series [58], although this has not been universally accepted.

Superficial incisional infections can typically be managed without the need for mesh removal, nor are they influenced by the use or choice of mesh [55]. Oral antibiotic therapy is frequently sufficient for management. However, deep prosthetic infections can have profound deleterious effects. While the initial infection is typically acute, it can be followed by a chronic inflammatory response that may generate further fibrosis, bowel entrapment, and ultimately fistulization with internal or external enterocutaneous fistulae formation. The use of open wound management with negative pressure wound therapy may often be able to salvage an onlay polypropylene prosthetic mesh (see below). Unfortunately, PTFE or dual-coated meshes have been reported to require complete excision and are not amenable to such attempts at conservation due to their innate characteristics [55].

2.4.3. Salvage of Infected Mesh

It has been conventionally taught that management of a PMI will mandate removal of the mesh [14,55]. In practice, however, this often equates to multiple reoperations, complex wound care, and the development of a recurrent hernia potentially larger than even the inciting defect [54,59]. Depending on the location and mesh type, it may be possible to salvage some meshes using antibiotics, interventional radiology, conservative surgical debridement, and negative pressure wound therapy [15,55,60]. Warren and colleagues concluded that mesh properties and position within the abdominal wall were the primary determinants regarding salvage of infected mesh. Notably, as demonstrated in one of the largest series of PMI, mesh in an intra-peritoneal position was more frequently associated with infection (58.7% of all PMI) and was rarely salvageable (2.4% of cases) [54]. Moreover, these infections were frequently associated with development of enteroprosthetic fistulae which occurred in 17.8% of cases (53). Macroporous polypropylene mesh was salvaged in 65% of cases (>72% when used extraperitoneally). Microporous mesh, however, was salvaged in only 7.7% of cases (53). When a PMI was associated with a composite or PTFE mesh, none were salvageable. Percutaneous drainage and antibiotics were able to salvage 34.5% of cases, all of which were microporous polypropylene or biological mesh. Local wound care salvaged only 18.8% of meshes, of which 80% were macroporous polypropylene [54]. The potential salvageability of polypropylene related to other prosthetic mesh formulations has been confirmed by others [55,60]. The relative difference in salvageability of a mesh is again related to the sizes of the pores, the weave of the mesh, and its anatomic position. If the pores are large enough to allow white blood cells (WBCs) to enter within the mesh, then bacteria can be eradicated by the body, and conversely if the pores are too small, bacteria may contaminate a mesh and be physically protected as the pore size will not admit leucocytes. A large review of vacuum-assisted closure therapy with infected mesh confirmed the highest salvage with polypropylene mesh (93.5%), intermediate with composite (83.3%), and none with PTFE. Furthermore, onlay (83%) and retromuscular (98.5%) had higher rates of salvage than IPOM (56%) [60].

Although not the most favorable anatomic position biomechanically [24], the onlay placement of a polypropylene mesh facilitates VAC therapy if necessary. Intra-peritoneal mesh placement does not allow for this salvage therapy and may make earlier detection of a mesh infection more difficult leading to a delay in therapy. We, therefore, question the wisdom of placing any prosthetic mesh inside the peritoneal cavity since, when infected, they frequently cannot be rescued and, perhaps even more significantly, can lead to highly morbid intraabdominal sequelae. Warren and colleagues similarly concluded their report on infected prosthetic mesh with the statement "the high proportion of patients in this study with an IPOM technique who developed secondary mesh infection after a subsequent abdominal operation should prompt special consideration of mesh selection and its position within the abdominal wall [54]".

When the decision has been made to remove infected mesh, the next question to consider is how much mesh to remove? Bueno-Lledo et al., published a relatively large series comparing complete mesh removal to partial removal for infected prosthetic mesh [55]. Partial mesh removal involved explantation of non-incorporated mesh and was less morbid for the patient. Not unsurprisingly, complete mesh removal led to more hernia recurrence (47.9%) and more frequent and severe post-operative complications, while persistent or recurrent infection was noted more frequently with partial removal [55]. Thus, translating the best evidence still requires surgical experience to balance morbidity versus benefit for every case of mesh infection requiring operation. However, infection is not the most concerning or serious risk of an intra-peritoneal prosthetic mesh.

2.4.4. Mesh Shrinkage, "Meshomas", and Bowel Obstruction after Incisional Hernia Repair with Mesh

Mesh shrinkage may have radically different implications depending on where a mesh is implanted and whether the mesh relies upon a protective coating to avoid visceral adhesion/erosion. A "meshoma" has recently been defined as the folding or balling up of mesh which contributes to chronic pain, hernia recurrence, and or nerve entrapment [14,61]. After the implantation of any foreign object, the immune system will react with an intensity and chronicity related to the chemical and morphological construction of the mesh [1,2,22,62,63]. It is reported that this can result in seroma formation and encapsulation as well as mesh shrinkage, sometimes by up to 60% or more [22,31,62]. Meshomas related to intra-peritoneal mesh are also associated with bowel entrapment, obstructions, enteroprosthetic and enterocutaneous fistulae [54]. One animal model documented that even with "protected" composite intra-peritoneal polypropylene-based mesh, 40% of animals still developed adhesions despite the protective barriers [2]. While the risk of bowel obstruction from adhesive disease following intraperitoneal violation is well documented, there has been sparse literature evaluating the specific risk of bowel obstruction following ventral hernia repair. It is highly likely that intraperitoneal placement of mesh will increase the risk of adhesion formation and subsequent bowel obstruction and should be taken into serious consideration when determining mesh position.

2.4.5. Enteroprosthetic and Enterocutaneous Fistula after Incisional Hernia Repair with Mesh

Perhaps the most feared complication of intra-peritoneal mesh placement is that of fistula development; yet, this highly morbid sequela is poorly documented in the medical literature. Fistula creation is facilitated by erosion of the mesh into the surrounding viscera [27]. The large series previously discussed from Warren noted that most (81%) of enteroprosthetic fistulae were associated with IPOM mesh [54]. Patients with enteroprosthetic fistulae tend to present much later; on average 4 years after incisional hernia repair or subsequent surgery. The fact that many of these complications frequently occur many years after implantation renders a five-year period of post-market surveillance for serious complications inadequate to truly understand the health implications of intra-peritoneal mesh. Thus, with a delayed mesh infection occurring years after the index surgery, an enteroprosthetic fistula should strongly be suspected or anticipated [54]. This may be partial thickness such that the mesh is adherent but with complete perforation or may be full-thickness resulting in intestinal perforation. As the result of surrounding inflammation and scarring, this typically does not result in acute intra-abdominal sepsis but rather in a chronic ongoing fistula to the skin and a resultant enterocutaneous fistula. All usual resuscitative and supportive measures for intra-abdominal sepsis may be required to support an acutely sick patient [64]. Standard measures to manage the enterocutaneous fistula are also appropriate in this setting, allowing time to prepare for a definitive solution. The only way to cure this complication is to perform a complete resection of the mesh and involved viscera which may be a very morbid and complex operation. Often elderly or comorbid patients will not be able to tolerate such surgery and a life-long acceptance of this debilitating condition may be the only, albeit suboptimal, solution. Thus, a corollary to the recommendation for IPOM in patients "not fit enough for open surgery" may be the recognition that they will certainly not be fit enough for any reconstructive surgery if required in the future.

2.4.6. Comparative Evidence Supporting the Use of Intra-Peritoneal Mesh for Incisional Hernia Repair

Soare and colleagues recently performed a contemporary systematic review of complications related to the intra-peritoneal placement of mesh [3]. They concluded that this technique lacks rigorous follow-up, thus missing major and previously unforeseen long-term complications. Indeed, more rigorous randomized studies are needed to justify whether to continue with the practice [3]. Notably, joint guidelines from the European and American Hernia Societies do not advise implanting a synthetic mesh prophylactically in the intra-peritoneal space given the increased risk of adhesive complications [19]. After a review of complications occurring with intraperitoneal prosthetic mesh placement, Halm and colleagues concluded that "intra-peritoneal placement of polypropylene mesh at incisional hernia repair should be avoided if possible" and noted that intra-peritoneal meshes were associated with complications in 77% of cases requiring a subsequent relaparotomy [4]. Alternatively, the most recent Italian national guidelines on laparoscopic treatment of ventral hernias recommended laparoscopic surgery with an intra-peritoneal mesh in defects less than 10 cm, in the elderly, obese, and in emergency settings, but noted generally very low evidence and commented that the uncertain risks of an intra-peritoneal prosthesis made all their guidelines conditional [9].

3. Discussion of the Gaps

3.1. The Surgeon–Patient Relationship and Implantable Devices

No matter how complex the manufacturing–evaluation–regulatory infrastructure, it is the individual surgeon and patient who take the irreversible leap of faith to permanently implant a mesh within a human body. Although it is assumed by both that this mesh protects the patient against the distress of a hernia recurrence, it also presents some degree of life-long risk of potential infection, mesh erosion, or mesh migration [4,6,51,65]. It has been noted that the involvement of patients in the decision-making process of embarking on hernia surgery can be limited [66]. Any surgeon involved in hernia surgery and utilizing mesh products in their repair must increasingly be aware of growing medicolegal concerns as well as the growth of patient support groups focused on problems related to the use of "mesh" in their repairs [66]. There is also an ever-increasing level of mistrust between patients and the "surgical industry" in general [66]. Further, the term "mesh-injured" has appeared in the lexicon, although it may functionally encompass many interrelated issues in the conduct of hernia repair that may have no relation to mesh whatsoever [66]. Thus, repairing hernias, long considered "bread and butter" general surgery, has become an increasingly politicized field of surgery where surgeons who simply want the best outcomes for their patients may unwittingly become the "bad guy/gal". Such challenges to this practice ought to call for increasing data collection and the output of high-quality research to make advising patients simple and logical. Unfortunately, the converse has proven true. Hernia research has unfortunately been referred to as an "oxymoron". When reviewing all the published studies concerning ventral hernias, less than 3% of published studies were randomized-controlled trials [10,11]. However, any attempt at an organized analysis of surgical techniques is admirably better than the analysis of surgical devices for which there is essentially no research (discussed below).

However, despite some notable efforts, the authors soberly contend that it is a blemish on both the profession and regulators that so little good research has been performed to inform surgeons how to best to treat these patients. Indeed, the most recent combined guidelines from the European and American Hernia societies noted "the limited quantity and/or quality of the studies available to answer key questions" [19]. The frequency of this condition, however, has provided a massive profit-making opportunity for medical device companies who have marketed an array of technical options that have little good science backing them. It is a further shame that regulatory bodies charged with the responsibility to protect patients have largely abandoned this responsibility and require little or no data regarding efficacy to approve medical devices. The authors are increasingly being required to perform complex and morbid abdominal wall repairs involving hernia recurrence, bowel obstructions, and the most feared complication, mesh-incorporated enterocutaneous and enteroprosthetic fistulae. This admittedly anecdotal experience thus prompts us to attempt to understand the Regulatory and Commercial background that complicates the best practice of ventral incisional hernia surgery.

3.2. Not Better, Not Even Safe, Just "Substantially Equivalent" (To What?)

The world is rife with unsubstantiated conspiracy theories. Many, for example, still believe that that the earth is flat. While it is certainly true that, historically, pharmaceutical manufacturers have grossly violated human rights and valued corporate profits over human well-being [67], there is now strict oversight of pharmaceutical development and marketing. Contemporary pharmaceutical companies should be complimented for having developed and appropriately tested many life-saving and life-improving drugs [68]. The public can also be reassured that any new pharmaceutical marketed will have undergone a rigorous process of testing and controlled study before being allowed on the marketplace. New pharmaceuticals must undergo Phase I, Phase II, and finally rigorous Phase III prospectively randomized adequately powered trials to conclusively demonstrate their benefit to patients [69].

However, one global conspiracy that actually appears to be a valid concern, and particularly affects the practice of surgery, relates to the release of medical devices for human use. Most surgeons and patients naturally assume that the device to be implanted will have been proven safe and efficacious. Unfortunately, this is not true [70]. Simply, the Emperor has no clothes; and surgeons may be left holding the bag as ignorance is not a valid legal defence. Under most existing regulations, implantable medical devices do not have to be shown to be efficacious, or even safe, but just to be "substantially equivalent" to some other device that has been historically used in surgery [71–75]. This means that as long as some surgeon previously believed that using some device was "a good idea," any corporation can introduce a new device to the market that is "substantially equivalent" to the older device that was "grandfathered" into practice. The United States Food and Drug Administration (FDA) standards of evidence relate to predicate devices (devices which can be legally marketed and serve as a point of comparison for new devices) marketed as part of interstate commerce prior to May 28, 1976. Beyond this "equivalence", minimal to no evidence of effectiveness, efficacy, or even usefulness is required to market a medical device in Canada or the United States [74,76]. In the United States, this process is known as the 510 (k) exemption. A "510 (k)" is a "premarket submission made to the FDA to demonstrate that the device to be marketed is as safe and effective, that is, substantially equivalent, to a legally marketed device [77]." With an exemption to this 510 (k) policy, the approval process no longer requires post-market surveillance for complications which ironically seems to put the onus on surgeons to report problems rather than ensuring safety prior to market release. Shah and colleagues recently reported that while few 510 (k)-exempt devices had any published research even 5 years after release, and 10% of these devices were actually subject to recalls [76]. All surgical meshes ever cleared for clinical use have been 510 (k)-exempt and have, therefore, not required any real research [71]. Zargar and Carr reported a remarkable analysis of the regulatory ancestral history of surgical meshes and noted that 97% of meshes introduced between 2013 and 2015, were descended through "substantial equivalence" from only 6 meshes present prior to 1976. Further alarming was the fact that 16% of recently approved meshes were connected through equivalence claims to 3 predicate devices that were actually recalled for flaws causing serious adverse events [71]. This is very concerning as a practicing surgeon will be subjected to a constant barrage of marketing pressure to use new devices with the reassurance that they are "approved". The result has been the relative uncontrolled proliferation of expensive medical devices marketed as "innovations" with the implied message that if surgeons do not use these devices, they are "laggards". All practicing surgeons will surely note the great irony that individual manufacturers will emphasize the uniqueness of their own proprietary mesh when advocating for market share, yet twist themselves 180 degrees to emphasize the monotony of similarity with previous mesh when applying for regularity approval. Upon review, Kahan concluded that there was "extreme under-reporting and lack of consistency of clinically important mesh properties" [78].

For example, the Kugel Patch consists of a product-line of hernia mesh products introduced in the 1990s. The manufacturer received reports that these devices were failing as early as 2002, but waited almost three years before recalling the mesh [79]. The Composix hernia patch was recalled once it was identified that the recoil ring may break, which could potentially lead to bowel perforation and or chronic enteric fistula [79]. This device was also approved by the FDA 510 (k) "workaround" strategy in 2001 as being "substantially equivalent" to a previous mesh [79]. Ultimately, the manufacturer recalled more than 137,000 of these devices between 2005 and 2007, and paid more than $180 million to settle litigation in 2011 in the United States and $1.4 million to settle related lawsuits in Canada in 2014 [80]. Some of the authors have personally removed entero-prosthetic fistula from our own patients related to this device. A further comment on the confusing regulatory science of recalled meshes on one continent is that they seem to still be available years afterwards on other continents with differing regulations [81,82]. Even more disturbing is that, as Zargar and colleagues have noted, recalled meshes associated with adverse effects may, indirectly, continue to serve as predicates for new devices, thus raising significant concerns over the safety of the regulatory approval process itself [71].

3.3. A Global Medicolegal Risk to a Hernia Surgeons

Any surgeon would be naïve to ignore the society within which they practice their craft. Although we have taken oaths to care for our patients and to do no harm, it is impossible to conduct ourselves according to that oath without scientific data. Scientific reports in the medical literature regarding mesh concerns are scant, yet there is an abundant, almost overwhelming amount of medicolegal and opinion advocacy online. Any search of the internet will reveal that the most prominently accessible websites will be those offering to commence legal action by a specially focused hernia mesh lawyer. Although accurate data are not available, the internet would suggest there are more lawyers specializing in litigating hernia mesh lawsuits than there are surgeons specializing in mesh hernia repair. Furthermore, these hernia mesh lawyers seem to enjoy a greater degree of confidence regarding evidence appraisal as they dramatically "inform" patients as to, for example, the symptoms that allergies to mesh produce while soliciting business [83]. Such conclusive but completely science-deprived legal communications contrast starkly with carefully appraised scientific studies that cautiously conclude that "there is little to no evidence that the use of polypropylene mesh can lead to autoimmunity" [51,52]. However, any patient accessing the internet will find the legal advertising rather than the appraised science.

As surgeons, we are taught to obtain our information from peer-reviewed medical journals, and to disregard the mass of "grey literature" or frank dis-information available on the Internet. However, such a purist approach will leave surgeons grossly unaware of the beliefs, understandings, and opinions of the populations we attempt to serve. In Canada, respected news media report that at least 12 brands of hernia mesh have been recalled or removed from the Canadian marketplace since 2000, but PubMed will not reveal this to surgeons. In fairness, the media also accurately reported that the majority of hernia mesh patients have no problems and that data show hernia mesh improves recovery and lowers recurrences [84]. It is thus very easy for patients to access legal websites providing them with some basic facts regarding proprietary meshes that have been removed over mesh-specific concerns. However, finding actual scientific data to better educate surgeons to be experts is impossible as the topic of mesh recall seems to have been ignored by Academia. The British Broadcasting Agency (BBC) has well stated the situation reporting that "currently, hernia mesh devices can be approved if they are similar to older products, which themselves may not have been required to undergo any rigorous testing or clinical trials in order to assess their safety or efficacy" [85]. Further, the BBC further voiced the opinion of the authors that "there is a lot of secrecy surrounding the approval of hernia mesh, with even doctors unable to access the clinical data" [85].

There may be the awakenings of initial consciousness in regulatory agencies, however. In 2014, after product recalls and ongoing compensation litigation, the FDA reclassified synthetic and non-synthetic meshes for pelvic organ prolapse from Class II to Class III devices, meaning that actual research would be required for future meshes in this category. Unsurprisingly, no new such meshes have been introduced since [71]. The authors (who practice hernia repair), believe that in order to enhance the protection of all patients, new devices must be proven safe and that prospective clinical trials must the minimal standard. We further suggest that, given the massive costs of healthcare, the safety of new devices must also be prospectively studied in the context of patient-centric outcomes and, ideally, economics to prove that any new device is actually "better." Otherwise, why are they needed in the first place?

4. Conclusions and Future Directions

Given the immense complexity of the use of mesh for incisional hernia repair, the authors are not able to answer many of the key questions surrounding this topic. We do conclude that prosthetic mesh repairs have benefited many patients globally. We continue to perform prosthetic mesh-augmented incisional hernia repair, but we believe it is prudent to avoid intra-peritoneal placement of any prosthetic mesh until adequate and conclusive scientific studies have been completed. We further warn all surgeons that in the current highly litigious climate, future medicolegal concerns regarding any use of mesh should be anticipated and that current regulatory bodies of many if not most First World nations do not appear to have prioritized the interests of patients, surgeons, or science as part of their framework. It is thus a complex but urgent responsibility for surgeons to try to understand the issues better and to advocate for good scientific data that will vindicate us when the judge states the obvious fact that "doctor, the operative reports clearly records that YOU made the decision to implant this device".

Author Contributions: Conceptualization, A.W.K., F.C. (Federico Coccolini), S.M., M.P., C.G.B., E.E.M. and J.M. (Jack Mather); methodology, A.W.K. and F.C. (Federico Coccolini); validation, all authors; formal analysis, A.W.K.; investigation, A.W.K.; data curation, A.W.K.; writing—original draft preparation, A.W.K.; writing—review and editing, all authors; visualization, A.W.K., F.F. and J.M. (Jack Mather); supervision, A.W.K.; project administration, A.W.K. and J.M. (Jack Mather). All authors have read and agreed to the published version of the manuscript.

Funding: This research received no external funding.

Institutional Review Board Statement: Not applicable.

Informed Consent Statement: Not applicable.

Data Availability Statement: No new data were created or analyzed in this study. Data sharing is not applicable to this article.

Conflicts of Interest: A.W.K. serves as the PI of the COOL trial, which previously was partially supported by the 3M/Acelity Corporation until August 2022. A.W.K. is also a member of the Canadian Forces Medical Services and has consulted for the 3m/Acelity Corporation, Zoll Medical, Innovative Trauma Care, and CSL Behring. He is the Director of the TeleMentored Ultrasound Supported Medical Interventions (TMUSMI) Research group and serves in the Canadian Forces Medical Services. S.M. received research support and speaking honorarium from COOK Biotech. M.S. reported consultancy for 3 M/Acelity and Novus Scientific. N.G.P. reported being a medical advisor for Front Line Medical Technologies—Cobra REBOA. J.L.M. reported consultancies with the Aceso, Innovative Trauma. Care, A.W.K., and Zoll Corporations, as well as consulting with the Geneva Foundation and South Trail Psychology. E.E.M. no relevant conflicts of interests, although currently the PI on studies funded by Prytime and Humacyte.

References

1. Serrano-Aroca, A.; Pous-Serrano, S. Prosthetic meshes for hernia repair: State of art, classification, biomaterials, antimicrobial approaches, and fabrication methods. *J. Biomed. Mater. Res. A* **2021**, *109*, 2695–2719. [CrossRef] [PubMed]
2. Novitsky, Y.W.; Harrell, A.G.; Cristiano, J.A.; Paton, B.L.; Norton, H.J.; Peindl, R.D.; Kercher, K.W.; Heniford, B.T. Comparative evaluation of adhesion formation, strength of ingrowth, and textile properties of prosthetic meshes after long-term intra-abdominal implantation in a rabbit. *J. Surg. Res.* **2007**, *140*, 6–11. [CrossRef] [PubMed]
3. Soare, A.M.; Cartu, D.; Nechita, S.L.; Andronic, O.; Surlin, V. Complications of Intraperitoneal Mesh Techniques for Incisional Hernia—A Systematic Review. *Chirurgia* **2021**, *116* (Suppl. S6), S36–S42. [PubMed]
4. Halm, J.A.; de Wall, L.L.; Steyerberg, E.W.; Jeekel, J.; Lange, J.F. Intraperitoneal polypropylene mesh hernia repair complicates subsequent abdominal surgery. *World J. Surg.* **2007**, *31*, 423–429, discussion 430. [CrossRef]
5. Aiolfi, A.; Bona, D.; Gambero, F.; Sozzi, A.; Bonitta, G.; Rausa, E.; Bruni, P.G.; Cavalli, M.; Campanelli, G. What is the ideal mesh location for incisional hernia prevention during elective laparotomy? A network meta-analysis of randomized trials. *Int. J. Surg.* **2023**, *109*, 1373–1381. [CrossRef]
6. Millas, S.G.; Mesar, T.; Patel, R.J. Chronic abdominal pain after ventral hernia due to mesh migration and erosion into the sigmoid colon from a distant site: A case report and review of literature. *Hernia* **2015**, *19*, 849–852. [CrossRef]
7. Howard, R.; Thumma, J.; Ehlers, A.; Englesbe, M.; Dimick, J.; Telem, D. Reoperation for Recurrence Up to 10 Years After Hernia Repair. *JAMA* **2022**, *327*, 872–874. [CrossRef]
8. Sanders, D.L.; Pawlak, M.M.; Simons, M.P.; Aufenacker, T.; Balla, A.; Berger, C.; Berrevoet, F.; de Beaux, A.C.; East, B.; Henriksen, N.A.; et al. Midline incisional hernia guidelines: The European Hernia Society. *Br. J. Surg.* **2023**, *110*, 1732–1768. [CrossRef]
9. Campanile, F.C.; Podda, M.; Pecchini, F.; Inama, M.; Molfino, S.; Bonino, M.A.; Ortenzi, M.; Silecchia, G.; Agresta, F.; Cinquini, M.; et al. Laparoscopic treatment of ventral hernias: The Italian national guidelines. *Updates Surg.* **2023**, *75*, 1305–1336. [CrossRef]
10. Sagar, A.; Tapuria, N. An Evaluation of the Evidence Guiding Adult Midline Ventral Hernia Repair. *Surg. J.* **2022**, *8*, e145–e156. [CrossRef]
11. Liang, M.K.; Holihan, J.L.; Itani, K.; Alawadi, Z.M.; Gonzalez, J.R.; Askenasy, E.P.; Ballecer, C.; Chong, H.S.; Goldblatt, M.I.; Greenberg, J.A.; et al. Ventral Hernia Management: Expert Consensus Guided by Systematic Review. *Ann. Surg.* **2017**, *265*, 80–89. [CrossRef]

12. Birindelli, A.; Sartelli, M.; Di Saverio, S.; Coccolini, F.; Ansaloni, L.; van Ramshorst, G.H.; Campanelli, G.; Khokha, V.; Moore, E.E.; Peitzman, A.; et al. 2017 update of the WSES guidelines for emergency repair of complicated abdominal wall hernias. *World J. Emerg. Surg.* **2017**, *12*, 37. [CrossRef]
13. Ventral Hernia Working, G.; Breuing, K.; Butler, C.E.; Ferzoco, S.; Franz, M.; Hultman, C.S.; Kilbridge, J.F.; Rosen, M.; Silverman, R.P.; Vargo, D. Incisional ventral hernias: Review of the literature and recommendations regarding the grading and technique of repair. *Surgery* **2010**, *148*, 544–558. [CrossRef]
14. Sharma, R.; Fadaee, N.; Zarrinkhoo, E.; Towfigh, S. Why we remove mesh. *Hernia* **2018**, *22*, 953–959. [CrossRef]
15. Shubinets, V.; Carney, M.J.; Colen, D.L.; Mirzabeigi, M.N.; Weissler, J.M.; Lanni, M.A.; Braslow, B.M.; Fischer, J.P.; Kovach, S.J. Management of Infected Mesh After Abdominal Hernia Repair: Systematic Review and Single-Institution Experience. *Ann. Plast. Surg.* **2018**, *80*, 145–153. [CrossRef]
16. Rastegarpour, A.; Cheung, M.; Vardhan, M.; Ibrahim, M.M.; Butler, C.E.; Levinson, H. Surgical mesh for ventral incisional hernia repairs: Understanding mesh design. *Plast. Surg.* **2016**, *24*, 41–50. [CrossRef]
17. Ansaloni, L.; Catena, F.; Coccolini, F.; Fini, M.; Gazzotti, F.; Giardino, R.; Pinna, A.D. Peritoneal adhesions to prosthetic materials: An experimental comparative study of treated and untreated polypropylene meshes placed in the abdominal cavity. *J. Laparoendosc. Adv. Surg. Tech. A* **2009**, *19*, 369–374. [CrossRef]
18. Delorme, T.; Cottenet, J.; Abo-Alhassan, F.; Bernard, A.; Ortega-Deballon, P.; Quantin, C. Does intraperitoneal mesh increase the risk of bowel obstruction? A nationwide French analysis. *Hernia* **2023**. [CrossRef] [PubMed]
19. Deerenberg, E.B.; Henriksen, N.A.; Antoniou, G.A.; Antoniou, S.A.; Bramer, W.M.; Fischer, J.P.; Fortelny, R.H.; Gok, H.; Harris, H.W.; Hope, W.; et al. Updated guideline for closure of abdominal wall incisions from the European and American Hernia Societies. *Br. J. Surg.* **2022**, *109*, 1239–1250. [CrossRef] [PubMed]
20. Sugrue, M.; Johnston, A.; Zeeshan, S.; Loughlin, P.; Bucholc, M.; Watson, A. The role of prophylactic mesh placement to prevent incisional hernia in laparotomy. Is it time to change practice? *Anaesthesiol. Intensive Ther.* **2019**, *51*, 323–329. [CrossRef] [PubMed]
21. Luijendijk, R.W.; Lemmen, M.H.; Hop, W.C.; Wereldsma, J.C. Incisional hernia recurrence following "vest-over-pants" or vertical Mayo repair of primary hernias of the midline. *World J. Surg.* **1997**, *21*, 62–65, discussion 66. [CrossRef]
22. Saiding, Q.; Chen, Y.; Wang, J.; Pereira, C.L.; Sarmento, B.; Cui, W.; Chen, X. Abdominal wall hernia repair: From prosthetic meshes to smart materials. *Mater. Today Bio* **2023**, *21*, 100691. [CrossRef] [PubMed]
23. Brown, R.H.; Subramanian, A.; Hwang, C.S.; Chang, S.; Awad, S.S. Comparison of infectious complications with synthetic mesh in ventral hernia repair. *Am. J. Surg.* **2013**, *205*, 182–187. [CrossRef] [PubMed]
24. Van Hoef, S.; Tollens, T. Primary non-complicated midline ventral hernia: Is laparoscopic IPOM still a reasonable approach? *Hernia* **2019**, *23*, 915–925. [CrossRef] [PubMed]
25. Luijendijk, R.W.; Hop, W.C.; van den Tol, M.P.; de Lange, D.C.; Braaksma, M.M.; IJzermans, J.N.M.; Boelhouwer, R.U.; de Vries, B.C.; Salu, M.K.; Wereldsma, J.C.; et al. A comparison of suture repair with mesh repair for incisional hernia. *N. Engl. J. Med.* **2000**, *343*, 392–398. [CrossRef] [PubMed]
26. Burger, J.W.; Luijendijk, R.W.; Hop, W.C.; Halm, J.A.; Verdaasdonk, E.G.; Jeekel, J. Long-term follow-up of a randomized controlled trial of suture versus mesh repair of incisional hernia. *Ann. Surg.* **2004**, *240*, 578–583, discussion 583–585. [CrossRef]
27. Voisard, G.; Feldman, L.S. An unusual cause of chronic anemia and abdominal pain caused by transmural mesh migration in the small bowel after laparoscopic incisional hernia repair. *Hernia* **2013**, *17*, 673–677. [CrossRef]
28. Cobb, W.S.; Carbonell, A.M.; Kalbaugh, C.L.; Jones, Y.; Lokey, J.S. Infection risk of open placement of intraperitoneal composite mesh. *Am. Surg.* **2009**, *75*, 762–767, discussion 767–768. [CrossRef]
29. Prasad, P.; Tantia, O.; Patle, N.M.; Khanna, S.; Sen, B. Laparoscopic ventral hernia repair: A comparative study of transabdominal preperitoneal versus intraperitoneal onlay mesh repair. *J. Laparoendosc. Adv. Surg. Tech. A* **2011**, *21*, 477–483. [CrossRef] [PubMed]
30. Paton, B.L.; Novitsky, Y.W.; Zerey, M.; Sing, R.F.; Kercher, K.W.; Heniford, B.T. Management of infections of polytetrafluoroethylene-based mesh. *Surg. Infect.* **2007**, *8*, 337–341. [CrossRef]
31. Amid, P.K. Classification of biomaterials and their related complications in abdominal wall hernia surgery. *Hernia* **1997**, *1*, 15–21. [CrossRef]
32. Sajid, M.S.; Leaver, C.; Baig, M.K.; Sains, P. Systematic review and meta-analysis of the use of lightweight versus heavyweight mesh in open inguinal hernia repair. *Br. J. Surg.* **2012**, *99*, 29–37. [CrossRef] [PubMed]
33. See, C.W.; Kim, T.; Zhu, D. Hernia mesh and hernia repair: A review. *Eng. Regen.* **2020**, *1*, 19–33. [CrossRef]
34. Costa, A.; Adamo, S.; Gossetti, F.; D'Amore, L.; Ceci, F.; Negro, P.; Bruzzone, P. Biological Scaffolds for Abdominal Wall Repair: Future in Clinical Application? *Materials* **2019**, *12*, 2375. [CrossRef] [PubMed]
35. King, K.S.; Albino, F.P.; Bhanot, P. Biologic mesh for abdominal wall reconstruction. *Chronic Wound Care Manag. Res.* **2014**, *1*, 57–65. [CrossRef]
36. Rosen, M.J.; Krpata, D.M.; Petro, C.C.; Carbonell, A.; Warren, J.; Poulose, B.K.; Costanzo, A.; Tu, C.; Blatnik, J.; Prabhu, A.S. Biologic vs Synthetic Mesh for Single-stage Repair of Contaminated Ventral Hernias: A Randomized Clinical Trial. *JAMA Surg.* **2022**, *157*, 293–301. [CrossRef]
37. Parker, S.G.; Halligan, S.; Liang, M.K.; Muysoms, F.E.; Adrales, G.L.; Boutall, A.; de Beaux, A.C.; Dietz, U.A.; Divino, C.M.; Hawn, M.T.; et al. International classification of abdominal wall planes (ICAP) to describe mesh insertion for ventral hernia repair. *Br. J. Surg.* **2020**, *107*, 209–217. [CrossRef]

38. Sorour, M.A. Interposition of the omentum and/or the peritoneum in the emergency repair of large ventral hernias with polypropylene mesh. *Int. J. Surg.* **2014**, *12*, 578–586. [CrossRef]
39. Sauerland, S.; Walgenbach, M.; Habermalz, B.; Seiler, C.M.; Miserez, M. Laparoscopic versus open surgical techniques for ventral or incisional hernia repair. *Cochrane Database Syst. Rev.* **2011**, *3*, CD007781. [CrossRef]
40. Tofolo Pasquini, M.; Medina, P.; Arrechea Antelo, R.; Cerutti, R.; Agustín Porto, E.; Enrique Pirchi, D. Ring closure outcome for laparoscopic ventral hernia repair (IPOM plus) in medium and large defects. Long-term follow-up. *Surg. Endosc.* **2023**, *37*, 2078–2084. [CrossRef]
41. Sanchez, V.M.; Abi-Haidar, Y.E.; Itani, K.M. Mesh infection in ventral incisional hernia repair: Incidence, contributing factors, and treatment. *Surg. Infect.* **2011**, *12*, 205–210. [CrossRef]
42. Al Chalabi, H.; Larkin, J.; Mehigan, B.; McCormick, P. A systematic review of laparoscopic versus open abdominal incisional hernia repair, with meta-analysis of randomized controlled trials. *Int. J. Surg.* **2015**, *20*, 65–74. [CrossRef]
43. Awaiz, A.; Rahman, F.; Hossain, M.B.; Yunus, R.M.; Khan, S.; Memon, B.; Memon, M.A. Meta-analysis and systematic review of laparoscopic versus open mesh repair for elective incisional hernia. *Hernia* **2015**, *19*, 449–463. [CrossRef]
44. Gurusamy, K.S.; Allen, V.B. Wound drains after incisional hernia repair. *Cochrane Database Syst. Rev.* **2013**, CD005570. [CrossRef]
45. Louis, V.; Diab, S.; Villemin, A.; Brigand, C.; Manfredelli, S.; Delhorme, J.B.; Rohr, S.; Romain, B. Do surgical drains reduce surgical site occurrence and infection after incisional hernia repair with sublay mesh? A non-randomised pilot study. *Hernia* **2023**, *27*, 873–881. [CrossRef] [PubMed]
46. Mohamedahmed, A.Y.Y.; Zaman, S.; Ghassemi, N.; Ghassemi, A.; Wuheb, A.A.; Abdalla, H.E.E.; Hajibandeh, S.; Hajibandeh, S. Should routine surgical wound drainage after ventral hernia repair be avoided? A systematic review and meta-analysis. *Hernia* **2023**, *27*, 781–793. [CrossRef] [PubMed]
47. Willemin, M.; Schaffer, C.; Kefleyesus, A.; Dayer, A.; Demartines, N.; Schafer, M.; Allemann, P. Drain Versus No Drain in Open Mesh Repair for Incisional Hernia, Results of a Prospective Randomized Controlled Trial. *World J. Surg.* **2023**, *47*, 461–468. [CrossRef] [PubMed]
48. Sahm, M.; Pross, M.; Hukauf, M.; Adolf, D.; Kockerling, F.; Mantke, R. Drain versus no drain in elective open incisional hernia operations: A registry-based analysis with 39,523 patients. *Hernia* **2023**, 1–15. [CrossRef] [PubMed]
49. Sartelli, M.; Weber, D.G.; Ruppe, E.; Bassetti, M.; Wright, B.J.; Ansaloni, L.; Catena, F.; Coccolini, F.; Abu-Zidan, F.M.; Coimbra, R.; et al. Antimicrobials: A global alliance for optimizing their rational use in intra-abdominal infections (AGORA). *World J. Emerg. Surg.* **2016**, *11*, 33. [CrossRef] [PubMed]
50. Cohen Tervaert, J.W. Autoinflammatory/autoimmunity syndrome induced by adjuvants (Shoenfeld's syndrome) in patients after a polypropylene mesh implantation. *Best. Pract. Res. Clin. Rheumatol.* **2018**, *32*, 511–520. [CrossRef] [PubMed]
51. Jisova, B.; Wolesky, J.; Strizova, Z.; de Beaux, A.; East, B. Autoimmunity and hernia mesh: Fact or fiction? *Hernia* **2023**, *27*, 741–749. [CrossRef]
52. Kowalik, C.R.; Zwolsman, S.E.; Malekzadeh, A.; Roumen, R.M.H.; Zwaans, W.A.R.; Roovers, J. Are polypropylene mesh implants associated with systemic autoimmune inflammatory syndromes? A systematic review. *Hernia* **2022**, *26*, 401–410. [CrossRef]
53. Dong, Z.; Kujawa, S.A.; Wang, C.; Zhao, H. Does the use of hernia mesh in surgical inguinal hernia repairs cause male infertility? A systematic review and descriptive analysis. *Reprod. Health* **2018**, *15*, 69. [CrossRef]
54. Warren, J.A.; Love, M.; Cobb, W.S.; Beffa, L.R.; Couto, F.J.; Hancock, B.H.; Morrow, D.; Ewing, J.A.; Carbonell, A.M. Factors affecting salvage rate of infected prosthetic mesh. *Am. J. Surg.* **2020**, *220*, 751–756. [CrossRef]
55. Bueno-Lledo, J.; Torregrosa-Gallud, A.; Carreno-Saenz, O.; Garcia-Pastor, P.; Carbonell-Tatay, F.; Bonafe-Diana, S.; Iserte-Hernandez, J. Partial versus complete removal of the infected mesh after abdominal wall hernia repair. *Am. J. Surg.* **2017**, *214*, 47–52. [CrossRef]
56. Engelsman, A.F.; van der Mei, H.C.; Ploeg, R.J.; Busscher, H.J. The phenomenon of infection with abdominal wall reconstruction. *Biomaterials* **2007**, *28*, 2314–2327. [CrossRef] [PubMed]
57. Leber, G.E.; Garb, J.L.; Alexander, A.I.; Reed, W.P. Long-term complications associated with prosthetic repair of incisional hernias. *Arch. Surg.* **1998**, *133*, 378–382. [CrossRef] [PubMed]
58. Houck, J.P.; Rypins, E.B.; Sarfeh, I.J.; Juler, G.L.; Shimoda, K.J. Repair of incisional hernia. *Surg. Gynecol. Obstet.* **1989**, *169*, 397–399. [PubMed]
59. Ober, I.; Stulenau, T.; Ball, C.g.; Nickerson, D.; Kirkpatrick, A.W. It all doesn't have to go: Abdominal wall reconstruction involving selective synthethic mesh explantation with bioilogic mesh salvage. *Can. J. Surg.* **2023**, in press. [CrossRef] [PubMed]
60. Li, J.; Wang, Y.; Shao, X.; Cheng, T. The salvage of mesh infection after hernia repair with the use of negative pressure wound therapy (NPWT), a systematic review. *ANZ J. Surg.* **2022**, *92*, 2448–2456. [CrossRef] [PubMed]
61. Amid, P.K. Radiologic images of meshoma: A new phenomenon causing chronic pain after prosthetic repair of abdominal wall hernias. *Arch. Surg.* **2004**, *139*, 1297–1298. [CrossRef]
62. Klinge, U.; Klosterhalfen, B.; Muller, M.; Schumpelick, V. Foreign body reaction to meshes used for the repair of abdominal wall hernias. *Eur. J. Surg. = Acta Chir.* **1999**, *165*, 665–673. [CrossRef]
63. Rosch, R.; Junge, K.; Schachtrupp, A.; Klinge, U.; Klosterhalfen, B.; Schumpelick, V. Mesh implants in hernia repair. Inflammatory cell response in a rat model. *Eur. Surg. Res.* **2003**, *35*, 161–166. [CrossRef] [PubMed]

64. Sartelli, M.; Coccolini, F.; Kluger, Y.; Agastra, E.; Abu-Zidan, F.M.; Abbas, A.E.S.; Ansaloni, L.; Adesunkanmi, A.K.; Atanasov, B.; Augustin, G.; et al. WSES/GAIS/SIS-E/WSIS/AAST global clinical pathways for patients with intra-abdominal infections. *World J. Emerg. Surg.* **2021**, *16*, 49. [CrossRef] [PubMed]
65. Zhang, Y.; Lin, H.; Liu, J.M.; Wang, X.; Cui, Y.F.; Lu, Z.Y. Mesh erosion into the colon following repair of parastomal hernia: A case report. *World J. Gastrointest. Surg.* **2023**, *15*, 294–302. [CrossRef] [PubMed]
66. East, B.; Hill, S.; Dames, N.; Blackwell, S.; Laidlaw, L.; Gok, H.; Stabilini, C.; de Beaux, A. Patient Views Around Their Hernia Surgery: A Worldwide Online Survey Promoted Through Social Media. *Front. Surg.* **2021**, *8*, 769938. [CrossRef] [PubMed]
67. Johnson, M.; Stokes, R.G.; Arndt, T. *The Thalidomide Catastrophe: How it Hapened, Who Was Responsible and Why the Search for Justice Continues after More Than Six Decades*; Onwards and Upwards Publishers: Cranbrook, UK, 2018.
68. Wikepedia. Big Pharma Conspiracy Theories. Available online: https://en.wikipedia.org/wiki/Big_Pharma_conspiracy_theories (accessed on 28 August 2022).
69. Darrow, J.J.; Dhruva, S.S.; Redberg, R.F. Changing FDA Approval Standards: Ethical Implications for Patient Consent. *J. Gen. Intern. Med.* **2021**, *36*, 3212–3214. [CrossRef] [PubMed]
70. Kirkpatrick, A.W.; Minor, S.; Coccolini, F. Why is there no data? Critically ill patients deserve better protection from both Regulatory Authorities and Surgeons. *J. Trauma Acute Care Surg.* **2023**, *95*, e61–e62. [CrossRef] [PubMed]
71. Zargar, N.; Carr, A. The regulatory ancestral network of surgical meshes. *PLoS ONE* **2018**, *13*, e0197883. [CrossRef]
72. Dietrich, E.M.; Sharfstein, J.M. Improving medical device regulation: A work in progress. *JAMA Intern. Med.* **2014**, *174*, 1779–1780. [CrossRef]
73. Dubin, J.R.; Simon, S.D.; Norrell, K.; Perera, J.; Gowen, J.; Cil, A. Risk of Recall Among Medical Devices Undergoing US Food and Drug Administration 510(k) Clearance and Premarket Approval, 2008–2017. *JAMA Netw Open* **2021**, *4*, e217274. [CrossRef]
74. Curfman, G.D.; Redberg, R.F. Medical devices—Balancing regulation and innovation. *N. Engl. J. Med.* **2011**, *365*, 975–977. [CrossRef]
75. Ashar, B.S.; Dang, J.M.; Krause, D.; Luke, M.C. Performing clinical studies involving hernia mesh devices: What every investigator should know about the FDA investigational device exemption (IDE) process. *Hernia* **2011**, *15*, 603–605. [CrossRef]
76. Shah, P.; Olavarria, O.; Dhanani, N.; Ciomperlik, H.; Mohr, C.; Bernardi, K.; Neela, N.; Coelho, R.; Ali, Z.; Prabhu, A.; et al. The Food and Drug Administration's (FDA's) 510(k) Process: A Systematic Review of 1000 Cases. *Am. J. Med.* **2023**, *136*, 172–178. [CrossRef] [PubMed]
77. Center for Devices and Radiological Health Food and Drug Administration. Premarket Notification 510(k). Available online: www.fda.gov/medical-devices/premarket-submissions-selecting-and-preparing-correct-submission/premarket-notification-510k (accessed on 28 December 2023).
78. Kahan, L.G.; Blatnik, J.A. Critical Under-Reporting of Hernia Mesh Properties and Development of a Novel Package Label. *J. Am. Coll. Surg.* **2018**, *226*, 117–125. [CrossRef] [PubMed]
79. US Food and Drug Administration. Medical Device Recalls. 2023. Available online: https://www.accessdata.fda.gov/scripts/cdrh/cfdocs/cfRes/res.cfm?start_search=1&event_id=&productdescriptiontxt=kugel&productcode=&IVDProducts=&rootCauseText=&recallstatus=%C2%A2erclassificationtypetext=&recallnumber=&postdatefrom=&postdateto=&productshortreasontxt=&firmlegalnam=&PMA_510K_Num=&pnumber=&knumber=&sortcolumn=cda (accessed on 24 August 2023).
80. Turner, T.; Miller, E.K. Kugel Patch. 2022. Available online: https://www.drugwatch.com/hernia-mesh/kugel-patch/ (accessed on 24 August 2023).
81. Yasuda, A.; Yasuda, T.; Kato, H.; Iwama, M.; Shiraishi, O.; Hiraki, Y.; Tanaka, Y.; Shinkai, M.; Imano, M.; Kimura, Y.; et al. A case of incisional hernia repair using Composix mesh prosthesis after antethoracic pedicled jejunal flap reconstruction following an esophagectomy. *Surg. Case Rep.* **2017**, *3*, 79. [CrossRef] [PubMed]
82. Yamagishi, S.; Aramaki, O.; Yoshida, N.; Mitsuka, Y.; Kawai, T.; Yamazaki, S.; Kang, W.; Nakayama, H.; Moriguchi, M.; Higaki, T.; et al. Laparoscopic-assisted modified Kugel herniorrhaphy for obturator hernia: A case report. *J. Surg. Case Rep.* **2022**, *2022*, rjac035. [CrossRef] [PubMed]
83. Miller, P. Hernia Mesh Complications: Allergy to Mesh and The Bodies' Response. 2017. Available online: https://herniameshlawsuit.ca/article/hernia-mesh-complications-allergy-mesh-bodies-response/ (accessed on 24 August 2023).
84. Favaro, A.; St Phillip, E. Growing Concerns in Canada Over Surgical Mesh Usage, Recalls: CTV News. 2017. Available online: https://www.ctvnews.ca/health/growing-concerns-in-canada-over-surgical-mesh-usage-recalls-1.3372733#:~:text=Figures%20from%20Health%20Canada%20show%20that%20some%2012,serious%20injury%20and%20other%20complications,%20including%20three%20deaths (accessed on 24 August 2023).
85. Collinson, R.; Furst, J. Hernia Mesh Implants Used 'With No Clinical Evidence': British Broadcasting Network. 2020. Available online: https://www.bbc.com/news/health-51024974?fbclid=IwAR3YX7TvYt30kiwsJ__QnClyYFshUZLIuzQRqZOFF1oHyiiWnHIaR7rGDeo (accessed on 24 August 2023).

Disclaimer/Publisher's Note: The statements, opinions and data contained in all publications are solely those of the individual author(s) and contributor(s) and not of MDPI and/or the editor(s). MDPI and/or the editor(s) disclaim responsibility for any injury to people or property resulting from any ideas, methods, instructions or products referred to in the content.

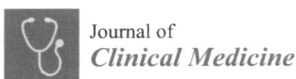 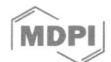

Systematic Review

Mesh Rectopexy or Resection Rectopexy for Rectal Prolapse; Is There a Gold Standard Method: A Systematic Review, Meta-Analysis and Trial Sequential Analysis

Georgios Koimtzis [1,*], Leandros Stefanopoulos [2], Georgios Geropoulos [3], Christopher G. Chalklin [4], Ioannis Karniadakis [4], Awad A. Alawad [4], Vyron Alexandrou [5], Nikos Tteralli [6], Eliot Carrington-Windo [7], Andreas Papacharalampous [8] and Kyriakos Psarras [9]

1. Department of Oesophageal and Gastric Surgery, University Hospital of Wales, Cardiff and Vale University Health Board, Cardiff CF14 4XW, UK
2. Department of Electrical and Computer Engineering, Northwestern University, 633 Clark St., Evanston, IL 60208, USA; leandros@northwestern.edu
3. Western General Hospital, NHS Lothian, Crewe Road South, Edinburgh EH4 2XU, UK; georgios.geropoulos@nhs.net
4. Cardiff Transplant Unit, University Hospital of Wales, Cardiff and Vale University Health Board, Cardiff CF14 4XW, UK; christopher.chalklin@wales.nhs.uk (C.G.C.); ioannis.karniadakis@wales.nhs.uk (I.K.); awad.alawad@wales.nhs.uk (A.A.A.)
5. Urology Department, General Hospital of Thessaloniki "G. Gennimata-Agios Dimitrios", Elenis Zografou 2, 54634 Thessaloniki, Greece; vyrwnal@hotmail.com
6. Department of General Surgery, North Hampshire NHS Foundation Trust, Basingstoke RG24 9NA, UK; nikos.tteralli@hhft.nhs.uk
7. Department of General Surgery, Grange University Hospital, Caerleon Road, Llanfrechfa, Cwmbran NP44 8YN, UK; eliot.carrington-windo@wales.nhs.uk
8. Department of Surgery Larnaca General Hospital Pandoras, Larnaca 6301, Cyprus; andreaspch96@hotmail.com
9. School of Medicine, Second Surgical Propedeutic Department, Ippokrateio General Hospital, Aristotle University of Thessaloniki, Konstantinoupoleos 49, 54642 Thessaloniki, Greece; psarrask@auth.gr
* Correspondence: georgios.koimtzis@wales.nhs.uk

Abstract: (1) Background: Rectal prolapse is a benign condition that mainly affects females and the elderly. The most common symptoms are constipation and incontinence. The treatment of choice is surgical, but so far, there has been no gold standard method. The aim of this study is to compare the two most common intrabdominal procedures utilized for treating rectal prolapse: the resection rectopexy and the mesh rectopexy. (2) Methods: In this study, we conducted a thorough systematic review and meta-analysis of the available literature and compared the two different approaches regarding their complication rate, recurrence rate, and improvement of symptoms rate. (3) Results: No statistically significant difference between the two methods was found regarding the operating time, the length of stay, the overall complication rate, the surgical site infection rate, the cardiopulmonary complication rate, the improvement in constipation and incontinence rates, and the recurrence rate. (4) Conclusions: Our study revealed that mesh rectopexy and resection rectopexy for rectal prolapse have similar short- and long-term outcomes. As a result, the decision for the procedure used should be individualized and based on the surgeon's preference and expertise.

Keywords: rectal prolapse; resection rectopexy; mesh rectopexy

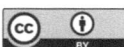

1. Introduction

Rectal prolapse is a rare, benign disease that has an incidence of 0.5% in the general population. It mainly affects females and the elderly. It is defined as the full-thickness protrusion of the rectal wall through the anus (external prolapse) [1]. On the other hand, internal rectal prolapse is defined as intussusception of the rectum above the level of the sphincteric mechanism [1]. The most predominant risk factors for rectal prolapse include old age, straining, traumatic vaginal delivery, or multiple vaginal deliveries. Nonetheless, in younger patients, the risk factors include chronic psychiatric diseases, previous pelvic surgery, redundant sigmoid colon, inflammatory bowel disease or colitis, irritable bowel syndrome, family history of gastrointestinal diseases, uterovaginal prolapse, solitary rectal ulcer, and Ehlers–Danlos syndrome [2]. Usually, rectal prolapse presents with fecal incontinence, constipation, or both, while it is also associated with blood and mucous discharge from the anus [3]. The diagnosis and assessment of external rectal prolapse do not usually require any specific diagnostic investigation, apart from the cases where fecal incontinence is present. Nonetheless, in the assessment of internal rectal prolapse, various diagnostic modalities may be useful, such as barium dynamic assessment and magnetic resonance or isotope defecography. Treatment of rectal prolapse is mainly surgical. Currently, there have been more than 120 techniques described in the literature, but there is a lack of consensus regarding the best available option, and no gold standard method has been suggested so far [4,5]. However, only a few procedures are routinely applied [1]. Generally, these procedures can be separated into two large categories: the ones that are carried out using a peritoneal approach and the ones that are performed through a perineal approach. The latest guidelines published by the American Society of Colorectal Surgeons suggest that for patients with satisfactory performance status and acceptable risk, a peritoneal approach should be used as it leads to lower recurrence rates and more satisfactory functional outcomes [1]. Nowadays, the most frequently used peritoneal procedures include the resection rectopexy and mesh rectopexy [4–8].

These operations can be carried out by open, laparoscopic, or robotic approach [9,10]. All of them include elevation of the rectum out of the pelvis in order to correct the protrusion, followed by stabilization (rectopexy) with different methods on the presacral fascia [2]. Resection rectopexy, also known as the Frykman–Goldberg procedure [11], consists of sigmoidectomy, tension-free anastomosis of the colon, and rectopexy with sutures on the presacral fascia [10]. During this procedure, the mesorectum is initially dissected to the level of the pelvic floor, both anteriorly and posteriorly. The level reached corresponds to the upper edge of the external sphincter, while the lateral ligaments are left completely intact. After the resection is complete, the Douglas' pouch or the rectovesical space is reconstructed by suturing the peritoneum to the right and left of the rectum. The rectopexy is completed by suturing the anterior rectal wall to the peritoneum. Mesh rectopexy without resection is another alternative that consists of a mesh or biological graft placement to reinforce either the anterior rectum or to fixate the rectum on the sacrum [12–15]. In this procedure, the initial dissection is similar to the one carried out for the resection rectopexy. However, after the level of the pelvic floor muscles is reached, a mesh is used to complete the rectopexy. The mesh is usually fashioned in a spatula shape and is placed anteriorly to the rectum. It is then fixated to the sides of the rectum using absorbable sutures and then fixated to the sacral promontory. The adhesive material can also be used to secure the mesh to the anterior rectal wall. Finally, the mesh is covered by approximating the pelvic peritoneum.

The purpose of our current study is to assess whether one of the above-mentioned procedures (resection rectopexy or mesh rectopexy) has better outcomes than the other. These procedures were compared regarding their complication rate, recurrence rate, and the patients' quality of life postoperatively (constipation and fecal incontinence improvement).

2. Materials and Methods

This systematic review and meta-analysis were carried out without a pre-existing registered protocol. It has been prepared by strictly adhering to the PRISMA checklist. A thorough and systematic literature search was performed to identify studies that compared the postoperative outcomes of resection rectopexy and mesh rectopexy for treating rectal prolapse. The databases that were looked into for relevant studies published in English were MEDLINE, Scopus, and Cochrane Library databases until 31 May 2023. An additional search to identify any available grey literature was carried out on the websites of international colorectal associations and on the abstract books of relevant conferences. The search of the MEDLINE database was carried out using the following search string: ((rectal prolapse[MeSH Terms]) AND (resection rectopexy)) AND (mesh rectopexy). Similar search strings were used for the other databases.

Firstly, two independent researchers (I.K. and G.G.) performed a detailed search of the above-mentioned databases. The inclusion criteria to which the generated studies were compared to were the following: (1) studies performed on human patients; (2) patients suffering from rectal prolapse undergoing operative treatment with either resection or mesh rectopexy; (3) articles written in English; and (4) articles having sufficient and extractable data on the operating time, length of stay, complication rate, recurrence rate and constipation and incontinence improvement rate. When there was a case of disagreement between the two reviewers, another experienced reviewer (N.T.) provided their opinion, and the ultimate decision on these studies was based on either a consensus or the majority opinion.

Data extraction was performed by two independent members of the research team (V.A. and E.C.-W.), and their findings were confirmed by a third assessor (A.P.). Extracted data from each article include the first author's name, the publication date, the study design, the number of patients included, the patients' demographics (age and sex), the type of procedure they underwent, the operating time, the length of stay, the overall complication rate, the surgical site infection rate, the cardiopulmonary complication rate, the recurrence rate, the improvement of constipation and improvement of incontinence rate and the mortality rate.

In this meta-analysis, all statistical analyses were conducted by utilizing Reviewer Manager 5.4.1 software [Review Manager (RevMan) (computer program) version 5.4.1, Copenhagen: The Nordic Cochrane Centre, Denmark, the Cochrane Collaboration, 2020] and STATA version 16.1. The data in this study are presented as mean ± standard deviation, while odds ratios (ORs) and weighted mean differences (WMDs) with a confidence interval (CI) of 95% were calculated for dichotomous and continuous variables, respectively. The level of statistical significance was set at a p-value of less than 0.05. When large heterogeneity among the studies ($I^2 \geq 50\%$) was present, a random effects model was applied, while in cases of low heterogeneity, a fixed effects model was utilized. When a random effects model was applied, sensitivity analysis was carried out at the levels of $I^2 = 50\%$ and $I^2 = 25\%$ to assess the effect of the large heterogeneity of the studies on the outcome of the meta-analysis. The publication bias was assessed by designing the respective Begg's funnel plot. Trial sequential analysis (TSA) was also carried out to evaluate whether the sample size in each analysis was enough to yield valid results or if further studies were needed. The software used to conduct TSA was Trial Sequential Analysis (TSA) (computer program) version 0.9.5.10 beta, Copenhagen Trial Unit, Centre for Clinical Intervention Research, Capital Region, Copenhagen University Hospital—Rigshospitalet, 2021.

The potential risk of bias across the studies that were included in this systematic review and meta-analysis was assessed using the 'Cochrane Collaboration tool for assessing the risk of bias' as integrated into the Review Manager 5.4.1 software, and the outcomes are presented in a risk of bias graph and a risk of bias summary.

3. Results

The initial literature search of the online archives resulted in a collective number of 160 articles, while one more was revealed through the search for grey literature. Following the removal of duplicates, the number of articles was brought down to 148. Afterward, the identified studies were screened according to their title and abstract, ultimately resulting in 48 articles eligible for full-text analysis. The remaining articles were not included because they investigated different research questions to the one of our study, or on the grounds of including non-adult patients, or because the required data were not extractable. Following the full-text analysis, eight studies in total [12–19] were eligible for inclusion in the qualitative and quantitative analysis. The selection process of the included articles can be found in Figure 1.

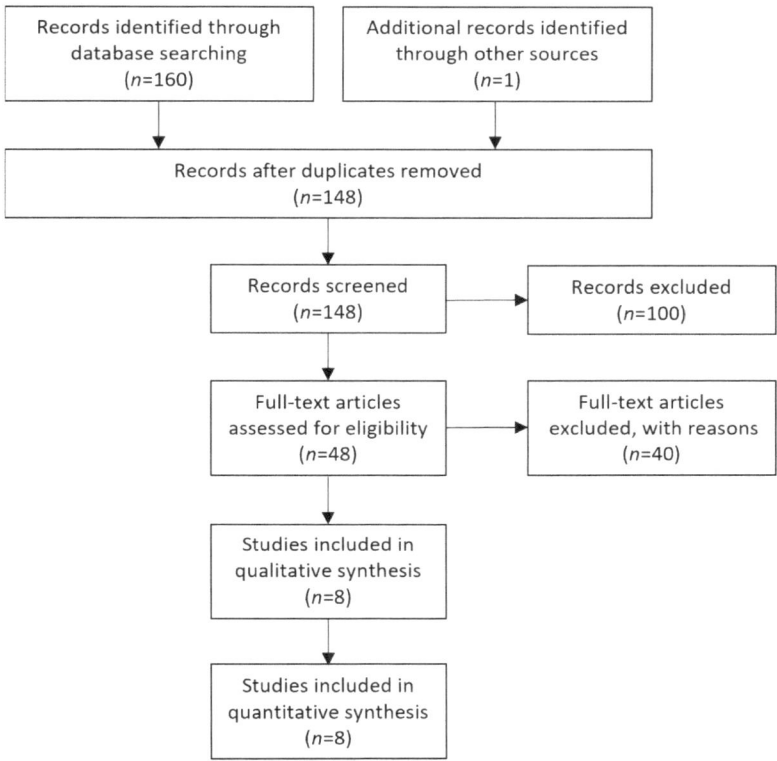

Figure 1. PRISMA flowchart depicting the study selection method.

The manuscripts included in the final analysis were published between 1992 and 2018. Three of these studies were prospective and randomized, while the rest were retrospective. The total number of patients included in these studies was 483, with 207 undergoing resection rectopexy and 276 undergoing mesh rectopexy. The basic characteristics of each individual article can be found in Table 1.

Two [11,12] out of the eight selected studies had extractable data on the operating time of the procedures carried out, and our statistical analysis showed that the two methods did not differ significantly (WMD 68.16, 95% CI −30.28 to 166.6). This analysis is shown in Figure 2. However, the sensitivity analysis of this random effect model with $I^2 = 50\%$ and $I^2 = 25\%$, revealed a statistically significant difference indicating longer operative time in cases of resection (WMD 53.15, 95% CI 24.37 to 81.93, $p < 0.001$ and WMD 44.85, 95% CI 23.22 to 66.48, $p < 0.001$, respectively). Similarly, two studies [11,16] provided data on the length of stay, and the meta-analysis revealed similar outcomes between the two methods (WMD 0.65, 95% CI −0.16 to 1.45). This outcome is shown in Figure 3.

Regarding the overall complication rate, six studies provided data [10–13,16,17], and the meta-analysis showed that the two methods did not differ significantly (OR 1.56, 95% CI 0.62 to 3.96). This finding is demonstrated in Figure 4. The sensitivity analysis of this random effects model meta-analysis with $I^2 = 50\%$ and $I^2 = 25\%$ confirmed the above findings (logOR −0.37, 95% CI −1.13 to 0.38, $p = 0.334$ and logOR −0.23, CI 95% −0.83 to 0.35, $p = 0.433$, respectively). Also, a statistical analysis of the rate of surgical site infections that was mentioned in three studies showed that the two methods under study had similar outcomes (OR 1.39, 95% CI 0.37 to 5.23). This outcome is shown In Figure 5. Furthermore, the comparison of the cardiopulmonary complication rate that was mentioned in five studies showed that the two methods under investigation did not differ significantly (OR

2.01, 95% CI 0.78 to 5.22). This outcome is shown in Figure 6. Moreover, only one case of death was reported by Luukkonen et al. in the resection group on the second postoperative day due to myocardial infarction.

Table 1. Primary characteristics of the selected articles [12–19].

Authors	Study Type	Resection Rectopexy (n)	Mesh Rectopexy (n)	Age in the Resection Group [Mean ± SD or Median (min, max)]	Age in the Mesh Group [Mean ± SD or Median (min, max)]	Sex (Male/Female)
McKee et al. [16]	Prospective, randomized	9	9	69 ± 4	70 ± 4	4/14
Luukkonen et al. [15]	Prospective, randomized	15	15	65.6	66.8	2/28
Benoist et al. [13]	Retrospective	18	14	53.5 ± 20.8	66.3 ± 17.3	3/29
Demirbas et al. [14]	Retrospective	13	20	25.3 (21–33)	24.7 (19–57)	31/2
Lechaux et al. [17]	Retrospective	13	35	53 (18–87)		4/44
Senapati et al. [19]	Prospective, randomized	32	35	58 ± 18	58 ± 16	10/68 (10 patients lost in follow-up)
Forminje Jonkers et al. [18]	Retrospective	28	40	50.1 ± 17.9	67.0 ± 15.4	4/64
Carvalho et al. [12]	Retrospective	79	108	53.86 ± 19.33	59.03 ± 17.0	12/175

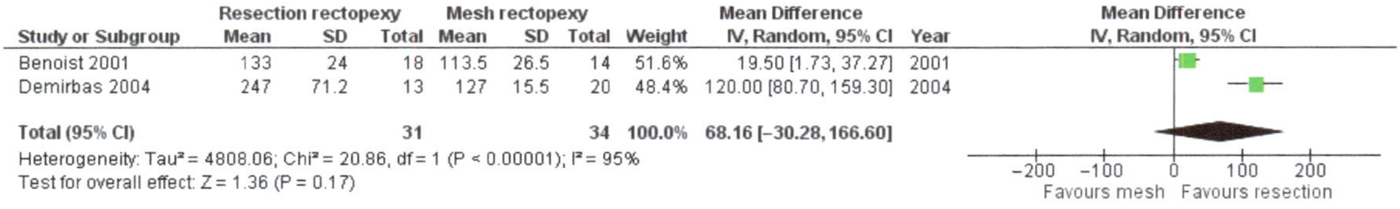

Figure 2. Forest plot of the analysis of the operative time of the compared procedures [13,14].

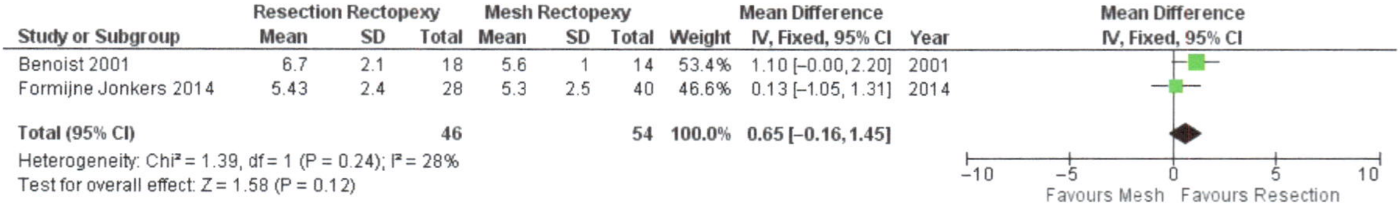

Figure 3. Forest plot of the analysis of the length of stay of the compared procedures [13,18].

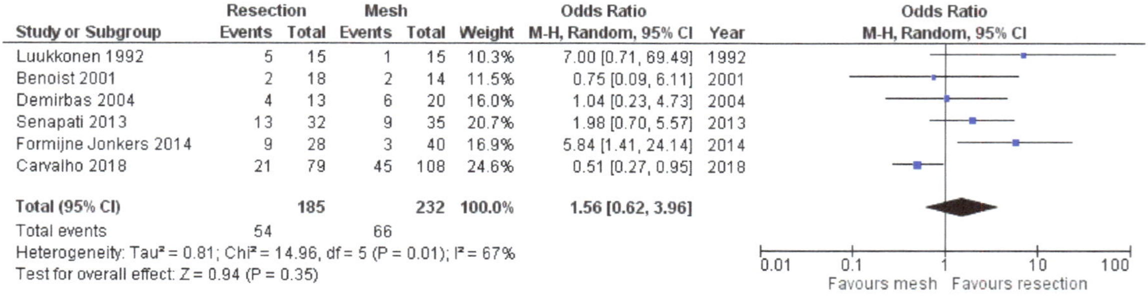

Figure 4. Forest plot demonstrating the comparison of the overall complication rate [12–15,18,19].

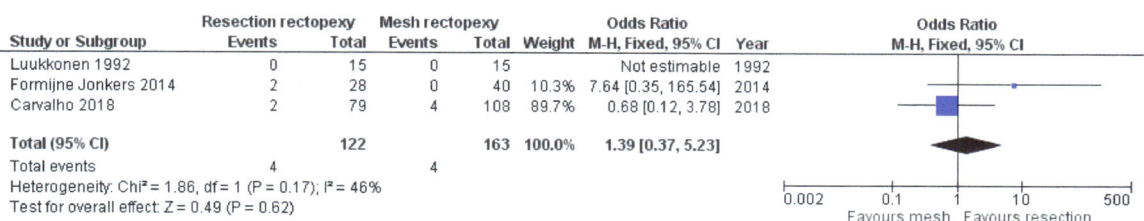

Figure 5. Forest plot demonstrating the comparison of the surgical site infection rate [12,15,18].

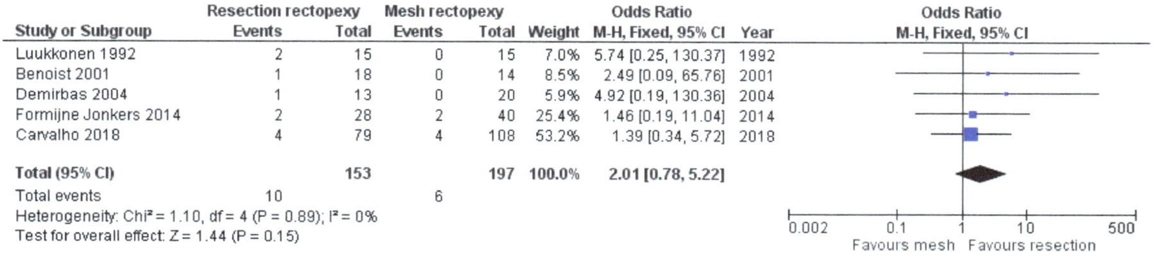

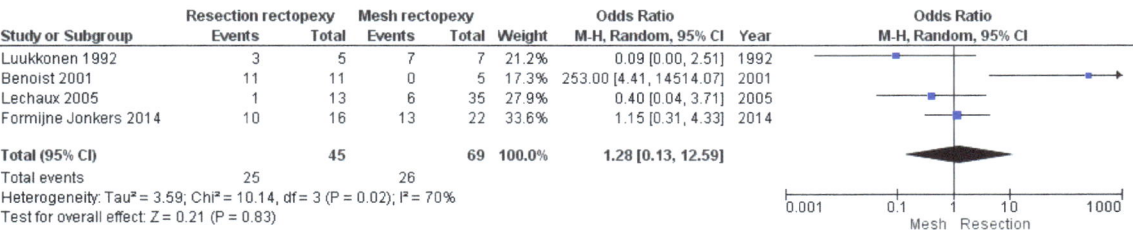

Figure 6. Forest plot demonstrating the comparison of the cardiopulmonary complication rate [12–15,18].

Regarding the long-term post-operative outcomes, there are comparable outcomes in the rate of constipation improvement between the two methods (OR 12.59, 95% CI 0.13 to 12.59). This outcome is shown in Figure 7. As this meta-analysis was carried out with an random effects model due to the large heterogeneity, we conducted a further sensitivity analysis with $I^2 = 50\%$ and $I^2 = 25\%$, which confirmed our findings (logOR -0.123, CI 95% -0.186 to 1.61 $p = 0.889$ and logOR -0.04, CI 95% -1.38 to 1.30, $p = 0.953$). Moreover, the two techniques had comparable outcomes in the rate of incontinence improvement (OR 1.60, 95% CI 0.65 to 3.91). This outcome is shown in Figure 8. Finally, no statistically significant difference between the two methods was identified when comparing the recurrence rate (OR 0.42, 95% CI 0.14 to 1.30). This comparison is demonstrated in Figure 9.

Based on the designed Funnel plots, no publication bias was identified across all the studies selected in all eight analyses performed. These outcomes are portrayed in Figure 10. Nonetheless, the trial sequential analysis performed revealed that more studies are required to corroborate our findings for all the comparisons made, apart from the operative time where the number of patients was sufficient to draw valid conclusions. The outcomes of the trial sequential analysis are shown in Figure 11.

Figure 7. Forest plot of the analysis of the constipation improvement rate [13,15,17,18].

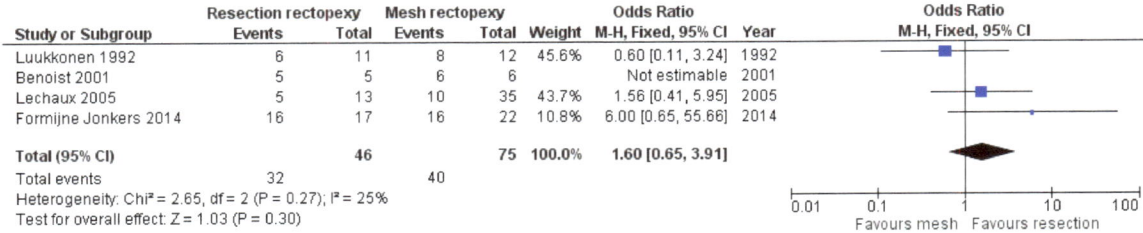

Figure 8. Forest plot of the comparison of the incontinence improvement rate [13,15,17,18].

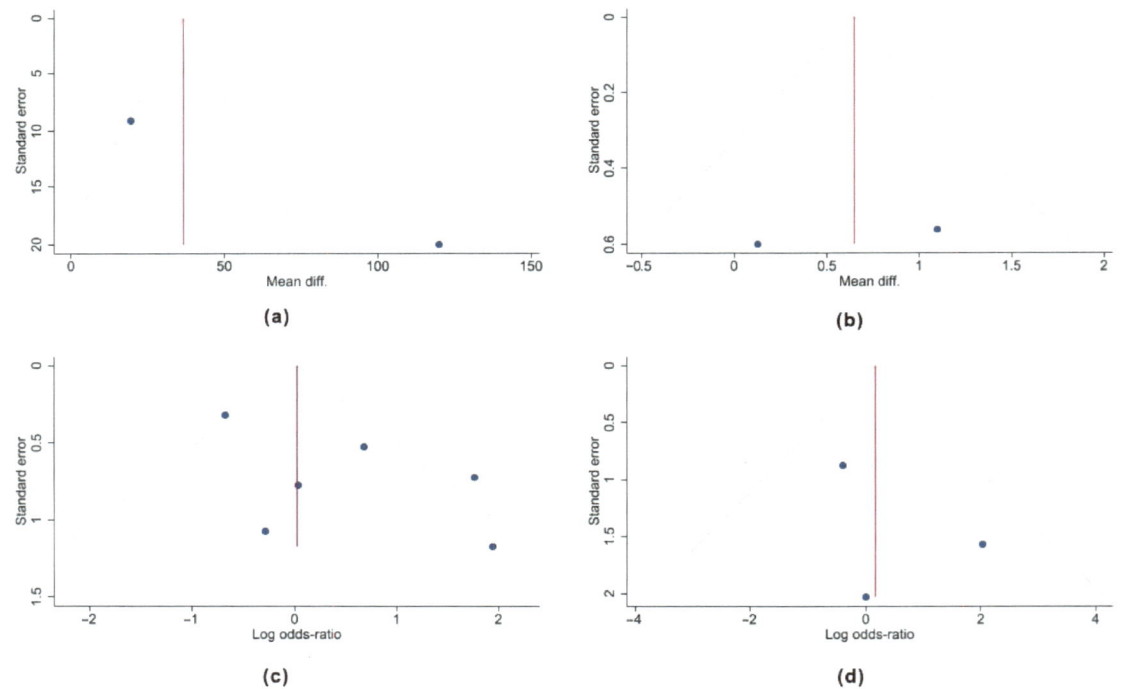

Figure 9. Forest plot of the comparison of the recurrence rate [12,15,16,18,19].

(a)

(b)

(c)

(d)

Figure 10. *Cont.*

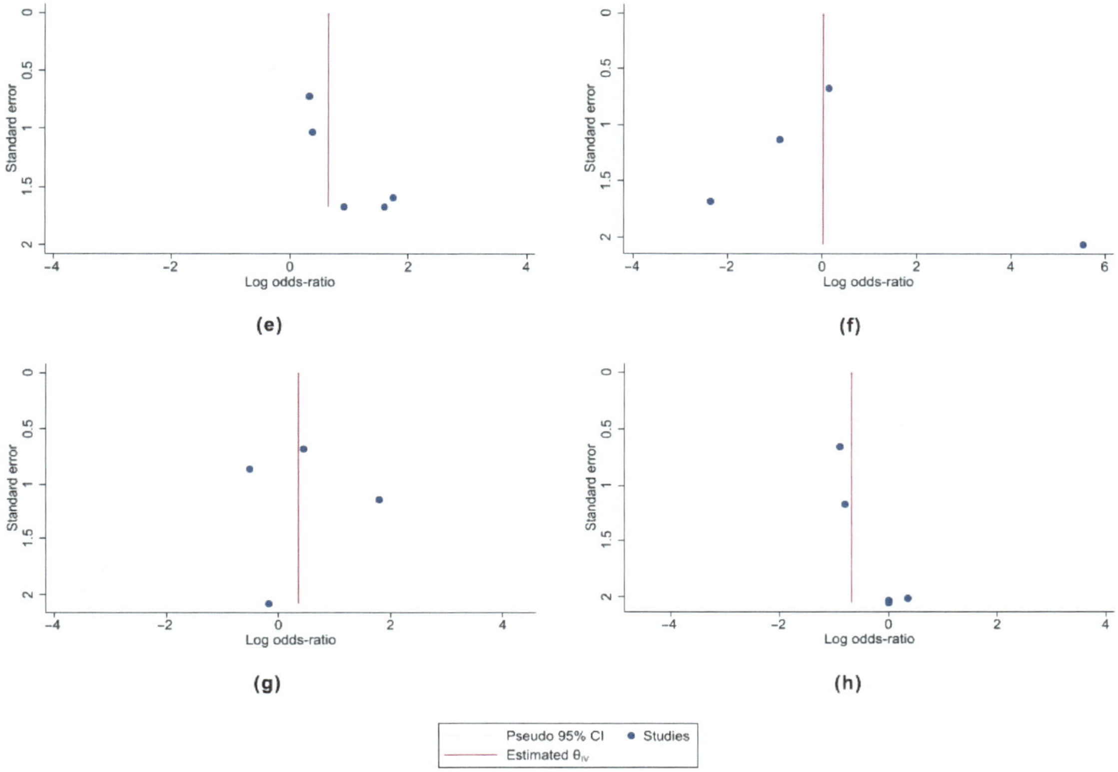

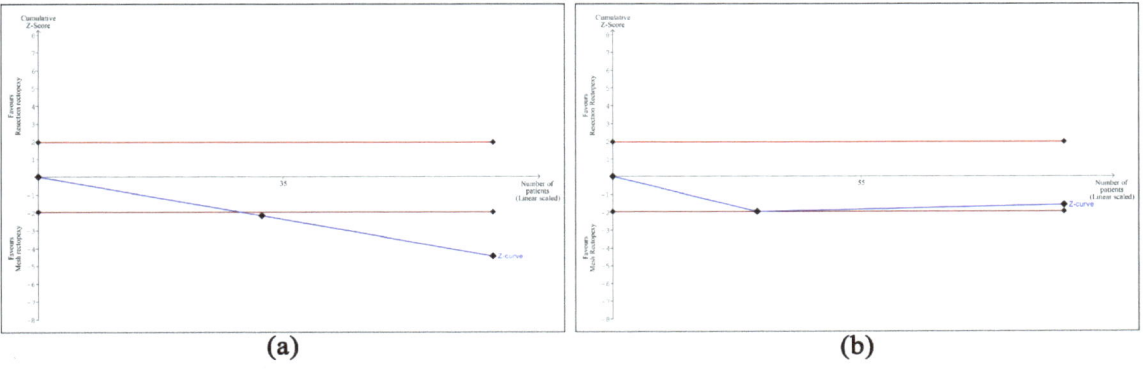

Figure 10. Funnel plots of the analyses performed indicating that there was no publication bias among the selected studies. (**a**) Funnel plot of comparison of operative time, (**b**) funnel plot of comparison of length of stay, (**c**) funnel plot of comparison of overall complication rate, (**d**) funnel plot of comparison of surgical site infection rate, (**e**) funnel plot of comparison of cardiopulmonary complication rate, (**f**) funnel plot of comparison of constipation improvement rate, (**g**) funnel plot of comparison of incontinence improvement rate, and (**h**) funnel plot of comparison of recurrence rate.

Figure 11. *Cont.*

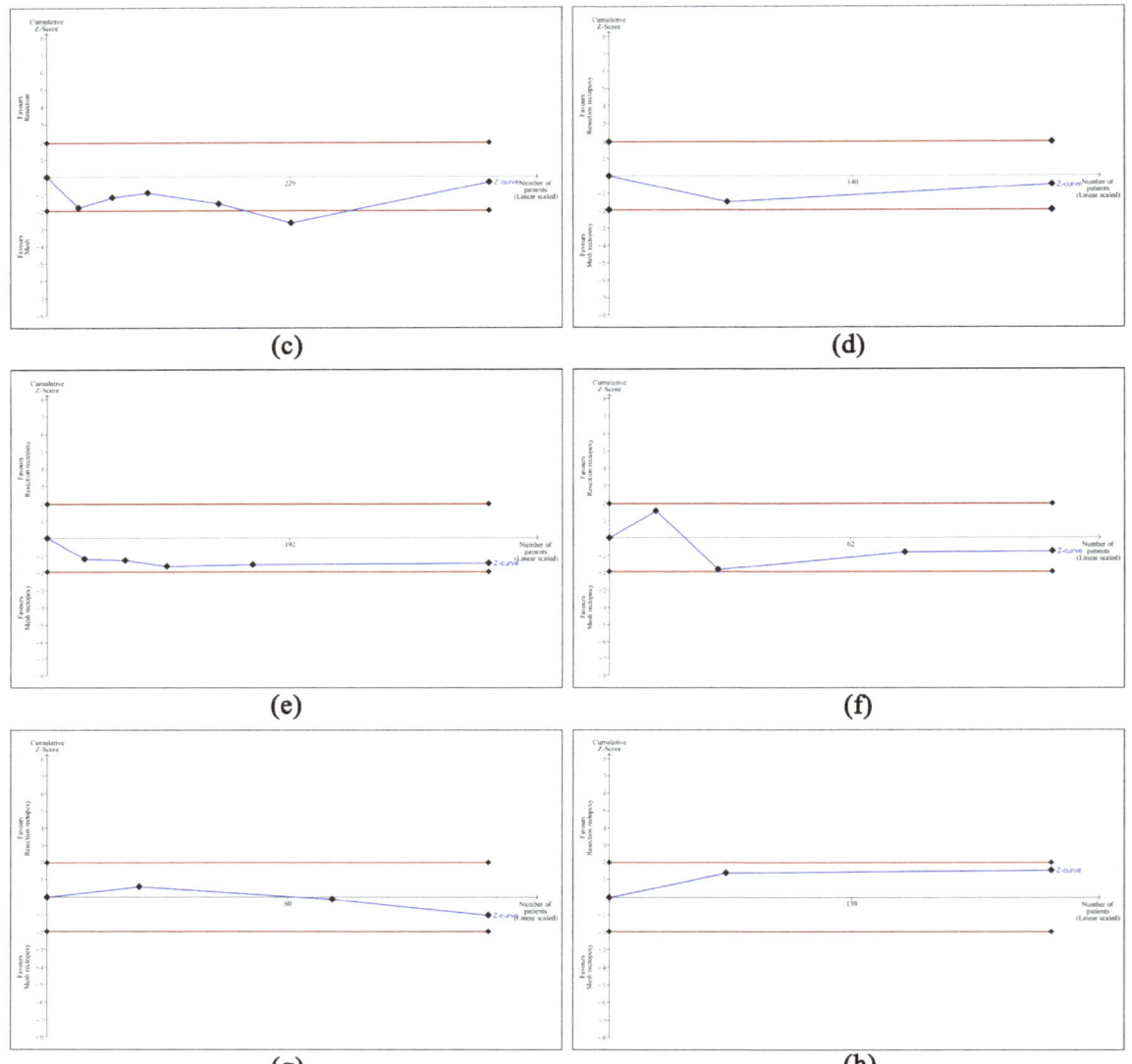

Figure 11. Outcomes of trial sequential analysis showing that the number of the included studies was sufficient to draw definite conclusions only for the first meta-analysis. (**a**) TSA of meta-analysis of operative time, (**b**) TSA of meta-analysis of length of stay, (**c**) TSA of meta-analysis of overall complication rate, (**d**) TSA of meta-analysis of surgical site infection rate, (**e**) TSA of meta-analysis of cardiopulmonary complication rate, (**f**) TSA of meta-analysis of constipation improvement rate, (**g**) TSA of meta-analysis of incontinence improvement rate, and (**h**) TSA of meta-analysis of recurrence rate.

Finally, the outcome of the assessment of potential bias in the included studies in this systematic review and meta-analysis is shown in Figures 12 and 13. According to this assessment, there is a significant risk of selection bias due to inadequate randomization and inadequate concealment prior to the intervention. This could have potentially affected the outcomes as the interventions were either based on availability, the surgeon's preference, or on the patient's specific symptoms as part of an individualized approach. Nonetheless, despite the lack of blindness, there is a low risk of performance and detection bias as the outcomes were judged using various valid scoring systems of post-operative performance or they were assessed using investigations such as anal manometry. Finally, there is a low risk of attrition, and as there were no missing outcome data, the risk of reporting bias is low to unclear as half of the included studies did not report all of the outcomes that were of interest in our systematic review and meta-analysis.

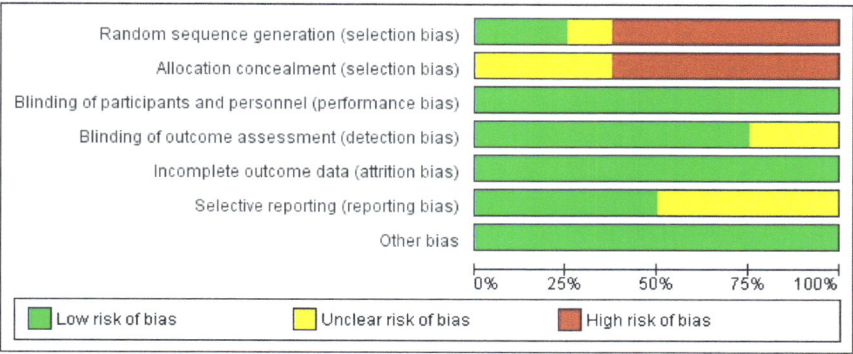

Figure 12. Risk of bias graph showing the percentage of bias that each study introduced in our meta-analysis.

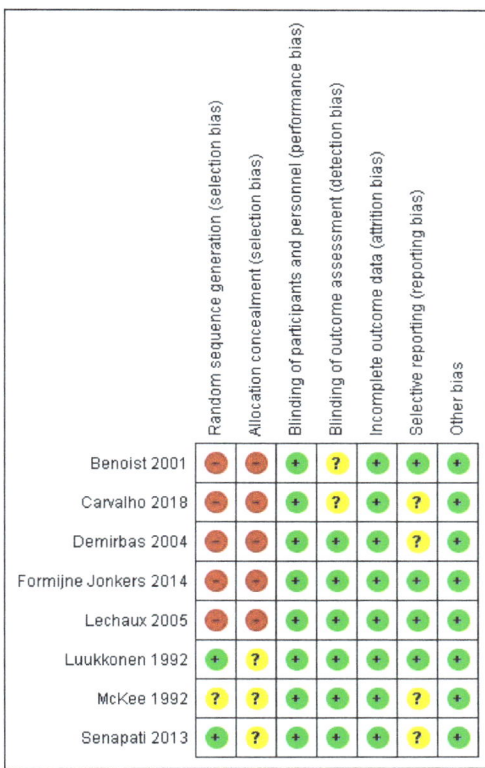

Figure 13. Risk of bias summary showing the level of risk of bias for each study included in the meta-analysis [12–19].

4. Discussion

Based on our review of the literature and as far as we can tell, this is the first meta-analysis that specifically compares the outcomes of resection rectopexy to mesh rectopexy for the management of rectal prolapse. Our results show that both procedures have similar outcomes regarding operative time, length of stay, recurrence rate, and complication rate, as well as similar outcomes regarding improvement of fecal incontinence and constipation. Nonetheless, the trial sequential analysis demonstrated that more studies will be required to confirm our findings. As a result, each patient will require an individualized approach, and the decision will ultimately rest with the operative surgeon and their personal experience and preference regarding the procedure of choice.

According to our review of the literature, so far, there have been some systematic reviews for the operative management of complete rectal prolapse that include abdominal approaches, but most of them compare other techniques, such as ventral mesh rectopexy and suture rectopexy (without sigmoidectomy), or they compare different approaches (mainly robotic and laparoscopic). From those that include abdominal approaches, Tou S. et al. [3] conclude that there are still not enough data to conclude which of the abdominal procedures is more effective. Although they conclude that bowel resection was associated with lower constipation rates, they believe that the usefulness of their results to guide clinical decisions is limited due to some limitations of the included studies. Another systematic review by Hotouras et al. in 2015 on the operative management of recurrent rectal prolapse was unable to come up with a management algorithm for recurrent rectal prolapse as a result of the wide variety of surgical procedures utilized and the low level of evidence within heterogeneous articles [20]. However, they report recurrence rates from 0% to 15% for abdominal procedures, with morbidity rates ranging from 0% to 32% and a mortality of 4%. Another systematic review by Faucheron et al. [21] included twelve case series with a total number of 574 patients that underwent laparoscopic anterior rectopexy and reported a mean recurrence rate of 4.7% with a median follow-up of 23 months. Also, constipation improved within a range of 3–72%, but deterioration or new appearance of constipation occurred in 0–20%. Incontinence improved in 31–84% of the patients. Moreover, in another meta-analysis of eight studies with a total number of 467 patients performed by Cadeddu et al., there were similar outcomes in recurrence, incontinence, and constipation improvement rates between laparoscopic and open abdominal rectopexy [22]. Also, regarding non-comparative trials, there was no statistically significant difference in recurrence rate in open and laparoscopic suture rectopexy studies and in open and laparoscopic mesh rectopexy trials [20]. Furthermore, another meta-analysis of 5 comparative studies by Hajibandeh et al. showed that laparoscopic mesh rectopexy has a lower recurrence rate but longer procedure time when compared to laparoscopic posterior suture rectopexy [23]. Finally, regarding the optimal method of approach, laparoscopic surgery has comparable outcomes with open in terms of morbidity and recurrence rate, while it has a shorter hospital stay [24]. The robotic approach has been revealed to have equal post-operative outcomes and an even shorter hospital stay [25,26].

Another interesting study that focused on the management of rectal prolapse in men was carried out by Poylin et al. in 2019 [27]. According to this multicenter retrospective review of 58 male patients who underwent surgical repair for rectal prolapse, thirty-nine (67%) patients underwent an abdominal procedure. These patients were younger and had a lower American Society of Anesthesiologists (ASA) score. The overall complication rate in this study was 26%, with the most common complication being urinary retention (16%). However, this was more common in perineal procedures. Also, the overall recurrence rate was 9%, with similar outcomes between the abdominal and perineal procedures. Regarding the long-term outcomes of this study, the constipation rate decreased from 59% to 36%, and fecal incontinence decreased from 40% to 14%. Nonetheless, 5% of the patients reported a new onset of constipation, and 7% developed new symptoms of incontinence. On top of that, 3% of the patients reported post-operative symptoms of sexual dysfunction. This study concludes that although surgical repair of rectal prolapse in men is a safe surgical procedure with a low recurrence rate, more studies are needed to identify which is the best surgical approach [26]. Another study that focused on the management of rectal prolapse in male patients was published in 2022 by Hu et al. [28]. This study performed a retrospective comparison between abdominal and perineal procedures for the management of external rectal prolapse. It included a total number of 51 patients and ultimately revealed that a perineal approach, either Altemeier or Delorme procedure, carries a higher complication and recurrence rate. Also, regarding the long-term functional outcomes, constipation was improved in both approaches, but fecal incontinence deteriorated with an abdominal approach. Nonetheless, patients in both groups reported an overall improvement in their quality of life, as assessed by the EuroQol 5-Dimension 5-Levels quality of life questionnaire. The matter of the management of rectal prolapse in male patients was also investigated by Ganapathi et al., who also published the outcomes of their study in 2022 [29]. They compared the outcomes of modified laparoscopic posterior mesh rectopexy (LPMR) to the ones of laparoscopic resection rectopexy (LRR) on a total number of 118 male patients. According to their findings, the mean operative time for LPMR was 102 ± 22 min and 121 ± 26 min for LRR, while the length of stay was 4.6 ± 1.4 days and 6.3 ± 1.2 days, respectively. Also, there were 12 cases of complications in the LPMR group and 5 cases of complications in the LRR group. Finally, two patients in each group reported post-operative constipation that improved with laxatives. The authors of this study conclude that randomized trials comparing these two methods will be required to establish if one of them is superior to the other.

Recently, an alternative to the classic operative approach for the management of rectal mucosal prolapse has been reported by Liu et al. [30]. The authors have reported the use of cap-assisted endoscopy sclerotherapy (CAES) to treat outlet obstructive constipation caused either by internal hemorrhoids or rectal mucosal prolapse. In this technique, a sclerosing agent is injected above the dental line at the area of loose submucosa via a colonoscope bearing a regular cap at its top. Based on the results of the pre- and post-operative anorectal manometry, CAES leads to a statistically significant increase in the maximum defecation pressure, a significant decrease in the rectal residual pressure, and a significant increase in the relaxation rate. There were no severe adverse side effects reported in this study. Another interesting aspect of rectal prolapse is the management of irreducible rectal prolapse that presents as a surgical emergency. In such a case, the rectum becomes edematous, it begins to ulcerate, and it cannot be reduced manually by the patient [31]. Seenivasagam et al. [31] reported a case series of 15 patients who presented with irreducible rectal prolapse from 2006 to 2010. In five of these patients, reduction was achieved by gentle manipulation under analgesia, while in two cases, reduction was achieved after applying sugar to the prolapsed rectum. The remaining cases were treated under general anesthesia with various techniques applied. In one case, general anesthesia was enough for successful reduction. One more patient underwent Delorme's procedure, and two more underwent laparotomy and Well's repair. The remaining cases were managed by either abdominal or perineal bowel resection.

In the latest guidelines published by the American Society of Colorectal Surgeons, it is mentioned that sigmoidectomy can be performed in patients who suffer from rectal prolapse and constipation, in addition to posterior suture rectopexy (recommendation: 1B) [1]. Furthermore, it is noted that improvement of fecal incontinence rate may be lower when sigmoidectomy is carried out [1]. Nonetheless, our results suggest that sigmoid resection does not affect the postoperative functional outcomes. While it is widely accepted that rectopexy is essential for the operative management of full-thickness rectal prolapse through the peritoneal approach, in the same guidelines, it is mentioned that there is no evidence that the use of different kinds of meshes for the rectopexy is superior to the sutures alone [1]. In our meta-analysis, mesh placement was found not to be superior to resection rectopexy. As a consequence, and taking into account the lack of consensus on the optimal surgical technique for the management of rectal prolapse, an individualized approach for each patient is required, while the surgeon's preference and expertise will also play a major role. Clinicians should take into account each patient's specific symptoms, anatomy, and bowel habits, as well as their pre-operative expectations. A thorough pre-operative workup will also be a deciding factor and should include physical examination, colonoscopy and proctoscopy, and, in specific cases, defecography and anal manometry.

This study has certain limitations. The articles included in the analysis were not randomized clinical trials, and there was no blinding of the researchers involved. This lack of randomization may have introduced a selection bias as, in such cases, patients tend to be allocated to the treatment that seems more beneficial to them. Other forms of bias that could have potentially affected our outcomes include bias due to missing data as a result of patients being lost to follow-up and bias in the selection of the reported results that prevents the estimate from being included in the meta-analysis. Moreover, lack of blinding could have introduced performance bias and bias in the measurement of the outcomes with an overestimation of the treatment effect as the assessors were aware of the intervention status. Also, despite including a total number of eight studies, not all of them provided extractable data to be included in every comparison performed.

5. Conclusions

The findings of our article show that mesh rectopexy and resection rectopexy for rectal prolapse have comparable outcomes, with neither of these methods demonstrating any superiority over the other in terms of complication rate, long-term outcomes, and recurrence rate. Therefore, the operative approach selected should mainly rely on the surgeon's preference and expertise. However, as indicated by the trial sequential analysis performed, more studies are required to consolidate our findings. We suggest that future researchers focus on performing randomized trials with independent assessors evaluating the outcomes of the procedures. We also suggest that these assessors are blinded to the original surgical technique that was utilized for each case.

Author Contributions: Conceptualization, G.K. and K.P.; methodology, L.S. and C.G.C.; software, L.S.; validation, G.K., G.G. and I.K.; formal analysis, G.K.; investigation, I.K. and G.G.; resources, A.P.; data curation, V.A. and N.T.; writing—original draft preparation, E.C.-W.; writing—review and editing, G.G.; visualization, L.S.; supervision, K.P.; project administration, G.K. and A.A.A.; funding acquisition, K.P. All authors have read and agreed to the published version of the manuscript.

Funding: This research received no external funding.

Institutional Review Board Statement: Not applicable.

Informed Consent Statement: Not applicable.

Data Availability Statement: The data supporting the findings of this study are available within the article.

Conflicts of Interest: The authors declare no conflicts of interest.

References

1. Kumar, N.; Kumar, D. Fecal incontinence and rectal prolapse. *Indian J. Gastroenterol.* **2019**, *38*, 465–469. [CrossRef]
2. Sun, C.; Hull, T.; Ozuner, G. Risk factors and clinical characteristics of rectal prolapse in young patients. *J. Visc. Surg.* **2014**, *151*, 425–429. [CrossRef]
3. Bordeianou, L.; Paquette, I.; Johnson, E.; Holubar, S.D.; Gaertner, W.; Feingold, D.L.; Steele, S.R. Clinical Practice Guidelines for the Treatment of Rectal Prolapse. *Dis. Colon Rectum* **2017**, *60*, 1121–1131. [CrossRef]
4. Wexner, S.D.; Cera, S.M. Procedures for rectal ProlaPse. In *Scientific American Surgery*; Decker Intellectual Properties Inc.: Toronto, ON, Canada, 2015; pp. 1–23.
5. Tou, S.; Brown, S.R.; Nelson, R.L. Surgery for complete (full-thickness) rectal prolapse in adults. *Cochrane Database Syst. Rev.* **2015**, *2015*. [CrossRef]
6. Emile, S.H.; Elfeki, H.A.; Youssef, M.; Farid, M.; Wexner, S.D. Abdominal rectopexy for the treatment of internal rectal prolapse: A systematic review and meta-analysis. *Colorectal. Dis.* **2017**, *19*, O13–O24. [CrossRef]
7. Manatakis, D.K.; Gouvas, N.; Pechlivanides, G.; Xynos, E. Ventral Prosthesis Rectopexy for obstructed defaecation syndrome: A systematic review and meta-analysis. *Updates Surg.* **2022**, *74*, 11–21. [CrossRef]
8. SA Shaikh, I.H. Surgical Approaches for Rectal Prolapse and their Comparative Study. *WJOLS* **2015**, *8*, 90–95. [CrossRef]

9. Li, Z.; Wang, S.H.; Li, G.B.; Lian, Y.G.; Gu, X.M.; Xia, K.K.; Yuan, W.T. Comparison of clinical efficacy of robotic, laparoscopic and open surgery in the treatment of severe rectal prolapse. *Zhonghua Wei Chang Wai Ke Za Zhi* **2020**, *23*, 1187–1193. [CrossRef]
10. Joubert, K.; Laryea, J. Abdominal Approaches to Rectal Prolapse. *Clin. Colon Rectal Surg.* **2016**, *30*, 057–062. [CrossRef]
11. Husa, A.; Sainio, P.; von Smitten, K. Abdominal rectopexy and sigmoid resection (Frykman-Goldberg operation) for rectal prolapse. *Acta Chir. Scand.* **1988**, *154*, 221–224.
12. Carvalho E Carvalho, M.E.; Hull, T.; Zutshi, M.; Gurland, B.H. Resection Rectopexy is Still an Acceptable Operation for Rectal Prolapse. *Am. Surg.* **2018**, *84*, 1470–1475. [CrossRef]
13. Benoist, S.; Taffinder, N.; Gould, S.; Chang, A.; Darzi, A. Functional results two years after laparoscopic rectopexy. *Am. J. Surg.* **2001**, *182*, 168–173. [CrossRef]
14. Demirbas, S.; Ogün, I.; Çelenk, T.; Akin, M.L.; Erenoglu, C.; Yldz, M. Early Outcomes of Laparoscopic Procedures Performed on Military Personnel With Total Rectal Prolapse and Follow-up. *Surg. Laparosc. Endosc. Percutaneous Tech.* **2004**, *14*, 194–200. [CrossRef]
15. Luukkonen, P.; Mikkonen, U.; Järvinen, H. Abdominal rectopexy with sigmoidectomy vs. rectopexy alone for rectal prolapse: A prospective, randomized study. *Int. J. Colorect. Dis.* **1992**, *7*, 219–222. [CrossRef]
16. McKee, R.F.; Lauder, J.C.; Poon, F.W.; Aitchison, M.A.; Finlay, I.G. A prospective randomized study of abdominal rectopexy with and without sigmoidectomy in rectal prolapse. *Surg. Gynecol. Obs.* **1992**, *174*, 145–148.
17. Lechaux, D.; Trebuchet, G.; Siproudhis, L.; Campion, J.P. Laparoscopic rectopexy for full-thickness rectal prolapse: A single-institution retrospective study evaluating surgical outcome. *Surg. Endosc.* **2005**, *19*, 514–518. [CrossRef]
18. Formijne Jonkers, H.A.; Maya, A.; Draaisma, W.A.; Bemelman, W.A.; Broeders, I.A.; Consten, E.C.J.; Wexner, S.D. Laparoscopic resection rectopexy versus laparoscopic ventral rectopexy for complete rectal prolapse. *Tech. Coloproctol.* **2014**, *18*, 641–646. [CrossRef]
19. Senapati, A.; Gray, R.G.; Middleton, L.J.; Harding, J.; Hills, R.K.; Armitage, N.C.M.; Buckley, L.; Northover, J.M.A.; the PROSPER Collaborative Group. PROSPER: A randomised comparison of surgical treatments for rectal prolapse. *Colorectal. Dis.* **2013**, *15*, 858–868. [CrossRef]
20. Hotouras, A.; Ribas, Y.; Zakeri, S.; Bhan, C.; Wexner, S.D.; Chan, C.L.; Murphy, J. A systematic review of the literature on the surgical management of recurrent rectal prolapse. *Colorectal. Dis.* **2015**, *17*, 657–664. [CrossRef]
21. Faucheron, J.-L.; Trilling, B.; Girard, E.; Sage, P.-Y.; Barbois, S.; Reche, F. Anterior rectopexy for full-thickness rectal prolapse: Technical and functional results. *World J. Gastroenterol.* **2015**, *21*, 5049–5055. [CrossRef]
22. Cadeddu, F.; Sileri, P.; Grande, M.; De Luca, E.; Franceschilli, L.; Milito, G. Focus on abdominal rectopexy for full-thickness rectal prolapse: Meta-analysis of literature. *Tech. Coloproctol.* **2012**, *16*, 37–53. [CrossRef]
23. Hajibandeh, S.; Hajibandeh, S.; Arun, C.; Adeyemo, A.; McIlroy, B.; Peravali, R. Meta-analysis of laparoscopic mesh rectopexy versus posterior sutured rectopexy for management of complete rectal prolapse. *Int. J. Colorectal. Dis.* **2021**, *36*, 1357–1366. [CrossRef]
24. Purkayastha, S.; Tekkis, P.; Athanasiou, T.; Aziz, O.; Paraskevas, P.; Ziprin, P.; Darzi, A. A Comparison of Open vs. Laparoscopic Abdominal Rectopexy for Full-Thickness Rectal Prolapse: A Meta-Analysis. *Dis. Colon Rectum* **2005**, *48*, 1930–1940. [CrossRef]
25. Flynn, J.; Larach, J.T.; Kong, J.C.H.; Warrier, S.K.; Heriot, A. Robotic versus laparoscopic ventral mesh rectopexy: A systematic review and meta-analysis. *Int. J. Colorectal. Dis.* **2021**, *36*, 1621–1631. [CrossRef]
26. Rondelli, F.; Bugiantella, W.; Villa, F.; Sanguinetti, A.; Boni, M.; Mariani, E.; Avenia, N. Robot-assisted or conventional laparoscoic rectopexy for rectal prolapse? Systematic review and meta-analysis. *Int. J. Surg.* **2014**, *12*, S153–S159. [CrossRef]
27. Poylin, V.Y.; Irani, J.L.; Rahbar, R.; Kapadia, M.R. Rectal-prolapse repair in men is safe, but outcomes are not well understood. *Gastroenterol. Rep.* **2019**, *7*, 279–282. [CrossRef]
28. Hu, B.; Zou, Q.; Xian, Z.; Su, D.; Liu, C.; Lu, L.; Luo, M.; Chen, Z.; Cai, K.; Gao, H.; et al. External rectal prolapse: Abdominal or perineal repair for men? A retrospective cohort study. *Gastroenterol. Rep.* **2022**, *10*, goac007. [CrossRef]
29. Ganapathi, S.K.; Subbiah, R.; Rudramurthy, S.; Kakkilaya, H.; Ramakrishnan, P.; Chinnusamy, P. Laparoscopic posterior rectopexy for complete rectal prolapse: Is it the ideal procedure for males? *J. Minim. Access Surg.* **2022**, *18*, 295–301. [CrossRef]
30. Liu, T.; He, S.; Li, Q.; Wang, H. Cap-assisted endoscopic sclerotherapy is effective for rectal mucosal prolapse associated outlet obstructive constipation. *Arab. J. Gastroenterol.* **2023**, *24*, 85–90. [CrossRef]
31. Seenivasagam, T. Irreducible Rectal Prolapse: Emergency Surgical Management of Eight Cases and A Review of the Literature. *Med. J. Malays.* **2011**, *66*, 105.

Disclaimer/Publisher's Note: The statements, opinions and data contained in all publications are solely those of the individual author(s) and contributor(s) and not of MDPI and/or the editor(s). MDPI and/or the editor(s) disclaim responsibility for any injury to people or property resulting from any ideas, methods, instructions or products referred to in the content.

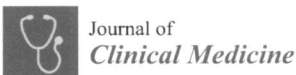 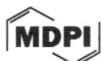

Article

Oncologic Outcomes of Salvage Abdominoperineal Resection for Anal Squamous Cell Carcinoma Initially Managed with Chemoradiation

Roni Rosen [1,†], Felipe F. Quezada-Diaz [1,†], Mithat Gönen [2], Georgios Karagkounis [1], Maria Widmar [1], Iris H. Wei [1], J. Joshua Smith [1], Garrett M. Nash [1], Martin R. Weiser [1], Philip B. Paty [1], Andrea Cercek [3], Paul B. Romesser [4], Francisco Sanchez-Vega [5], Mohammad Adileh [1], Diana Roth O'Brien [4], Carla Hajj [4], Vonetta M. Williams [4], Marina Shcherba [3], Ping Gu [3], Christopher Crane [4], Leonard B. Saltz [3], Julio Garcia Aguilar [1] and Emmanouil Pappou [1,*]

1. Department of Surgery, Memorial Sloan Kettering Cancer Center, New York, NY 10065, USA; ffquezad@gmail.com (F.F.Q.-D.); smithj5@mskcc.org (J.J.S.)
2. Department of Epidemiology and Biostatistics, Memorial Sloan Kettering Cancer Center, New York, NY 10065, USA
3. Department of Medicine, Memorial Sloan Kettering Cancer Center, New York, NY 10065, USA; gup@mskcc.org (P.G.)
4. Department of Radiation Oncology, Memorial Sloan Kettering Cancer Center, New York, NY 10065, USA; romessep@mskcc.org (P.B.R.)
5. Department of Computational Oncology, Memorial Sloan Kettering Cancer Center, New York, NY 10065, USA
* Correspondence: pappoue@mskcc.org
† These authors contributed equally to this work.

Citation: Rosen, R.; Quezada-Diaz, F.F.; Gönen, M.; Karagkounis, G.; Widmar, M.; Wei, I.H.; Smith, J.J.; Nash, G.M.; Weiser, M.R.; Paty, P.B.; et al. Oncologic Outcomes of Salvage Abdominoperineal Resection for Anal Squamous Cell Carcinoma Initially Managed with Chemoradiation. *J. Clin. Med.* **2024**, *13*, 2156. https://doi.org/10.3390/jcm13082156

Academic Editor: Goran Augustin

Received: 24 February 2024
Revised: 1 April 2024
Accepted: 3 April 2024
Published: 9 April 2024

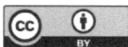

Copyright: © 2024 by the authors. Licensee MDPI, Basel, Switzerland. This article is an open access article distributed under the terms and conditions of the Creative Commons Attribution (CC BY) license (https://creativecommons.org/licenses/by/4.0/).

Abstract: Background: Abdominoperineal resection (APR) has been advocated for persistent or recurrent disease after failure of chemoradiation (CRT) for anal squamous cell cancer (SCC). Treatment with salvage APR can potentially achieve a cure. This study aimed to analyze oncological outcomes for salvage APR in a recent time period at a comprehensive cancer center. **Methods:** A retrospective review of all patients who underwent APR for biopsy-proven persistent or recurrent anal SCC between 1 January 2007 and 31 December 2020 was performed. Patients with stage IV disease at the time of initial diagnosis and patients with missing data were excluded. Univariate analysis was used with a chi-square test for categorical variables, and non-parametric tests were used for continuous variables. Kaplan–Meier survival analysis was performed to evaluate disease-specific (DSS), post-APR local recurrence-free (RFS), and disease-free survival (DFS). **Results:** A total of 96 patients were included in the analysis: 39 (41%) with persistent disease and 57 (59%) with recurrent SCC after chemoradiation had been completed. The median follow-up was 22 months (IQR 11–47). Forty-nine patients (51%) underwent extended APR and/or pelvic exenteration. Eight (8%) patients developed local recurrence, 30 (31%) developed local and distant recurrences, and 16 (17%) developed distant recurrences alone. The 3-year DSS, post-APR local recurrence-free survival, and disease-free survival were 53.8% (95% CI 43.5–66.5%), 54.5% (95% CI 44.4–66.8%), and 26.8% (95% CI 18.6–38.7%), respectively. In multivariate logistic regression analysis, positive microscopic margin (OR 10.0, 95% CI 2.16–46.12, $p = 0.003$), positive nodes in the surgical specimen (OR 9.19, 95% CI 1.99–42.52, $p = 0.005$), and lymphovascular invasion (OR 2.61 95% CI 1.05–6.51, $p = 0.04$) were associated with recurrence of disease. Gender, indication for APR (recurrent vs. persistent disease), HIV status, extent of surgery, or type of reconstruction did not influence survival outcomes. Twenty patients had targeted tumor-sequencing data available. Nine patients had PIK3CA mutations, seven of whom experienced a recurrence. **Conclusions:** Salvage APR for anal SCC after failed CRT was associated with poor disease-specific survival and low recurrence-free survival. Anal SCC patients undergoing salvage APR should be counseled that microscopic positive margins, positive lymph nodes, or the presence of lymphovascular invasion in the APR specimen are prognosticators for disease relapse. Our results accentuate the necessity for additional treatment strategies for the ongoing treatment challenge of persistent or recurrent anal SCC after failed CRT.

Keywords: anal cancer; salvage APR; combined modality treatment

1. Introduction

Anal cancers are rare, comprising about 0.5% of all new cancer diagnoses in the United States in 2023, with squamous cell carcinoma being the most common subtype [1]. Prior to the 1980s, patients with anal SCC would routinely undergo abdominoperineal resections (APR), with considerable morbidity. Since the Nigro protocol was first published in 1974, multiple trials have shown improved disease-free survival and colostomy-free survival with combined modality therapy, making chemoradiation with mitomycin-c and 5-FU the standard of care for locoregional disease today [2–6]. Combined modality therapy offers a long-term survival of up to 90% for patients without distant metastases [7,8]. As the incidence of anal squamous cell carcinoma increased over time, the treatment of local recurrence and persistent disease after combined modality therapy has become a treatment challenge [9].

After multimodal therapy, local failure—defined as persistent disease after 6 months, progression of disease, or recurrent disease—has been described in up to 30% of patients [2,5,10,11]. Currently, the mainstay of treatment for locoregional failure after chemoradiation for anal SCC is APR, with little proven benefit of adjuvant chemotherapy or radiation. Surgical outcomes feature high morbidity rates of up to 80%, with patients commonly experiencing complications like perineal dehiscence or infection [12]. Due to the rarity of the disease, reports of the oncologic outcomes of salvage APR are sparse and heterogenous due to small sample sizes and varying CRT regimens [11,13–15].

The aim of the present report is to analyze oncological outcomes for salvage APR for persistent/recurrent anal SCC in a contemporary timeframe at a comprehensive cancer center and identify potential predictors of poor prognosis.

2. Methods

2.1. Patient Selection

This retrospective review was approved by the institutional review board of Memorial Sloan Kettering Cancer Center (MSK) with a waiver of informed consent. A retrospective review identified patients who underwent APR for biopsy-proven anal SCC at MSK from January 2007 to December 2020. Patients with stage IV disease, synchronous cancer, or lack of follow-up were excluded. Demographic and treatment data were obtained via chart review, including age, surgery type, indication for surgery, HIV status, treatment regimen, pathology results, and oncologic outcomes.

2.2. Treatment

Patients were treated with chemoradiation therapy (CRT), and the primary tumor intended radiation dose varied from 50 Gy to 58 Gy depending on T stage and nodal size. Patients predominantly received mitomycin (MMC) and fluorouracil (5-FU) infusion or oral capecitabine as concurrent chemotherapy. MMC was administered during weeks 1 and 5 of treatment, infusional 5-FU was administered during weeks 1 and 5, and capecitabine was administered orally twice daily on radiation treatment days. Following CRT, patients were surveilled with anoscopy every 6 to 12 months and annual imaging with CT or MRI for 3 years. Local failure after CRT was defined as persistent disease at 6 months after CRT, local recurrence, and progression of disease during therapy. Patients who had persistent disease within 6 months of finishing chemoradiation were recommended to undergo surgery.

Surgical treatment of local failure included APR, extended APR, or pelvic exenteration. Extended APR involved performing a standard APR procedure with the resection of contents from one additional pelvic compartment or a lateral or inguinal lymph node dissection. Surgeries that included a cystectomy and APR were considered total pelvic exenterations. Indications for an extended APR were tumor extension to the pelvic sidewall or adjacent organs such as the posterior vaginal wall or the prostate. Involvement or close proximity (within 1–2 mm) of the tumor to the urethra or bladder was an indication of pelvic exenteration.

2.3. Statistical Analysis

Statistical analysis was performed using SPSS version 27 (IBM). Frequencies and percentages were calculated for categorical variables, and medians and ranges were calculated for continuous variables.

A Kaplan–Meier analysis was performed to estimate 3-year disease-specific survival (DSS), post-APR relapse-free survival (RFS), and disease-free survival (DFS) of the cohort. Multivariate logistic regression analysis was performed to evaluate the effect of several clinical and pathological variables on RFS; a p-value < 0.05 was considered statistically significant.

This paper was prepared in accordance with the Strengthening the Reporting of Observational Studies in Epidemiology guidelines [16].

3. Results

3.1. Patients and Tumor Characteristics

A total of 104 patients with anal SCC underwent APR during the study period, 96 of whom were included in the analysis. Patients with synchronous tumors (n = 2), stage IV disease (n = 2), missing follow-up information (n = 2), or who had upfront surgery (n = 2) were excluded. Patient and tumor characteristics are summarized in Table 1.

Table 1. Patient and tumor characteristics.

Characteristics	N = 96 (%)
Median age in years (range)	63 (33.87)
No. (%) male	39 (40.6)
No. (%) HIV [a] (+)	17 (17.7)
Primary tumor treatment regimen, n (%)	
5-FU/capecitabine + MMC [b]/cisplatin+ RT	86 (89.6)
5-FU + RT	6 (6.2)
RT alone	4 (4.2)
Indication for surgery	
Persistent	39 (40.6)
Recurrent	57 (59.4)
AJCC [c] pathological stage, n (%)	
0	7 (7.3)
is	1 (1.0)
I	7 (7.7)
II	32 (33.3)
III	49 (51.0)
Pathological T classification, n (%)	
pT0/Tis	9 (9.4)
pT1	7 (7.3)
pT2	31 (32.3)
pT3	18 (18.7)
pT4	31 (32.3)
Pathological N classification, n (%)	
pN−	77 (80.2)
pN+	19 (19.8)

[a] HIV, Human Immunodeficiency Virus; [b] Mitomycin C; [c] AJCC, American Joint Committee on Cancer.

The median age was 63 years (range 33–87), and 39 (40.6%) patients were male. Seventeen (17.7%) of the patients tested positive for the human immunodeficiency virus (HIV). The indication for salvage APR was persistent disease in 39 (40.6%) patients and local recurrence in 57 (59.4%) patients. All but 10 patients received MMC or cisplatin and 5-FU or capecitabine-based CRT. The remaining patients had either RT alone or 5-FU and

CRT (Table 1). The median radiation dose was 54 Gy (range 28–70 Gy), and the median follow-up time was 22 months (IQR 11–47). Seven (7.3%) of the patients had a complete pathologic response after CRT, yet most patients had pathologic stage III disease (n = 49; 51.0%) in their surgical specimens. Twenty (20.8%) patients had microscopic tumors or R1 disease, and 19 (19.8%) patients had positive lymph nodes in their surgical specimens. Six (6.3%) patients underwent adjuvant chemotherapy with or without radiation.

Of the patients in our cohort, 20 had targeted tumor-sequencing genetic testing available (MSK-IMPACT), 15 of which were from primary anal SCC, and 5 were from recurrent sites. Nine patients had PIK3CA mutations, seven of whom experienced a recurrence.

3.2. Surgical Technique and Complications

The majority of patients underwent an APR alone (n = 43, 44.8%) or an extended APR combined with a posterior vaginectomy, prostatectomy, coccygectomy, pelvic sidewall dissection, or inguinal lymph node dissection (n = 44; 45.8%). Five (5.2%) patients underwent a posterior pelvic exenteration, and four (4.2%) had a total pelvic exenteration. Two patients (2%) underwent inguinal lymph node resection due to PET-avidity on preoperative imaging, both of which were confirmed to be metastatic lymphadenopathy on final pathology. Six (6.3%) patients had intraoperative radiation therapy. Most patients had a vertical rectus abdominis musculocutaneous (VRAM) flap for perineal reconstruction (Table 2).

Table 2. Surgical Intervention and Complications.

Characteristics	N = 96 (%)
No. (%) type surgical approach	
APR	43 (44.8)
Extended APR [a]	44 (45.8)
Pelvic Exenteration, posterior [b]	5 (5.2)
Pelvic Exenteration, Total	4 (4.2)
No. (%) type perineal wound closure	
Primary	15 (15.6)
Gluteal Flap	8 (8.3)
Gracilis Flap	4 (4.2)
VRAM	69 (71.9)
No. (%) surgical complications by Clavien–Dindo grade	
1–2	8 (8.3)
3–5	19 (19.8)
No. (%) positive margin resection	20 (20.8)

[a] Includes rectum and any of the following: partial vaginectomy, prostatectomy, pelvic sidewall dissection, coccygectomy, or inguinal lymph node dissection. [b] Includes APR with a total hysterectomy and bilateral salpingo–oophorectomy.

The thirty-day morbidity rate was 28.1% (n = 27), with 20.8% (n = 20) of the cohort experiencing at least a grade 3 complication. The most common adverse event was wound dehiscence, occurring in 10 (10.4%) patients (Table 2). The rate of serious (Clavien–Dindo grade $\geq$ 3) was unrelated to the extent of surgery; in other words, patients who underwent APR had similar 30-day complication rates to those who had a more extensive operation (OR 0.88, 95% CI 0.321–2.40, p = 0.801).

3.3. Disease-Specific, Recurrence-Free, and Disease-Free Survival

A Kaplan–Meier Survival analysis was performed to evaluate DSS, RFS, and DFS. With a median follow-up of 22 months (IQR 11 to 47), the 3-year disease-specific survival (DSS), post-APR local recurrence-free survival (RFS), and disease-free survival (DFS) were 53.8% (95% CI 43.5 to 66.5%), 54.5% (95% CI 44.4 to 66.8%), and 26.8% (95% CI 18.6 to 38.7%), respectively (Figures 1–3, respectively). Patients who had a complete pathologic response upon surgical resection did not experience a local recurrence or disease-related death. Three (50%) of the six patients who underwent IORT experienced local recurrence. According to multivariate logistic regression analysis, positive microscopic margin

(OR 10.0, 95% CI 2.16–46.12, p = 0.003), positive lymph nodes (OR 9.19, 95% CI 1.99–42.52, p = 0.005), and presence of lymphovascular invasion (OR 2.61, 95% CI 1.05–6.51, p = 0.04) in the surgical specimen were associated with recurrence of disease after salvage APR. Gender, indication for APR (recurrent vs. persistent disease), HIV status, and extent of surgery or type of reconstruction did not influence survival outcomes.

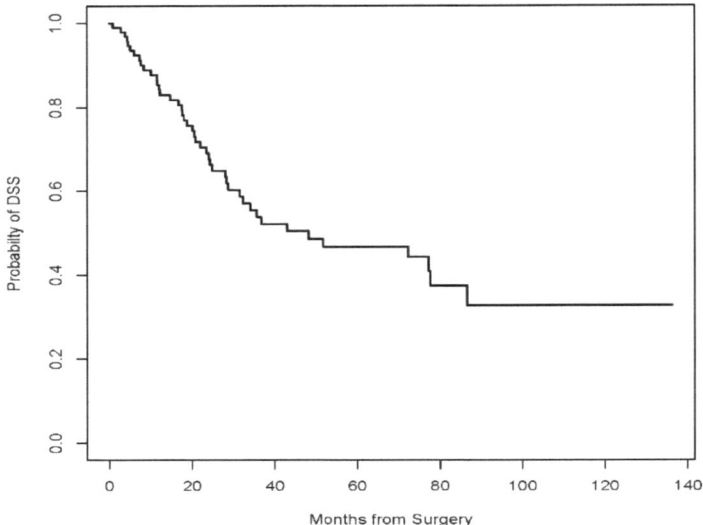

Figure 1. Kaplan–Meier curve for Disease-Specific Survival (DSS).

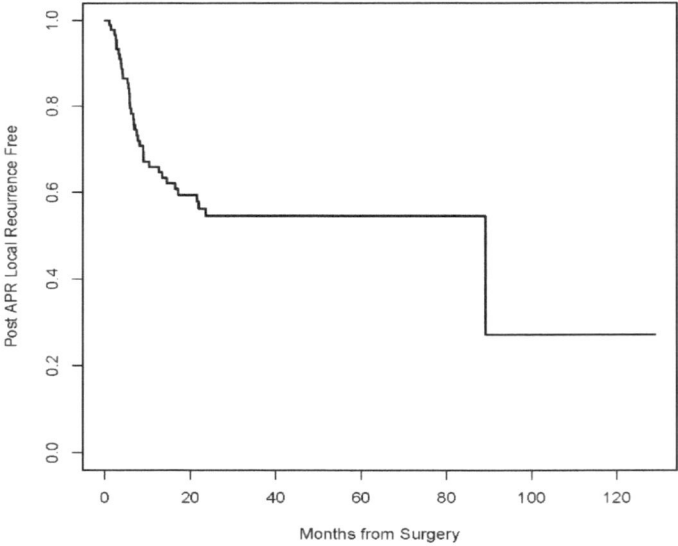

Figure 2. Kaplan–Meier curve for post-APR local recurrence-free survival (RFS).

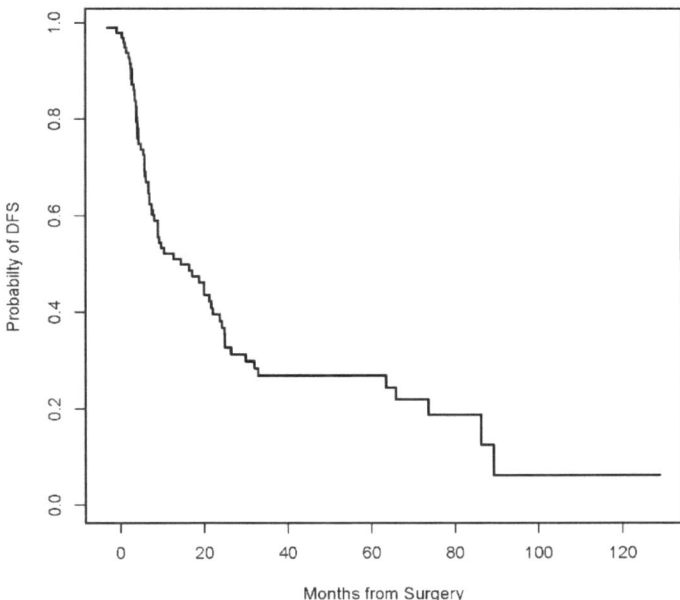

Figure 3. Kaplan–Meier curve for Disease-free survival (DFS).

4. Discussion

This is among the largest single institutional studies to present the morbidity, oncological, and survival outcomes after salvage APR for anal SCC in patients who underwent combined modality treatment at a comprehensive cancer center. Positive microscopic margins, positive nodes, and the presence of lymphovascular invasion in the surgical specimen were associated with the recurrence of disease after salvage APR. Gender, indication for APR (recurrent vs. persistent disease), HIV status, extent of surgery, and type of reconstruction did not influence survival outcomes. The results in this study demonstrate a poor 3-year DFS rate of 26.8%, with a 3-year RFS of 54.5% and a 3-year DSS of 53.8%, which fall within the range of overall survival rates reported in the literature, ranging between 30% and 78% [12,17–24].

Anal squamous cell carcinoma is a rare disease with excellent long-term survival rates of up to 90% in patients who respond to combined modality therapy. Locoregional failure rates, however, are up to 30%, and the effectiveness of salvage APR for anal SCC remains limited [19,22]. Despite refinements in technique and advances in surgical care, oncologic outcomes of salvage APR have remained similar at our center over the past three decades [25–27]. Surgical complications in our study were similar to those reported in the literature, with 20% of patients in our cohort experiencing at least a grade 3 complication and wound dehiscence occurring in 53% of patients, despite a high proportion of patients (84%) undergoing flap reconstruction of the perineum [28].

Previous studies have identified heterogeneous risk factors for local and distant recurrence after salvage APR, with some reporting persistent disease as a risk factor while others do not [13,22,29,30]. The largest cohort to address the timing of salvage APR was collected from the National Cancer Database (NCDB) by Fields et al. and included 437 patients treated between 2004 and 2013. The results yielded no significant differences in overall survival between patients who underwent salvage APR within 6 months of CRT (early) and beyond 6 months of treatment (late) [31]. Our present study corroborates this finding as an indication that APR (recurrent vs. persistent disease) did not influence survival outcomes.

While studies are discordant on certain predictors of oncologic outcomes, most recognize positive lymph nodes and positive resection margins as risk factors for recurrence and poor survival. In our cohort, these factors were independently associated with a two to tenfold risk of local recurrence. Perhaps the most important prognostic indicator in the setting of salvage surgery for locoregional failure, however, is surgery resulting in negative resection margins. Interestingly, the extent of surgery in our study was unrelated to oncologic outcomes and was not correlated to higher morbidity rates when compared to APR alone. Rather, negative resection margins were strongly associated with improved overall and local recurrence-free survival in this study, as addressed in previous reports [22,24,32]. These results suggest that salvage surgery, including extended resection or pelvic exenteration, is justified, especially when negative margins are expected with a more aggressive surgical intervention [19]. Additionally, consideration for preoperative imaging, such as pelvic MRI to assess local tumor extent prior to surgical resection, may guide surgical planning and predict the need for exenteration, which can lead to higher rates of negative resection margins. Furthermore, in cases of advanced disease, consideration for reirradiation can be made; however, further studies are needed to determine the feasibility, efficacy, and optimal regimen for reirradiation.

Another common prognosticator for post-resection recurrence, identified in the present study as well as others, is positive lymph nodes, serving as a major treatment challenge for this rare disease. Previous trials, including RTOG 92-08 and ACCORD3, showed no improvement in local control with radiation dose escalation in combination with MMC or cisplatin-based CRT [33–36]. Few retrospective series exist examining adjuvant or multimodal therapies for salvaging local failure of anal SCC, especially in node-positive patients. A few small retrospective reviews examined intraoperative radiation with salvage APR for locoregional failure of anal SCC and found little to no oncologic benefit [27,37,38]. More recent work has described the use of immune checkpoint inhibitors and targeted therapy for primary anal SCC; however, no results have been published as supplements to surgery [39]. Although a small sample, almost half of the patients in our study who had genomic data available had a PIK3CA mutation, speaking to the need for further genomic studies that may help identify high-risk patients and target treatment. Activating mutations in PIK3CA have been reported to arise in 20–25% of human anal cancers, suggesting that this pathway may be a relevant target for therapeutic interventions in the future [40,41].

Like comparable studies of its kind, this study is limited by its retrospective nature and sample size. Information regarding genomic testing was limited. While it is one of the larger single institutional studies of its kind, a larger sample size would have provided greater power to this study. Ultimately, locoregional failure of anal SCC remains a treatment challenge, and further, more robust studies are required to identify potentially beneficial treatments in addition to surgical resection.

5. Conclusions

Salvage APR for the locoregional failure of anal SCC has poor oncologic outcomes. Positive resection margins, positive lymph nodes, and the presence of lymphovascular invasion in the resected specimen were risk factors for recurrence and decreased survival. Careful preoperative planning, including pelvic MRI to assess tumor extent, extended surgery such as exenteration in order to achieve negative resection margins, and additional salvage therapies, including preoperative reirradiation or targeted therapies, should be explored to improve the oncologic outcomes in the case of recurrent or persistent anal SCC.

Author Contributions: E.P.: Conceptualization, data curation, Investigation, Supervision, Writing—original draft, Methodology, Writing—review & editing; R.R.: Conceptualization, data curation, Investigation, Supervision, Methodology, Writing—original draft, Writing—review & editing; F.F.Q.-D.: Conceptualization, data curation, Investigation, Supervision, Writing—original draft, Writing—review & editing; M.G.: Conceptualization, Supervision, Writing—original draft, Methodology, Writing—review & editing, Validation; G.K.: Conceptualization, Writing—review & editing; M.W.: Conceptualization, Writing—review & editing; I.H.W.: Conceptualization, Writing—review & editing; J.J.S.: Conceptualization, Supervision, Writing—review & editing; G.M.N.: Conceptualization, Supervision, Writing—review & editing; M.R.W.: Conceptualization, Supervision, Writing—review & editing; P.B.P.: Conceptualization, Supervision, Writing—review & editing; A.C.: Conceptualization, Supervision, Writing—review & editing; P.B.R.: Conceptualization, Supervision, Writing—original draft, Writing—review & editing; F.S.-V.: Conceptualization, Supervision, Writing—review & editing; M.A.: Conceptualization, Writing—review & editing; D.R.O.: Conceptualization, Supervision, Writing—review & editing; C.H.: Conceptualization, Writing—review & editing; V.M.W.: Conceptualization, Writing—review & editing; M.S.: Conceptualization, Supervision, Writing—review & editing; P.G.: Conceptualization, Supervision, Writing—review & editing; C.C.: Conceptualization, Writing—review & editing; L.B.S.: Conceptualization, Supervision, Writing—original draft, Methodology, Writing—review & editing; J.G.A.: Conceptualization, Supervision, Writing—review & editing. All authors have read and agreed to the published version of the manuscript.

Funding: This work was supported in part by the National Institutes of Health/National Cancer Institute (NIH/NCI) Memorial Sloan Kettering Cancer Center (MSK) Support Grant (P30 CA008748).

Institutional Review Board Statement: The study was approved by the institutional review board of MSKCC.

Informed Consent Statement: The study was approved by the institutional review board of MSKCC, and a waiver of informed consent was obtained.

Data Availability Statement: Data is stored in a secure institutional server. It is not publicly available.

Conflicts of Interest: Julio Garcia Aguilar receives honoraria from Johnson & Johnson, Medtronic, and Intuitive Surgical and owns stock in Intuitive Surgical. Joshua Smith received travel support for fellow education from Intuitive Surgical (2015), served as a clinical advisor for Guardant Health (2019), served as a clinical advisor for Foundation Medicine (2022), served as a consultant and speaker for Johnson & Johnson (2022), serves as a clinical advisor and consultant for GSK (2023). Paul B. Romesser received research funding (2019) and serves as a consultant for EMD Serono (2018-present), receives research funding from XRAD Therapeutics (2022–present), is a consultant for Faeth Therapeutics (2022–present), is a consultant for Natera (2022–present), and is a volunteer on the advisory board for the HPV Alliance and Anal Cancer Foundation non-profit organizations. The remaining authors declare no conflict of interest.

References

1. Siegel, R.L.; Miller, K.D.; Wagle, N.S.; Jemal, A. Cancer statistics, 2023. *CA Cancer J. Clin.* **2023**, *73*, 17–48. [CrossRef] [PubMed]
2. UKCCCR Anal Cancer Trial Working Party. Epidermoid anal cancer: Results from the UKCCCR randomised trial of radiotherapy alone versus radiotherapy, 5-fluorouracil, and mitomycin. UKCCCR Anal Cancer Trial Working Party. UK Co-ordinating Committee on Cancer Research. *Lancet* **1996**, *348*, 1049–1054. [CrossRef]
3. Bartelink, H.; Roelofsen, F.; Eschwege, F.; Rougier, P.; Bosset, J.F.; Gonzalez, D.G.; Peiffert, D.; van Glabbeke, M.; Pierart, M. Concomitant radiotherapy and chemotherapy is superior to radiotherapy alone in the treatment of locally advanced anal cancer: Results of a phase III randomized trial of the European Organization for Research and Treatment of Cancer Radiotherapy and Gastrointestinal Cooperative Groups. *J. Clin. Oncol. Off. J. Am. Soc. Clin. Oncol.* **1997**, *15*, 2040–2049. [CrossRef]
4. Flam, M.; John, M.; Pajak, T.F.; Petrelli, N.; Myerson, R.; Doggett, S.; Quivey, J.; Rotman, M.; Kerman, H.; Coia, L.; et al. Role of mitomycin in combination with fluorouracil and radiotherapy, and of salvage chemoradiation in the definitive nonsurgical treatment of epidermoid carcinoma of the anal canal: Results of a phase III randomized intergroup study. *J. Clin. Oncol. Off. J. Am. Soc. Clin. Oncol.* **1996**, *14*, 2527–2539. [CrossRef] [PubMed]
5. Gunderson, L.L.; Winter, K.A.; Ajani, J.A.; Pedersen, J.E.; Moughan, J.; Benson, A.B., 3rd; Thomas, C.R., Jr.; Mayer, R.J.; Haddock, M.G.; Rich, T.A.; et al. Long-term update of US GI intergroup RTOG 98-11 phase III trial for anal carcinoma: Survival, relapse, and colostomy failure with concurrent chemoradiation involving fluorouracil/mitomycin versus fluorouracil/cisplatin. *J. Clin. Oncol. Off. J. Am. Soc. Clin. Oncol.* **2012**, *30*, 4344–4351. [CrossRef] [PubMed]

6. James, R.D.; Glynne-Jones, R.; Meadows, H.M.; Cunningham, D.; Myint, A.S.; Saunders, M.P.; Maughan, T.; McDonald, A.; Essapen, S.; Leslie, M.; et al. Mitomycin or cisplatin chemoradiation with or without maintenance chemotherapy for treatment of squamous-cell carcinoma of the anus (ACT II): A randomised, phase 3, open-label, 2 × 2 factorial trial. *Lancet Oncol.* **2013**, *14*, 516–524. [CrossRef] [PubMed]
7. Ko, G.; Sarkaria, A.; Merchant, S.J.; Booth, C.M.; Patel, S.V. A systematic review of outcomes after salvage abdominoperineal resection for persistent or recurrent anal squamous cell cancer. *Color. Dis. Off. J. Assoc. Coloproctol. Great Br. Irel.* **2019**, *21*, 632–650. [CrossRef]
8. Park, I.J.; Chang, G. Survival and Operative Outcomes After Salvage Surgery for Recurrent or Persistent Anal Cancer. *Ann. Coloproctol.* **2020**, *36*, 361–373. [CrossRef] [PubMed]
9. Deshmukh, A.A.; Suk, R.; Shiels, M.S.; Sonawane, K.; Nyitray, A.G.; Liu, Y.; Gaisa, M.M.; Palefsky, J.M.; Sigel, K. Recent Trends in Squamous Cell Carcinoma of the Anus Incidence and Mortality in the United States, 2001–2015. *J. Natl. Cancer Inst.* **2020**, *112*, 829–838. [CrossRef]
10. Glynne-Jones, R.; Northover, J.M.; Cervantes, A.; ESMO Guidelines Working Group. Anal cancer: ESMO Clinical Practice Guidelines for diagnosis, treatment and follow-up. *Ann. Oncol. Off. J. Eur. Soc. Med. Oncol.* **2010**, *21* (Suppl. 5), v87–v92. [CrossRef]
11. van der Wal, B.C.; Cleffken, B.I.; Gulec, B.; Kaufman, H.S.; Choti, M.A. Results of salvage abdominoperineal resection for recurrent anal carcinoma following combined chemoradiation therapy. *J. Gastrointest. Surg. Off. J. Soc. Surg. Aliment. Tract* **2001**, *5*, 383–387. [CrossRef] [PubMed]
12. Papaconstantinou, H.T.; Bullard, K.M.; Rothenberger, D.A.; Madoff, R.D. Salvage abdominoperineal resection after failed Nigro protocol: Modest success, major morbidity. *Color. Dis. Off. J. Assoc. Coloproctol. Great Br. Irel.* **2006**, *8*, 124–129. [CrossRef] [PubMed]
13. Hagemans, J.A.W.; Blinde, S.E.; Nuyttens, J.J.; Morshuis, W.G.; Mureau, M.A.M.; Rothbarth, J.; Verhoef, C.; Burger, J.W.A. Salvage Abdominoperineal Resection for Squamous Cell Anal Cancer: A 30-Year Single-Institution Experience. *Ann. Surg. Oncol.* **2018**, *25*, 1970–1979. [CrossRef] [PubMed]
14. Patel, S.V.; Ko, G.; Raphael, M.J.; Booth, C.M.; Brogly, S.B.; Kalyvas, M.; Li, W.; Hanna, T. Salvage Abdominoperineal Resection for Anal Squamous Cell Carcinoma: Use, Risk Factors, and Outcomes in a Canadian Population. *Dis. Colon Rectum* **2020**, *63*, 748–757. [CrossRef] [PubMed]
15. Smith, A.J.; Whelan, P.; Cummings, B.J.; Stern, H.S. Management of persistent or locally recurrent epidermoid cancer of the anal canal with abdominoperineal resection. *Acta Oncol.* **2001**, *40*, 34–36. [CrossRef] [PubMed]
16. von Elm, E.; Altman, D.G.; Egger, M.; Pocock, S.J.; Gøtzsche, P.C.; Vandenbroucke, J.P. The Strengthening the Reporting of Observational Studies in Epidemiology (STROBE) statement: Guidelines for reporting observational studies. *Lancet* **2007**, *370*, 1453–1457. [CrossRef] [PubMed]
17. Alamri, Y.; Buchwald, P.; Dixon, L.; Dobbs, B.; Eglinton, T.; McCormick, J.; Wakeman, C.; Frizelle, F.A. Salvage surgery in patients with recurrent or residual squamous cell carcinoma of the anus. *Eur. J. Surg. Oncol. J. Eur. Soc. Surg. Oncol. Br. Assoc. Surg. Oncol.* **2016**, *42*, 1687–1692. [CrossRef] [PubMed]
18. Allal, A.S.; Laurencet, F.M.; Reymond, M.A.; Kurtz, J.M.; Marti, M.C. Effectiveness of surgical salvage therapy for patients with locally uncontrolled anal carcinoma after sphincter-conserving treatment. *Cancer* **1999**, *86*, 405–409. [CrossRef]
19. Brown, K.G.M.; Solomon, M.J.; Steffens, D.; Ng, K.S.; Byrne, C.M.; Austin, K.K.S.; Lee, P.J. Pelvic Exenteration for Squamous Cell Carcinoma of the Anus: Oncological, Morbidity, and Quality-of-Life Outcomes. *Dis. Colon Rectum* **2023**, *66*, 1427–1434. [CrossRef]
20. Ferenschild, F.T.; Vermaas, M.; Hofer, S.O.; Verhoef, C.; Eggermont, A.M.; de Wilt, J.H. Salvage abdominoperineal resection and perineal wound healing in local recurrent or persistent anal cancer. *World J. Surg.* **2005**, *29*, 1452–1457. [CrossRef]
21. Guerra, G.R.; Kong, J.C.; Bernardi, M.P.; Ramsay, R.G.; Phillips, W.A.; Warrier, S.K.; Lynch, A.C.; Ngan, S.Y.; Heriot, A.G. Salvage Surgery for Locoregional Failure in Anal Squamous Cell Carcinoma. *Dis. Colon Rectum* **2018**, *61*, 179–186. [CrossRef] [PubMed]
22. Lefèvre, J.H.; Corte, H.; Tiret, E.; Boccara, D.; Chaouat, M.; Touboul, E.; Svrcek, M.; Lefrancois, M.; Shields, C.; Parc, Y. Abdominoperineal resection for squamous cell anal carcinoma: Survival and risk factors for recurrence. *Ann. Surg. Oncol.* **2012**, *19*, 4186–4192. [CrossRef] [PubMed]
23. Mullen, J.T.; Rodriguez-Bigas, M.A.; Chang, G.J.; Barcenas, C.H.; Crane, C.H.; Skibber, J.M.; Feig, B.W. Results of surgical salvage after failed chemoradiation therapy for epidermoid carcinoma of the anal canal. *Ann. Surg. Oncol.* **2007**, *14*, 478–483. [CrossRef] [PubMed]
24. Schiller, D.E.; Cummings, B.J.; Rai, S.; Le, L.W.; Last, L.; Davey, P.; Easson, A.; Smith, A.J.; Swallow, C.J. Outcomes of salvage surgery for squamous cell carcinoma of the anal canal. *Ann. Surg. Oncol.* **2007**, *14*, 2780–2789. [CrossRef] [PubMed]
25. Ellenhorn, J.D.; Enker, W.E.; Quan, S.H. Salvage abdominoperineal resection following combined chemotherapy and radiotherapy for epidermoid carcinoma of the anus. *Ann. Surg. Oncol.* **1994**, *1*, 105–110. [CrossRef] [PubMed]
26. Beal, K.P.; Wong, D.; Guillem, J.G.; Paty, P.B.; Saltz, L.L.; Wagman, R.; Minsky, B.D. Primary adenocarcinoma of the anus treated with combined modality therapy. *Dis. Colon Rectum* **2003**, *46*, 1320–1324. [CrossRef]
27. Wright, J.L.; Gollub, M.J.; Weiser, M.R.; Saltz, L.B.; Wong, W.D.; Paty, P.B.; Temple, L.K.; Guillem, J.G.; Minsky, B.D.; Goodman, K.A. Surgery and high-dose-rate intraoperative radiation therapy for recurrent squamous-cell carcinoma of the anal canal. *Dis. Colon Rectum* **2011**, *54*, 1090–1097. [CrossRef] [PubMed]

28. Chessin, D.B.; Hartley, J.; Cohen, A.M.; Mazumdar, M.; Cordeiro, P.; Disa, J.; Mehrara, B.; Minsky, B.D.; Paty, P.; Weiser, M.; et al. Rectus flap reconstruction decreases perineal wound complications after pelvic chemoradiation and surgery: A cohort study. *Ann. Surg. Oncol.* **2005**, *12*, 104–110. [CrossRef] [PubMed]
29. Kitaguchi, D.; Tsukada, Y.; Ito, M.; Horasawa, S.; Bando, H.; Yoshino, T.; Yamada, K.; Ajioka, Y.; Sugihara, K. Survival outcomes following salvage abdominoperineal resection for recurrent and persistent anal squamous cell carcinoma. *Eur. J. Surg. Oncol. J. Eur. Soc. Surg. Oncol. Br. Assoc. Surg. Oncol.* **2023**, *49*, 106929. [CrossRef]
30. Severino, N.P.; Chadi, S.A.; Rosen, L.; Coiro, S.; Choman, E.; Berho, M.; Wexner, S.D. Survival following salvage abdominoperineal resection for persistent and recurrent squamous cell carcinoma of the anus: Do these disease categories affect survival? *Color. Dis.* **2016**, *18*, 959–966. [CrossRef]
31. Fields, A.C.; Melnitchouk, N.; Senturk, J.; Irani, J.; Bleday, R.; Goldberg, J. Early versus late salvage abdominoperineal resection for anal squamous cell carcinoma: Is there a difference in survival? *J. Surg. Oncol.* **2019**, *120*, 287–293. [CrossRef] [PubMed]
32. Correa, J.H.; Castro, L.S.; Kesley, R.; Dias, J.A.; Jesus, J.P.; Olivatto, L.O.; Martins, I.O.; Lopasso, F.P. Salvage abdominoperineal resection for anal cancer following chemoradiation: A proposed scoring system for predicting postoperative survival. *J. Surg. Oncol.* **2013**, *107*, 486–492. [CrossRef] [PubMed]
33. Ajani, J.A.; Winter, K.A.; Gunderson, L.L.; Pedersen, J.; Benson, A.B., 3rd; Thomas, C.R., Jr.; Mayer, R.J.; Haddock, M.G.; Rich, T.A.; Willett, C. Fluorouracil, mitomycin, and radiotherapy vs fluorouracil, cisplatin, and radiotherapy for carcinoma of the anal canal: A randomized controlled trial. *JAMA* **2008**, *299*, 1914–1921. [CrossRef] [PubMed]
34. John, M.; Pajak, T.; Flam, M.; Hoffman, J.; Markoe, A.; Wolkov, H.; Paris, K. Dose escalation in chemoradiation for anal cancer: Preliminary results of RTOG 92-08. *Cancer J. Sci. Am.* **1996**, *2*, 205–211.
35. Konski, A.; Garcia, M., Jr.; John, M.; Krieg, R.; Pinover, W.; Myerson, R.; Willett, C. Evaluation of planned treatment breaks during radiation therapy for anal cancer: Update of RTOG 92-08. *Int. J. Radiat. Oncol. Biol. Phys.* **2008**, *72*, 114–118. [CrossRef] [PubMed]
36. Peiffert, D.; Tournier-Rangeard, L.; Gérard, J.P.; Lemanski, C.; François, E.; Giovannini, M.; Cvitkovic, F.; Mirabel, X.; Bouché, O.; Luporsi, E.; et al. Induction chemotherapy and dose intensification of the radiation boost in locally advanced anal canal carcinoma: Final analysis of the randomized UNICANCER ACCORD 03 trial. *J. Clin. Oncol. Off. J. Am. Soc. Clin. Oncol.* **2012**, *30*, 1941–1948. [CrossRef]
37. Hallemeier, C.L.; You, Y.N.; Larson, D.W.; Dozois, E.J.; Nelson, H.; Klein, K.A.; Miller, R.C.; Haddock, M.G. Multimodality therapy including salvage surgical resection and intraoperative radiotherapy for patients with squamous-cell carcinoma of the anus with residual or recurrent disease after primary chemoradiotherapy. *Dis. Colon Rectum* **2014**, *57*, 442–448. [CrossRef]
38. Osborne, M.C.; Maykel, J.; Johnson, E.K.; Steele, S.R. Anal squamous cell carcinoma: An evolution in disease and management. *World J. Gastroenterol.* **2014**, *20*, 13052–13059. [CrossRef]
39. Carr, R.M.; Jin, Z.; Hubbard, J. Research on Anal Squamous Cell Carcinoma: Systemic Therapy Strategies for Anal Cancer. *Cancers* **2021**, *13*, 2180. [CrossRef]
40. Cacheux, W.; Rouleau, E.; Briaux, A.; Tsantoulis, P.; Mariani, P.; Richard-Molard, M.; Buecher, B.; Dangles-Marie, V.; Richon, S.; Lazartigues, J.; et al. Mutational analysis of anal cancers demonstrates frequent PIK3CA mutations associated with poor outcome after salvage abdominoperineal resection. *Br. J. Cancer* **2016**, *114*, 1387–1394. [CrossRef]
41. Cacheux, W.; Dangles-Marie, V.; Rouleau, E.; Lazartigues, J.; Girard, E.; Briaux, A.; Mariani, P.; Richon, S.; Vacher, S.; Buecher, B.; et al. Exome sequencing reveals aberrant signalling pathways as hallmark of treatment-naive anal squamous cell carcinoma. *Oncotarget* **2018**, *9*, 464–476. [CrossRef] [PubMed]

Disclaimer/Publisher's Note: The statements, opinions and data contained in all publications are solely those of the individual author(s) and contributor(s) and not of MDPI and/or the editor(s). MDPI and/or the editor(s) disclaim responsibility for any injury to people or property resulting from any ideas, methods, instructions or products referred to in the content.

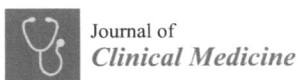 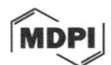

Systematic Review

The Reduction of Anastomosis-Related Morbidity Using the Kono-S Anastomosis in Patients with Crohn's Disease: A Meta-Analysis

Ioannis Baloyiannis [1], Konstantinos Perivoliotis [2,*], Chamaidi Sarakatsianou [1], Charito Chatzinikolaou [2] and George Tzovaras [1]

1 Department of Surgery, University Hospital of Larissa, 41110 Larissa, Greece; balioan@hotmail.com (I.B.); heidisarak@gmail.com (C.S.); geotzovaras@gmail.com (G.T.)
2 Department of Surgery, General Hospital of Volos, 38222 Volos, Greece; xaritoxatz@gmail.com
* Correspondence: kperi19@gmail.com

Abstract: (1) **Background**: we conducted this study to evaluate the effect of Kono-S anastomosis on postoperative morbidity after bowel resection for Crohn's disease. (2) **Methods**: This study adhered to the PRISMA guidelines and the Cochrane Handbook for Systematic Reviews of Interventions. The primary endpoint was the overall complications rate. Secondary outcomes included specific complications analyses, disease recurrence and efficiency endpoints. A systematic literature screening was performed in major electronic scholar databases (Medline, Scopus, Web of Science), from inception to 17 January 2024. Both Random (RE) and Fixed Effects (FE) models were estimated; the reported analysis was based on the Cochran Q test results. (3) **Results**: Overall, eight studies and 913 patients were included in this meta-analysis. Pooled analyses confirmed that Kono-S was not superior in terms of overall morbidity (OR: 0.69 [0.42, 1.15], $p = 0.16$). Kono-S displayed a reduced risk for anastomotic leakage (OR: 0.34 [0.16, 0.71], $p = 0.004$) and reoperation (OR: 0.12 [0.05, 0.27], $p < 0.001$), and a shortened length of hospital stay (WMD: -0.54 [-0.73, -0.34], $p < 0.001$). On the contrary, Kono-S results in higher rates of postoperative SSIs (OR: 1.85 [1.02, 3.35], $p = 0.04$). (4) **Conclusions**: This study confirms a comparable morbidity, but a lower risk of anastomotic leak and reoperation of Kono-S over conventional anastomoses. Further high quality studies are required to validate these findings.

Keywords: Kono-S; Crohn; anastomosis; complications; morbidity; meta-analysis

Citation: Baloyiannis, I.; Perivoliotis, K.; Sarakatsianou, C.; Chatzinikolaou, C.; Tzovaras, G. The Reduction of Anastomosis-Related Morbidity Using the Kono-S Anastomosis in Patients with Crohn's Disease: A Meta-Analysis. *J. Clin. Med.* **2024**, *13*, 2461. https://doi.org/10.3390/jcm13092461

Academic Editors: Byron Vaughn and Angelo Viscido

Received: 22 February 2024
Revised: 21 April 2024
Accepted: 22 April 2024
Published: 23 April 2024

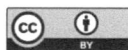

Copyright: © 2024 by the authors. Licensee MDPI, Basel, Switzerland. This article is an open access article distributed under the terms and conditions of the Creative Commons Attribution (CC BY) license (https://creativecommons.org/licenses/by/4.0/).

1. Introduction

1.1. Rationale

Crohn's disease (CD) is a chronic idiopathic disorder that is characterized of transmural inflammation of the gastrointestinal tract, alongside extraintestinal manifestations [1]. Current epidemiologic studies suggest that CD has an increasing prevalence, especially in industrialized countries, with a peaked incidence in young adults [2,3].

Despite recent advances in overall management, CD has a detrimental impact on patients' health-related quality of life due to work disability, disease relapse, treatment side-effects and repeated hospitalizations [4]. In addition to these, in most cases, the administration of immunosuppressors and biologic therapies fails to control the natural course of the disease [5,6]; indeed, almost 80% of CD patients will ultimately be submitted to bowel resection [3]. However, removing the affected bowel segment is not curative and, due to 50% clinical recurrence rates, many patients will require multiple resections [3,7].

The anastomotic site is of pivotal importance, and almost 90% of patients will have an endoscopic recurrence at 3 years postoperatively [6]. Several risk factors have been identified as early anastomotic recurrence predictors, including smoking, disease behavior, perianal involvement, prior resections, histologic characteristics, patient demographics, disease location, and postoperative complications [8–11]. Moreover, the optimal anastomotic technique has been a matter of debate, with handsewn end-to-end and stapled side-to-side configurations being the most frequently performed techniques [12]. Previous pooled analyses reported conflicting results regarding anastomotic leakage, morbidity, hospitalization duration, and recurrence risk between the two anastomotic approaches [13,14].

In 2011, Kono et al. [15] described a novel anastomotic technique after bowel resection for CD, acknowledging the role of mesenteric inflammation and attempting to prevent early disease recurrence. In this technique, the mesentery is excluded through the construction of supporting columns [16]. The latter allows the orientation of the anastomosis to be maintained, and secures a wide lumen [6,15,17]. Kono-S is completed by the performance of an antimesenteric handsewn anastomosis in a single-layer Gambee manner with 3/0 Vicryl running sutures [6,15,17].

The initial report by Kono et al. [15] suggested a significantly lower endoscopic recurrence score at 5 years postoperative, with no increase in postoperative morbidity. Subsequent trials, though, failed to confirm this superiority of Kono-S over conventional anastomoses [16,18,19]. On the contrary, a recent pooled analysis [20] reported a 24.7% incidence of endoscopic recurrence in the Kono-S arm, compared to the respective 42.6% in the comparison group.

However, current evidence regarding the effect of the novel anastomotic technique on perioperative morbidity is still inconclusive [16,18,19]. More specifically, a meta-analysis by Ng et al. [12] estimated a significantly lower risk (1%) of anastomotic leak when Kono-S was performed. Similarly, Shimada et al. [6] reported that Kono-S resulted in a significant reduction in anastomotic leakage rates, while Kelm et al. [18] associated the new approach with a higher risk of surgical site infections. In addition to these, recently published comparative studies [17,19] provided contradictive results regarding the comparability of Kono-S and conventional anastomotic techniques in terms of postoperative complications. Therefore, the need for updated evidence and ranking of the two approaches considering morbidity and perioperative efficacy, is thoroughly justified.

1.2. Objectives

Taking into consideration the above-mentioned evidence, we designed and conducted the present meta-analysis to evaluate the role of the Kono-S anastomosis in postoperative morbidity and efficiency after bowel resection for CD.

2. Materials and Methods

2.1. Study Protocol

This meta-analysis was conducted according to the PRISMA guidelines [21] and the Cochrane Handbook for Systematic Reviews of Interventions [22]. The review protocol was not pre-registered.

2.2. Endpoints

The primary endpoint of this study was the comparison of Kono-S and conventional (CONV) anastomosis regarding the overall complications rate, in patients submitted to surgical resection for CD. Secondary outcomes included specific complication analyses (Clavien–Dindo $\geq$ III, intraabdominal abscess, surgical site infection-SSI, ileus, bleeding, anastomotic leakage, readmission, and reoperation), disease recurrence (clinical recurrence and Rutgeerts score > i2 [23]), and efficiency endpoints (operation duration and length of hospital stay (LOS)). Conventional anastomosis was considered any standardized anastomotic technique, besides Kono-S, regardless of its layout (end-to-side, end-to-end, side-to-side) and technique (handsewn, stapled).

2.3. Eligibility Criteria

All clinical studies that compared the two anastomotic techniques after any bowel resection, in patients with CD, whose data were extractable, and the original report was written in English were considered as eligible. The following exclusion criteria were applied: (1) non-human studies, (2) no outcomes of interest, (3) no comparison group, (4) article not written in English, (5) irretrievable data, and (6) manuscripts in the form of editorials, case reports, expert opinions, or conference abstracts. There was no restriction in terms of bowel resection type.

2.4. Literature Search

After the removal of duplicate entries, the titles and abstracts of the search results were screened based on the eligibility criteria. Consequently, a full text evaluation of the remaining manuscripts was performed. All literature searches, data extractions, and quality assessments were performed in duplicate and blindly by two independent researchers (P.K. and B.I.). In case of a discrepancy that was not resolved by mutual revision, the opinion of a third investigator was considered (T.G.).

Methodological assessment was based on the ROBINS-I [24] and RoB 2 tool [25] (Website: https://www.riskofbias.info/, access on date: 21 January 2024) for non-randomized and randomized controlled trials (RCTs), respectively. Interrater agreement was estimated through the calculation of Cohen's k statistic.

2.5. Study Selection and Data Collection

To identify eligible studies, a systematic literature screening was performed in major electronic scholar databases (Medline, Scopus, Web of Science) from inception to 17 January 2024. The following keywords were introduced as search terms: "Kono-S". To avoid missing any study, a broad search strategy was introduced, with minimum restrictive terms.

After the identification of the eligible studies the data extraction process was initiated. Besides the analyzed endpoints, the following data were recorded: included studies' characteristics (first author, country, study type, number of centers, publication year, study period, sample per arm, gender, age and Body Mass Index (BMI) allocation, follow-up period), patient characteristics (American Society of Anesthesiologists (ASA) score, smoking, previous operations, perianal disease and Vienna classification), previous treatment characteristics (type of medications), and surgical approach characteristics (previous surgical experience, number of surgeons, emergency operations, resection site, type of approach, anastomotic technique, length of resected bowel).

2.6. Statistical Analysis

Statistical analyses were performed in Cochrane Collaboration RevMan (Version 5.4.1 Copenhagen: The Cochrane Collaboration, 2020) and IBM SPSS Statistics for Windows (Version 29.0.2.0 Armonk, NY: IBM Corp). Categorical and continuous endpoints were reported as odds ratio (OR) and weighted mean difference (WMD), respectively. All variables were provided with the corresponding 95% confidence interval (95%CI).

In cases where the mean or the standard deviation (SD) of a variable was not reported, they were estimated from the respective median, range, or interquartile range (IQR), based on the formula described by Hozo et al. [26]. Meta-analysis estimations utilized the Mantel–Haenszel (MH) and inverse variance (IV) algorithms. Heterogeneity estimation included the calculation of I^2. Both random -RE and fixed effects -FE models were estimated; the reported analysis was based on the Cochran Q test results (Q $p < 0.1$). Explanatory analyses included subgroup analysis and meta-regression. Meta-regression was based on the RE model and utilized a DerSimonian–Laird estimator. Statistical significance was considered at the level of $p < 0.05$.

2.7. Risk of Bias across Studies

The funnel plot of all outcomes was visually evaluated for the presence of publication bias.

3. Results

The application of the screening algorithm resulted to the retrieval of 2325 entries (Figure 1). After the removal of 731 duplicates, the titles and abstracts of the remaining articles were reviewed. Overall, 1578 records (reviews and meta-analyses: 187; single armed study: 17; non-English article: 3; letters, expert opinions, or conference abstracts: 17; experimental studies: 2; irrelevant records: 1352) were excluded during this step. Full text assessment identified four studies with no comparison group and four irrelevant articles. Consequently, eight studies [5,6,15,17–19,27] were included in the qualitative and quantitative synthesis.

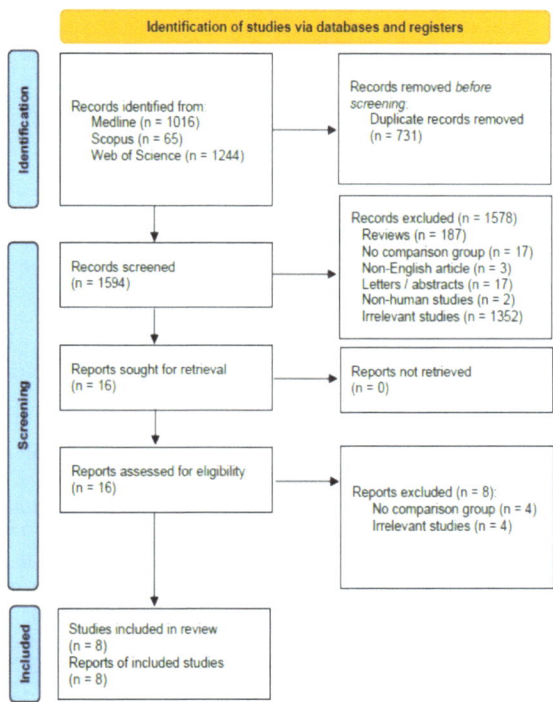

Figure 1. PRISMA study flow diagram. For more information, visit: https://www.prisma-stataement.org (accessed on 18 January 2024).

Overall, 913 patients were included in this meta-analysis (Table 1). There was only one RCT [5]; the remaining trials applied either a prospective or a retrospective methodology. Most studies were performed in a single center [5,6,16–18,27], and the publication period spanned from 2011 to 2023. Data regarding gender, age, and BMI allocation are also provided in Table 1. Mean follow up spanned from 6.55 to 89 months.

Data regarding the ASA status of the patients were provided only in three [16,17,19] studies (Supplementary Materials). Overall, 141 patients had received a previous operation. In total, 71 patients displayed perianal disease manifestations. Furthermore, 89, 279 and 242 CD cases were classified as inflammatory (B1), stricturing (B2) and penetrating (B3) disease behavior, respectively. Biologics were administered in 403 patients.

Table 1. Included studies.

Author	Country	Study Type	Center	Year	Study Period	Group	Sample	Gender (M)	Age	BMI	Follow Up
Alibert et al. [19]	France	prospective	multi	2023	2020–2022	KONO-S	61	26	37 (4.75)	21.9 (1.17)	6.7 (0.41)
						CONV	122	55	34 (3)	20.9 (0.90)	
Holubar et al. [16]	USA	retrospective	single	2023	2015–2022	KONO-S	74	36	38.2 (16.3)	25.1 (5.6)	n/a
						CONV	66	33	37.9 (15.5)	25.4 (5.6)	
Obi et al. [27]	USA	retrospective	single	2023	2019–2022	KONO-S	9	4	15.4	21.6	6.55
						CONV	9	3	16.2	20	7.57
Tyrode et al. [17]	France	retrospective	single	2023	2020–2022	KONO-S	30	13	32.2 (13.4)	22.3 (3.92)	12
						CONV	55	24	36.1 (15.6)	23.5 (6)	
Kelm et al. [18]	Germany	retrospective	single	2022	2019–2021	KONO-S	22	14	37.4 (10.5)	24.3	8.8 (2.5)
						CONV	29	14	36.8 (13.7)	22.8	
Luglio et al. [5]	Italy	RCT	single	2020	2015–2017	KONO-S	36	18	34 (6.25)	n/a	24
						CONV	43	22	43 (8.25)		
Shimada et al. [6]	Japan	retrospective	single	2019	2006–2016	KONO-S	117	84	39 (11.8)	18.9 (2.51)	38 (23.7)
						CONV	98	74	34 (11.1)	18.6 (2.44)	89 (34)
Kono et al. [15]	Japan	retrospective	multi	2011	2003–2009	KONO-S	69	57	31 (10.7)	n/a	42 (18.7)
						CONV	73	58	28 (12)		52 (29.7)

n/a: not available.

Overall, three studies [17,18,27] confirmed previous surgical expertise (Supplementary Materials Tables S1–S5). Similarly, data regarding the number of operating surgeons were scarce. Only 19 resections were performed in an emergency setting. All studies, except two [6,15], reported data on ileocolic anastomoses (Supplementary Materials). Most operations were performed in a laparoscopic approach. Open conversion was required in 22 cases. Finally, 162 stapled conventional anastomoses were included in the comparative analyses.

Quality assessment of the eligible studies highlighted moderate to serious methodological deficits in most non-RCTs. The RCT by Luglio et al. [5] was graded as having some concerns regarding the overall risk of bias. There was an adequate level of agreement in both tools (RoB 2 Cohen k statistic:1 $p = 0.025$, ROBINS-I Cohen k statistic: 0.85 $p < 0.001$).

All eligible studies provided data regarding the primary outcome (Figure 2, Table 2). Pooled evidence did not confirm a superiority (OR: 0.69 [0.42, 1.15], $p = 0.16$) of Kono-S over conventional anastomosis after bowel resection in patients with CD. Due to significant heterogeneity levels (I^2: 46%, $p = 0.08$), further explanatory analyses were performed. The results of meta-regression (Supplementary Materials) could not confirm a significant effect of any analyzed variable (publication year, sample size, gender, age, BMI, follow up, smoking, previous operation, perianal disease, anti-TNF medication, laparoscopic approach, stapled conventional anastomosis, and resected length of bowel). Stratifying for ileocolic anastomoses (OR: 0.83 [0.4, 1.73], $p = 0.61$) and side-to-side conventional anastomoses only (OR: 0.89 [0.29, 2.75], $p = 0.84$) did not alter the overall outcome. A non-significant result was also estimated in the experienced surgeons' subgroup (OR: 1.67 [0.37, 7.64], $p = 0.51$). A significant superiority of Kono-S (Supplementary Materials) was confirmed in the prospective (OR: 0.47 [0.24, 0.89], $p = 0.02$), but not in the retrospective studies subgroup. Exclusion of high risk of bias studies resulted in a significant effect of the experimental technique (OR: 0.47 [0.24, 0.89], $p = 0.02$).

In terms of secondary outcomes (Table 2, Supplementary Materials), Kono-S displayed comparable rates of Clavien–Dindo $\geq$ III complications ($p = 0.18$), intraabdominal abscesses ($p = 0.18$), postoperative ileus ($p = 0.87$) and bleeding ($p = 0.1$). Similarly, there was no difference in terms of readmission rates ($p = 0.21$). On the contrary, Kono-S was associated with a significantly higher risk of SSIs (OR: 1.85 [1.02, 3.35], $p = 0.04$). Anastomotic leakage (OR: 0.34 [0.16, 0.71], $p = 0.004$) and reoperation rates (OR: 0.12 [0.05, 0.27], $p < 0.001$) were significantly decreased when Kono-S was applied.

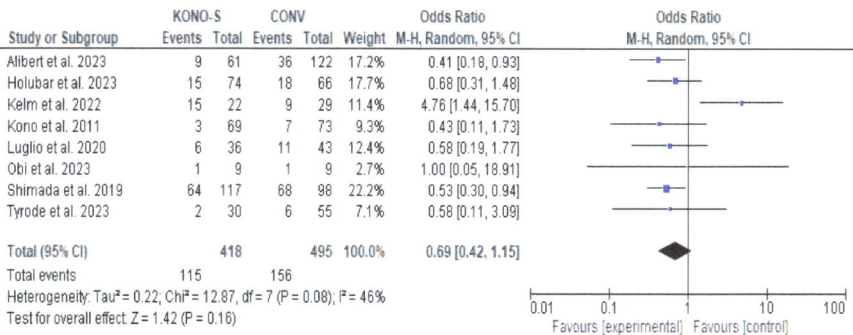

Figure 2. Overall complications forest plot [5,6,15–19,27].

Table 2. Primary and secondary outcomes.

Outcome	Studies	Participants	Statistical Method	Effect Estimate 95%CI	p	I²	Heterogeneity p
Overall Complications	8	913	Random Effects	0.69 [0.42, 1.15]	0.16	46%	0.08
CD ≥ III	4	459	Fixed Effects	0.54 [0.22, 1.32]	0.18	14%	0.32
Intrabdominal Abscess	6	624	Fixed Effects	0.62 [0.31, 1.25]	0.18	0%	0.68
SSI	7	730	Fixed Effects	1.85 [1.02, 3.35]	0.04	0%	0.71
Ileus	6	645	Fixed Effects	0.95 [0.55, 1.66]	0.87	0%	0.88
Bleeding	4	446	Fixed Effects	0.34 [0.09, 1.25]	0.1	0%	0.82
Leakage	7	828	Fixed Effects	0.34 [0.16, 0.71]	0.004	0%	0.66
Readmission	4	453	Fixed Effects	0.59 [0.26, 1.35]	0.21	5%	0.37
Reoperation	4	515	Fixed Effects	0.12 [0.05, 0.27]	<0.001	0%	0.66
>i2	5	540	Random Effects	0.66 [0.33, 1.29]	0.22	68%	0.01
Clinical Recurrence	4	562	Random Effects	0.42 [0.14, 1.24]	0.12	75%	0.007
Operation Duration [minutes]	5	702	Random Effects	5.71 [−4.93, 16.36]	0.29	83%	<0.001
LOS [days]	4	487	Fixed Effects	−0.54 [−0.73, −0.34]	<0.001	0%	0.48

Pooled analyses could not confirm an improvement in clinical ($p = 0.12$) or endoscopic recurrence ($p = 0.22$) with Kono-S. Furthermore, the introduction of Kono-S as an anastomotic technique did not alter the procedure duration ($p = 0.29$); however, it resulted in a significant reduction in LOS by a mean of 0.54 days (WMD: -0.54 [-0.73, -0.34], $p < 0.001$).

Inspection of the primary endpoint funnel plot (Supplementary Materials) showed a symmetrical distribution of the studies over the combined effect size line. The funnel plots of the secondary outcomes are also provided in Supplementary Materials.

4. Discussion

4.1. Summary of Evidence

Our study is an effort to provide updated evidence regarding the efficacy of the novel Kono-S anastomotic technique in reducing postoperative morbidity and recurrence rates after bowel resection in CD patients. Our results suggest that Kono-S is not effective in minimizing clinical and endoscopic recurrence, and does not provide an enhanced overall safety profile. Despite these, a lower risk of anastomotic leakage and reoperation was confirmed.

Optimal therapeutic management of CD is based on disease staging, patient risk stratification and preferences, and clinical characteristics [28]. In most cases, the initial approach includes the administration of steroids to alleviate the symptoms and the subsequent introduction of biologics to control and reduce the risk of disease flares [28]. A significant proportion of patients, though, will ultimately undergo bowel resection due to the development of stenoses, fistulas or disease refractory to conventional immunomodulatory therapy [28]. Additionally, in specific disease phenotypes, including inflammatory ileocolic CD, upfront surgery is considered as a valid option due to optimal results [3,29,30]. In the LIR!C RCT [31], laparoscopic ileocecal resection was compared to infliximab for limited non-stricturing ileocecal CD, with comparable results in terms of restoring quality of life and overall morbidity. A significant finding of this study was that one-third of patients in the biologic group required resection compared to one fourth of the surgical arm that received infliximab [31].

Consequently, it became apparent that, to enhance postoperative outcomes, the surgical approach, including the anastomotic technique, should be optimized. In the CAST trial [32], side-to-side was compared to end-to-end anastomosis after ileocecal resection; no significant difference in the endoscopic and symptomatic recurrence rates was found during follow-up. Comparability of the two techniques in early postoperative outcomes was also reported by the ISRCTN-45665492 study [33]. Contrary to these, a recent network meta-analysis [34] suggested the superiority of side-to-side anastomosis in terms of overall morbidity, clinical recurrence, and reoperation. Furthermore, the role of mesenteric resection in disease outcome has also attracted the interest of researchers [35]. As an answer to these, Kono et al. [15] described the homonymous anastomotic layout with specific technical features, and also reported promising postoperative results.

Despite being a side-to-side handsewn anastomosis, Kono-S incorporates several technical features that render it a complex procedural step [18]. As such, to minimize postoperative morbidity, structured training should be considered prior to performing Kono-S [18]. More specifically, based on recent studies, approximately 20 cases are required to overcome the learning curve of this new technique [18]. This further highlights the need to properly assess the safety of this new approach, prior to extensively applying it to CD patients. In a recent cohort by Tyrode et al. [17], Kono-S did not have a higher morbidity profile compared to conventional handsewn, side-to-side anastomoses. This was also confirmed in a meta-analysis by Ng et al. [12], where minimal rates of complications were reported. Our pooled analyses calculated a 27.5% and 31.5% overall morbidity rate for Kono-S and a control group, respectively. This was reduced to 3.7% and 6.6% when assessing severe (Clavien–Dindo $\geq$ III) complications. Statistical significance was not reached in any of these comparisons, and the influencing factors were not identified.

Previous experimental and clinical studies confirmed that the bowel segments affected by CD have an over 50% decrease in blood flow [15]. The imaging quantification of this clinical parameter is currently under evaluation with novel techniques, including shear wave and strain elastography [36]. Due to its configuration, the novel anastomotic technique presents several advantages, including the preservation of bowel perfusion and innervation, factors directly associated with optimal anastomotic healing [15]. Initial reports did not suggest a superiority of Kono-S over conventional techniques in terms of anastomotic healing [15]. In a large cohort by Shimada et al. [6], Kono-S displayed a lower rate (5.1% vs. 17.3%) of anastomotic leakage when compared to layer-to-layer end-to-end anastomosis; this, though, did not reach statistical significance. Interestingly, our pooled estimations suggested a significant difference in favor of Kono-S regarding the risk of postoperative anastomotic leakage.

Our meta-analysis confirmed a higher rate of SSIs in patients submitted to Kono-S anastomosis after bowel resection. In addition to this, a low heterogeneity level was identified. Although no single study had a significant effect size, the trials of Kelm et al. [18] and Shimada et al. [6] reported a higher incidence of infections in the experimental group. As mentioned by Kelm et al. [18], a possible explanation for this could be the access routes used for the anastomoses after different approaches (suprapubic for conventional and periumbilical for Kono-S).

The mesentery in CD develops characteristic macroscopic and microscopic changes, including fat thickening and hyperplasia of adipocytes and connective tissue [19]. Several researchers suggested that the mesentery has a pivotal role in the pathogenesis and recurrence of the disease, given the fact that mucosal inflammation is usually located in the mesenteric side and has a positive association with the mesenteric inflammation [19]. To prevent this, Kono et al. [15] proposed the creation of a supporting column and the formation of the anastomosis on the antimesenteric axis [15]. Besides the biomechanistic properties, Kono-S may also prevent early recurrence through the preservation of gut flora [12]; the isoperistaltic layout and the supporting column minimizes microbiome changes, especially in cases of ileocecal resections [12].

The potential of Kono-S in reducing recurrence rates has been extensively evaluated in multiple clinical scenarios [12]. Comparing Kono-S to conventional anastomoses, Kono et al. [15] found that, although 1-year endoscopic recurrence rates were comparable, the experimental group displayed a lower mean Rutgeert score at 5 years. In the SuPREMe-CD RCT [5], Kono-S was compared to a conventional side-to-side stapled anastomosis and had a lower risk for endoscopic recurrence at 6 and 18 months postoperatively. Logistic regression also confirmed the anastomotic technique as the sole predictor of endoscopic recurrence and a lower recurrence-free survival was reported in the conventional study arm [5]. On the contrary, in the propensity score matched cohort of the KoCoRICCO study [19], Kono-S was not associated with lower endoscopic recurrence events. In our study, the two approaches did not differ in terms of clinical and endoscopic recurrence (Rutgeert score $\geq$ i2). However, when evaluating such outcomes, several factors should be acknowledged, including time endpoints, disease behavior, definition of recurrence and control technique. Regarding the latter, it has been confirmed that the mechanical staple line may falsely be diagnosed with endoscopic recurrence, whereas handsewn anastomoses heal without ulcerations [19].

In the Kono-S technique, a complex handsewn anastomosis is performed; thus, theoretically, prolonging the operative time [16]. Indeed, previous studies suggested that due to the additional hand-sewing, Kono-S resulted to an average 30 min longer operation duration [16]. In the previous meta-analysis by Ng et al. [12], the mean operative time of resection and restoration of bowel continuity was 179 min, which was comparable to the respective control group. Our results were like the latter, since no significant difference was found between the Kono-S and conventional anastomosis groups. It must be noted, though, that this estimation was plagued by high heterogeneity levels; thus, suggesting that factors like the Kono-S learning curve status and the conventional technique that was used as comparator could have influenced the results.

We confirmed that patients submitted to resection and restoration of bowel continuity with this novel technique, were discharged earlier compared to the conventional group. Previous cohorts, though, did not identify a hospitalization duration benefit of Kono-S [5,16]. Moreover, data regarding postoperative bowel function and patient mobilization were scarce and, therefore, no analysis of other recovery endpoints was available. Therefore, this significant effect could be associated with the previously reported lower rates of anastomotic complications and reoperation in the Kono-S group.

4.2. Limitations

Prior to the appraisal of the results of this study, several limitations should be acknowledged. First, most of the eligible studies did not include an adequate randomization or blinding algorithm, thus reducing the validity of the pooled analyses. Furthermore, the quality assessment highlighted several methodological deficits that could have contributed to the overall bias. Moreover, the small sample size in the included trials reduced the power of the pooled statistical calculations. Additionally, the inherent heterogeneity in terms of patient characteristics, disease stage, perioperative treatment regimens, and the conventional anastomotic technique, further impacted the significance of the estimate endpoints. Finally, the divergence in the reported follow-up period could have affected several time-related endpoints including morbidity and disease recurrence.

5. Conclusions

This meta-analysis failed to estimate a significant effect of Kono-S over conventional anastomoses, in reducing the overall postoperative morbidity rates, after bowel resection for CD. Kono-S displayed a reduced risk for anastomotic leakage and reoperation, and a shortened length of hospital stay. On the contrary, Kono-S resulted in higher rates of postoperative SSIs. Due to several study limitations, further higher quality RCTs are required to delineate the exact role of Kono-S in patients submitted to surgery for Crohn's disease.

Supplementary Materials: The following supporting information can be downloaded at: https://www.mdpi.com/article/10.3390/jcm13092461/s1, Table S1. Included patient characteristics; Table S2. Previous treatment characteristics; Table S3. Surgical approach characteristics; Table S4. Overall Morbidity Meta-Regression; Table S5. Subgroup Analysis Based on Study Type; Figure S1. Risk of Bias 2 traffic light plot; Figure S2. ROBINS-I traffic light plot; Figure S3. CD>III forest plot; Figure S4. Intraabdominal abscess forest plot; Figure S5. SSI forest plot; Figure S6. Ileus forest plot; Figure S7. Bleeding forest plot; Figure S8. Leakage forest plot; Figure S9. Readmission forest plot; Figure S10. Reoperation forest plot; Figure S11. >i2 forest plot; Figure S12. Clinical recurrence forest plot; Figure S13. Operation duration forest plot; Figure S14. LOS forest plot; Figure S15. Overall complications funnel plot; Figure S16. CD>III funnel plot; Figure S17. Intraabdominal abscess funnel plot; Figure S18. SSI funnel plot; Figure S19. Ileus funnel plot; Figure S20. Bleeding funnel plot; Figure S21. Leakage funnel plot; Figure S22. Readmission funnel plot; Figure S23. Reoperation funnel plot; Figure S24. >i2 funnel plot; Figure S25. Clinical recurrence funnel plot; Figure S26. Operation duration funnel plot; Figure S27. LOS funnel plot.

Author Contributions: Conceptualization, K.P. and I.B.; methodology, K.P.; formal analysis, K.P.; investigation, I.B. and K.P.; writing—original draft preparation, K.P. and C.S.; writing—review and editing, I.B. and C.C.; supervision, G.T.; project administration, G.T. All authors have read and agreed to the published version of the manuscript.

Funding: This research received no external funding.

Institutional Review Board Statement: Not applicable.

Informed Consent Statement: Not applicable.

Data Availability Statement: Data sharing not applicable to this article as no datasets were generated or analyzed during the current study.

Conflicts of Interest: The authors declare no conflicts of interest.

References

1. Torres, J.; Mehandru, S.; Colombel, J.F.; Peyrin-Biroulet, L. Crohn's Disease. *Lancet* **2017**, *389*, 1741–1755. [CrossRef] [PubMed]
2. Feuerstein, J.D.; Cheifetz, A.S. Crohn Disease: Epidemiology, Diagnosis, and Management. *Mayo Clin. Proc.* **2017**, *92*, 1088–1103. [CrossRef]
3. Meima-van Praag, E.M.; Buskens, C.J.; Hompes, R.; Bemelman, W.A. Surgical Management of Crohn's Disease: A State of the Art Review. *Int. J. Color. Dis.* **2021**, *36*, 1133–1145. [CrossRef] [PubMed]
4. Van der Have, M.; van der Aalst, K.S.; Kaptein, A.A.; Leenders, M.; Siersema, P.D.; Oldenburg, B.; Fidder, H.H. Determinants of Health-Related Quality of Life in Crohn's Disease: A Systematic Review and Meta-Analysis. *J. Crohns Colitis* **2014**, *8*, 93–106. [CrossRef] [PubMed]
5. Luglio, G.; Rispo, A.; Imperatore, N.; Giglio, M.C.; Amendola, A.; Tropeano, F.P.; Peltrini, R.; Castiglione, F.; De Palma, G.D.; Bucci, L. Surgical Prevention of Anastomotic Recurrence by Excluding Mesentery in Crohn's Disease: The SuPREMe-CD Study—A Randomized Clinical Trial. *Ann. Surg.* **2020**, *272*, 210–217. [CrossRef] [PubMed]
6. Shimada, N.; Ohge, H.; Kono, T.; Sugitani, A.; Yano, R.; Watadani, Y.; Uemura, K.; Murakami, Y.; Sueda, T. Surgical Recurrence at Anastomotic Site after Bowel Resection in Crohn's Disease: Comparison of Kono-S and End-to-End Anastomosis. *J. Gastrointest. Surg.* **2019**, *23*, 312–319. [CrossRef] [PubMed]
7. Colombo, F.; Frontali, A.; Baldi, C.; Cigognini, M.; Lamperti, G.; Manzo, C.A.; Maconi, G.; Ardizzone, S.; Foschi, D.; Sampietro, G.M. Repeated Surgery for Recurrent Crohn's Disease: Does the Outcome Keep Worsening Operation after Operation? A Comparative Study of 1224 Consecutive Procedures. *Updates Surg.* **2022**, *74*, 73. [CrossRef]
8. De Cruz, P.; Hamilton, A.L.; Burrell, K.J.; Gorelik, A.; Liew, D.; Kamm, M.A. Endoscopic Prediction of Crohn's Disease Postoperative Recurrence. *Inflamm. Bowel Dis.* **2022**, *28*, 680–688. [CrossRef] [PubMed]

9. Navaratne, L.; Hurndall, K.H.; Richardson, D.M.; Stephenson, R.; Power, N.; Gillott, H.; Ruiz Sánchez, S.; Khodatars, K.; Chan, C.L.H. Risk Factors for Symptomatic Anastomotic Postoperative Recurrence Following Ileo-Colic Resection in Crohn's Disease. *Color. Dis.* **2021**, *23*, 1184–1192. [CrossRef]
10. Aaltonen, G.; Keränen, I.; Carpelan-Holmström, M.; Lepistö, A. Risk Factors for Anastomotic Recurrence after Primary Ileocaecal Resection in Crohn's Disease. *Eur. J. Gastroenterol. Hepatol.* **2018**, *30*, 1143–1147. [CrossRef]
11. Gklavas, A.; Dellaportas, D.; Papaconstantinou, I. Risk Factors for Postoperative Recurrence of Crohn's Disease with Emphasis on Surgical Predictors. *Ann. Gastroenterol.* **2017**, *30*, 598–612. [CrossRef] [PubMed]
12. Ng, C.H.; Chin, Y.H.; Lin, S.Y.; Koh, J.W.H.; Lieske, B.; Koh, F.H.-X.; Chong, C.S.; Foo, F.J. Kono-S Anastomosis for Crohn's Disease: A Systemic Review, Meta-Analysis, and Meta-Regression. *Surg. Today* **2021**, *51*, 493–501. [CrossRef] [PubMed]
13. Simillis, C.; Purkayastha, S.; Yamamoto, T.; Strong, S.A.; Darzi, A.W.; Tekkis, P.P. A Meta-Analysis Comparing Conventional End-to-End Anastomosis vs. Other Anastomotic Configurations after Resection in Crohn's Disease. *Dis. Colon Rectum* **2007**, *50*, 1674–1687. [CrossRef] [PubMed]
14. Guo, Z.; Li, Y.; Zhu, W.; Gong, J.; Li, N.; Li, J. Comparing Outcomes between Side-to-Side Anastomosis and Other Anastomotic Configurations after Intestinal Resection for Patients with Crohn's Disease: A Meta-Analysis. *World J. Surg.* **2013**, *37*, 893–901. [CrossRef] [PubMed]
15. Kono, T.; Ashida, T.; Ebisawa, Y.; Chisato, N.; Okamoto, K.; Katsuno, H.; Maeda, K.; Fujiya, M.; Kohgo, Y.; Furukawa, H. A New Antimesenteric Functional End-to-End Handsewn Anastomosis: Surgical Prevention of Anastomotic Recurrence in Crohn's Disease. *Dis. Colon Rectum* **2011**, *54*, 586–592. [CrossRef]
16. Holubar, S.D.; Lipman, J.; Steele, S.R.; Uchino, T.; Lincango, E.P.; Liska, D.; Ban, K.; Rosen, D.; Sommovilla, J.; Gorgun, E.; et al. Safety & Feasibility of Targeted Mesenteric Approaches with Kono-S Anastomosis and Extended Mesenteric Excision in Ileocolic Resection and Anastomosis in Crohn's Disease. *Am. J. Surg.* **2023**, *230*, 16–20. [CrossRef]
17. Tyrode, G.; Lakkis, Z.; Vernerey, D.; Falcoz, A.; Clairet, V.; Alibert, L.; Koch, S.; Vuitton, L. KONO-S Anastomosis Is Not Superior to Conventional Anastomosis for the Reduction of Postoperative Endoscopic Recurrence in Crohn's Disease. *Inflamm. Bowel Dis.* **2023**, izad214. [CrossRef]
18. Kelm, M.; Reibetanz, J.; Kim, M.; Schoettker, K.; Brand, M.; Meining, A.; Germer, C.-T.; Flemming, S. Kono-S Anastomosis in Crohn's Disease: A Retrospective Study on Postoperative Morbidity and Disease Recurrence in Comparison to the Conventional Side-To-Side Anastomosis. *J. Clin. Med.* **2022**, *11*, 6915. [CrossRef]
19. Alibert, L.; Betton, L.; Falcoz, A.; Manceau, G.; Benoist, S.; Zerbib, P.; Podevin, J.; Maggiori, L.; Brouquet, A.; Tyrode, G.; et al. Does KONO-S Anastomosis Reduce Recurrence in Crohn's Disease Compared to Conventional Ileocolonic Anastomosis? A Nationwide Propensity Score-Matched Study from GETAID Chirurgie Group (KoCoRICCO Study). *J. Crohns Colitis* **2023**, jjad176. [CrossRef]
20. Nardone, O.M.; Calabrese, G.; Barberio, B.; Giglio, M.C.; Castiglione, F.; Luglio, G.; Savarino, E.; Ghosh, S.; Iacucci, M. Rates of Endoscopic Recurrence In Postoperative Crohn's Disease Based on Anastomotic Techniques: A Systematic Review and Meta-Analysis. *Inflamm. Bowel Dis.* **2023**, izad252. [CrossRef]
21. Page, M.J.; McKenzie, J.E.; Bossuyt, P.M.; Boutron, I.; Hoffmann, T.C.; Mulrow, C.D.; Shamseer, L.; Tetzlaff, J.M.; Akl, E.A.; Brennan, S.E.; et al. The PRISMA 2020 Statement: An Updated Guideline for Reporting Systematic Reviews. *BMJ* **2021**, *372*, n71. [CrossRef] [PubMed]
22. Higgins, J.P.T.; Cochrane Collaboration. *Cochrane Handbook for Systematic Reviews of Interventions*, 2nd ed.; Wiley-Blackwell Publishing Ltd.: Hoboken, NJ, USA, 2019; ISBN 9781119536628.
23. Narula, N.; Wong, E.C.L.; Dulai, P.S.; Marshall, J.K.; Jairath, V.; Reinisch, W. The Performance of the Rutgeerts Score, SES-CD, and MM-SES-CD for Prediction of Postoperative Clinical Recurrence in Crohn's Disease. *Inflamm. Bowel Dis.* **2023**, *29*, 716–725. [CrossRef]
24. Schünemann, H.J.; Cuello, C.; Akl, E.A.; Mustafa, R.A.; Meerpohl, J.J.; Thayer, K.; Morgan, R.L.; Gartlehner, G.; Kunz, R.; Katikireddi, S.V.; et al. GRADE Guidelines: 18. How ROBINS-I and Other Tools to Assess Risk of Bias in Nonrandomized Studies Should Be Used to Rate the Certainty of a Body of Evidence. *J. Clin. Epidemiol.* **2019**, *111*, 105–114. [CrossRef]
25. Sterne, J.A.C.; Savović, J.; Page, M.J.; Elbers, R.G.; Blencowe, N.S.; Boutron, I.; Cates, C.J.; Cheng, H.-Y.; Corbett, M.S.; Eldridge, S.M.; et al. RoB 2: A Revised Tool for Assessing Risk of Bias in Randomised Trials. *BMJ* **2019**, *366*, l4898. [CrossRef]
26. Hozo, S.P.; Djulbegovic, B.; Hozo, I. Estimating the Mean and Variance from the Median, Range, and the Size of a Sample. *BMC Med. Res. Methodol.* **2005**, *5*, 13. [CrossRef] [PubMed]
27. Obi, M.; DeRoss, A.L.; Lipman, J. Use of the Kono-S Anastomosis in Pediatric Crohn's Disease: A Single-Institution Experience. *Pediatr. Surg. Int.* **2023**, *39*, 290. [CrossRef]
28. Cushing, K.; Higgins, P.D.R. Management of Crohn Disease: A Review. *JAMA* **2021**, *325*, 69. [CrossRef]
29. Torres, J.; Bonovas, S.; Doherty, G.; Kucharzik, T.; Gisbert, J.P.; Raine, T.; Adamina, M.; Armuzzi, A.; Bachmann, O.; Bager, P.; et al. ECCO Guidelines on Therapeutics in Crohn's Disease: Medical Treatment. *J. Crohns Colitis* **2020**, *14*, 4–22. [CrossRef] [PubMed]
30. Adamina, M.; Bonovas, S.; Raine, T.; Spinelli, A.; Warusavitarne, J.; Armuzzi, A.; Bachmann, O.; Bager, P.; Biancone, L.; Bokemeyer, B.; et al. ECCO Guidelines on Therapeutics in Crohn's Disease: Surgical Treatment. *J. Crohns Colitis* **2020**, *14*, 155–168. [CrossRef] [PubMed]
31. Ponsioen, C.Y.; de Groof, E.J.; Eshuis, E.J.; Gardenbroek, T.J.; Bossuyt, P.M.M.; Hart, A.; Warusavitarne, J.; Buskens, C.J.; van Bodegraven, A.A.; Brink, M.A.; et al. Laparoscopic Ileocaecal Resection versus Infliximab for Terminal Ileitis in Crohn's Disease: A Randomised Controlled, Open-Label, Multicentre Trial. *Lancet Gastroenterol. Hepatol.* **2017**, *2*, 785–792. [CrossRef]

32. McLeod, R.S.; Wolff, B.G.; Ross, S.; Parkes, R.; McKenzie, M. Recurrence of Crohn's Disease after Ileocolic Resection Is Not Affected by Anastomotic Type: Results of a Multicenter, Randomized, Controlled Trial. *Dis. Colon Rectum* **2009**, *52*, 919–927. [CrossRef] [PubMed]
33. Zurbuchen, U.; Kroesen, A.J.; Knebel, P.; Betzler, M.H.; Becker, H.; Bruch, H.P.; Senninger, N.; Post, S.; Buhr, H.J.; Ritz, J.P. Complications after End-to-End vs. Side-to-Side Anastomosis in Ileocecal Crohn's Disease—Early Postoperative Results from a Randomized Controlled Multi-Center Trial (ISRCTN-45665492). *Langenbecks Arch. Surg.* **2013**, *398*, 467–474. [CrossRef] [PubMed]
34. Feng, J.S.; Li, J.Y.; Yang, Z.; Chen, X.Y.; Mo, J.J.; Li, S.H. Stapled Side-to-Side Anastomosis Might Be Benefit in Intestinal Resection for Crohn's Disease: A Systematic Review and Network Meta-Analysis. *Medicine* **2018**, *97*, e0315. [CrossRef] [PubMed]
35. Alshantti, A.; Hind, D.; Hancock, L.; Brown, S.R. The Role of Kono-S Anastomosis and Mesenteric Resection in Reducing Recurrence after Surgery for Crohn's Disease: A Systematic Review. *Color. Dis.* **2021**, *23*, 7–17. [CrossRef]
36. Grażyńska, A.; Kufel, J.; Dudek, A.; Cebula, M. Shear Wave and Strain Elastography in Crohn's Disease—A Systematic Review. *Diagnostics* **2021**, *11*, 1609. [CrossRef]

Disclaimer/Publisher's Note: The statements, opinions and data contained in all publications are solely those of the individual author(s) and contributor(s) and not of MDPI and/or the editor(s). MDPI and/or the editor(s) disclaim responsibility for any injury to people or property resulting from any ideas, methods, instructions or products referred to in the content.

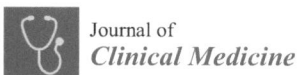 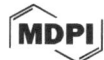

Systematic Review

The Effects of Sarcopenia on Overall Survival and Postoperative Complications of Patients Undergoing Hepatic Resection for Primary or Metastatic Liver Cancer: A Systematic Review and Meta-Analysis

Alexandros Giakoustidis [1,*], Menelaos Papakonstantinou [1], Paraskevi Chatzikomnitsa [1], Areti Danai Gkaitatzi [1], Petros Bangeas [1], Panagiotis Dimitrios Loufopoulos [1], Eleni Louri [1], Athanasia Myriskou [1], Ioannis Moschos [2], Diomidis Antoniadis [3], Dimitrios Giakoustidis [1] and Vasileios N. Papadopoulos [1]

[1] A' Department of Surgery, General Hospital Papageorgiou, School of Medicine, Faculty of Medical Sciences, Aristotle University of Thessaloniki, 56429 Thessaloniki, Greece; menelaospap.md@gmail.com (M.P.); voula.hatzikomnitsa@gmail.com (P.C.); aretidanaegtz24@gmail.com (A.D.G.); pbangeas@gmail.com (P.B.); loufopoulosp@gmail.com (P.D.L.); elenilouri@gmail.com (E.L.); myriskou@gmail.com (A.M.); dgiakoustidis@gmail.com (D.G.); papadvas@auth.gr (V.N.P.)
[2] International Hellenic University, 56429 Thessaloniki, Greece; gutgutgut2011@gmail.com
[3] School of Medicine, Aristotle University of Thessaloniki, 56429 Thessaloniki, Greece; dio_psych@yahoo.gr
* Correspondence: alexgiakoustidis@gmail.com

Abstract: Background: Colorectal cancer is the third most common cancer worldwide, and 20–30% of patients will develop liver metastases (CRLM) during their lifetime. Hepatocellular carcinoma (HCC) is also one of the most common cancers worldwide with increasing incidence. Hepatic resection represents the most effective treatment approach for both CRLM and HCC. Recently, sarcopenia has gained popularity as a prognostic index in order to assess the perioperative risk of hepatectomies. The aim of this study is to assess the effects of sarcopenia on the overall survival (OS), complication rates and mortality of patients undergoing liver resections for HCC or CRLM. **Methods:** A systematic literature search was performed for studies including patients undergoing hepatectomy for HCC or CRLM, and a meta-analysis of the data was performed. **Results:** Sarcopenic patients had a significantly lower 5-year OS compared to non-sarcopenic patients (43.8% vs. 63.6%, respectively; $p < 0.01$) and a significantly higher complication rate (35.4% vs. 23.1%, respectively; $p = 0.002$). Finally, no statistical correlation was found in mortality between sarcopenic and non-sarcopenic patients ($p > 0.1$). **Conclusions:** Sarcopenia was significantly associated with decreased 5-year OS and increased morbidity, but no difference was found with regard to postoperative mortality.

Keywords: sarcopenia; liver resection; overall survival; complications

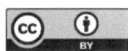

1. Introduction

Hepatocellular carcinoma (HCC) is one of the most common cancers worldwide, with an increasing incidence, rapid progression and frequent tumor recurrence and metastasis [1–3]. Colorectal cancer is the third most common cancer worldwide, and approximately 20%–30% of these patients will develop liver metastasis during their lifetime [4,5]. For both hepatocellular carcinoma and colorectal liver metastases (CRLM), hepatic resection (hepatectomy) remains the mainstay intervention with curative intent, followed by modern techniques, such as orthotopic liver transplantation or transarterial chemoembolization, which emerge nowadays. According to Furukawa et al., hepatic resection can provide a prolonged survival for patients with CRLM, with a 5-year survival rate up to 30%–60%. However, even in patients with curative hepatic resections, there is still a high recurrence rate postoperatively (up to 70% in a 5-year follow-up) and a high morbidity rate (approximately

40%–50%) [1,2,6,7]. Many risk factors, such as sarcopenia, are closely related to high incidence of postoperative complications and poor long-term outcomes for patients with cancer [3]. Therefore, early preoperative recognition of perioperative risk factors is crucial in avoiding adverse consequences after hepatectomy and improving overall survival (OS) and disease-free survival (DFS) for these patients.

Sarcopenia is a term first introduced by Rosenberg in 1989 to describe the involuntary age-related loss of skeletal muscle mass [4,8,9]. It was initially noticed in elderly people and had a negative impact on health. In 2010, The European Working Group on Sarcopenia in Older People (EWGSOP) published a clinical definition of sarcopenia, which described it as a syndrome characterized by progressive and generalized loss of skeletal muscle mass (quality and quantity), strength and function [4,6–8,10,11].

Sarcopenia is strongly associated with nutritional health/malnutrition and is of great prognostic significance in patients with cancer [1,6]. Malnutrition is very common in these patients due to the combination of malignant disease progress and anticancer treatment, and in severe cases, it can lead to cachexia, a syndrome characterized by the loss of skeletal muscle mass. It is highly associated with tumor aggressiveness, longer hospitalization, and it is identified as a poor prognostic factor with reduced overall, disease-free and recurrence-free survival rate for patients with cancer undergoing surgery [1,4,10,12–14]. Sarcopenia also carries a risk of increased short-term and long-term adverse outcomes, such as major postoperative complications, physical disability, poor health-related quality of life, postoperative morbidity and death [2,10,15,16]. According to Hou et al.'s retrospective study published in 2021 comparing sarcopenic and non-sarcopenic patients with HCC and cholangiocarcinoma undergoing liver resection, sarcopenia has been proven to be an independent prognostic indicator for overall survival and disease-free survival for these patients after surgery. This finding agrees with other previous studies indicating that sarcopenia is related to adverse postoperative results and poor prognosis for cancer patients, as described in a study by Bernardi et al. in 2020, in which sarcopenic patients undergoing hepatectomies presented a higher 90-day morbidity rate compared to non-sarcopenic patients, as well as a higher complication incidence.

Body composition profiling plays a valuable role in preoperative risk assessment and in predicting the short-term and long-term outcomes of patients undergoing oncologic liver surgery [17,18]. Based on parameters obtained from diagnostic preoperative imaging with computed tomography (CT) or magnetic resonance imaging (MRI), such as the measurement of psoas area, muscle density at the third lumbar vertebra (L3) and intramuscular adipose tissue in Hounsfield units, it is possible to accurately quantify intra-abdominal fat and muscle mass in order to reveal sarcopenia and predict postoperative survival rate after surgical resection for colorectal cancer, hepatocellular carcinoma and colorectal liver metastasis [5,10]. Any abnormalities in these parameters are associated with poor postoperative outcomes and prognosis.

This systematic review aims to summarize the current evidence available from the literature on the effects of sarcopenia on overall survival and postoperative complications regarding liver resections in patients suffering from primary liver or metastatic colorectal cancer.

2. Materials and Methods

2.1. Study Selection

A thorough literature search was conducted on PubMed for articles including patients with sarcopenia undergoing liver resection for primary or metastatic liver cancer. The terms "sarcopenia", "liver resection", "hepatectomy", "metastasis", "metastases", "hepatocellular carcinoma", "hcc", "laparoscopic liver resection" and "complications" were used in various combinations. The search was conducted manually by two independent reviewers and yielded 209 results. Any conflict during the selection process was resolved through discussion. All articles were scrutinized against predetermined inclusion and exclusion criteria, and after excluding duplicates and irrelevant studies, 86 were eligible for further assessment. After full-text screening, 60 studies were excluded and 26 were finally included in our systematic review. The study selection algorithm is shown on the Preferred Reporting Items of Systematic Reviews and Meta-Analyses (PRISMA) flow chart (Figure 1) [19]. The systematic review protocol was registered in the International Prospective Register of Systematic Reviews (PROSPERO ID CRD42023426589).

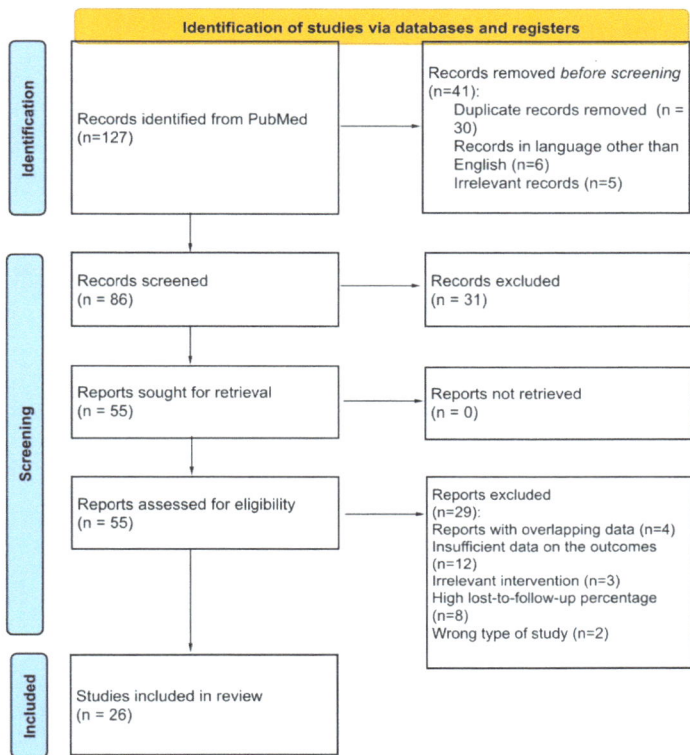

Figure 1. PRISMA flow diagram.

2.2. Inclusion and Exclusion Criteria

The following inclusion criteria were applied: cohort studies with adult patients published over the last decade in the English language; studies including patients undergoing open or laparoscopic hepatic resections for HCC or CRLM; studies including patients with sarcopenia, as defined above, prior to any intervention related to the hepatic disease; studies having overall survival or complications after hepatectomy as primary outcomes.

Case reports, case series, commentaries and letters to the editor were excluded from this review.

2.3. Definition

The International Working Group on Sarcopenia (IWGS) has published a consensus in which sarcopenia is defined as the presence of low skeletal muscle mass and low muscle function [20]. However, other associations, such as the European Working Group on Sarcopenia in Older People (EWGSOP) and the European Society for Clinical Nutrition and Metabolism—Special Interest Groups (ESPEN—SIG), have proposed their own sarcopenia definitions, defining it, respectively, as (i) the presence of low skeletal muscle mass and either low muscle strength (assessed by handgrip) or low muscle performance (assessed by measuring the walking speed) and (ii) the presence of low skeletal muscle mass and low muscle strength (assessed by handgrip) [21,22]. In our review, the skeletal muscle mass was assessed with preoperative CT scans at the L3 level, except for one study that measured the cross-sectional muscle area at the L4 level [5]. The total muscle area was then normalized for height, generating the skeletal muscle index (SMI). Sarcopenia was finally defined based on the SMI cut-off values that each study set according to international consensuses or statistical analyses, which differed among the studies and between men and women.

2.4. Data Extraction

The following data were extracted in a preformed datasheet: author, year, institution and study period, type of operation, patient population, age, sex, BMI, primary disease, staging, administration of neoadjuvant chemotherapy (NAC), follow-up, overall survival, morbidity, mortality and postoperative complications.

2.5. Risk of Bias and Quality Assessment

The risk of bias and the quality of each individual study were assessed using the Cochrane Tool to Assess Risk of Bias in Cohort Studies and the Newcastle–Ottawa Quality Assessment Scale (NOS), respectively [23]. The Cochrane Tool consists of 7 questions, and according to the answers, a cohort study can be categorized as having low or high risk of bias. The NOS consists of 8 items regarding the selection of subjects, the comparability and the outcomes of each individual cohort study (Table 1).

Table 1. Newcastle–Ottawa Scale scores for the included studies. * is a star awarded for each item.

Study	Selection				Comparability	Outcomes			Total
	Representativeness of the Exposed Cohort	Selection of the Non-Exposed Cohort	Ascertainment of Exposure	Outcome of Interest Not Present at the Start of the Study	Assessment of Outcome	Length of Follow-Up	Adequacy of Follow-Up	[24]
Bajric et al. [24]	*	*	*	*	*	*	*	*	8/8
Harimoto et al. [2]	*	*	*	*	*	*		*	7/8
Harimoto et al. [11]	*		*	*		*			4/8
Hayashi et al. [3]	*	*	*	*	*	*	*	*	8/8
Hu et al. [16]	*	*	*	*	*	*	*		7/8
Kobayashi et al. [4]	*	*	*	*	*	*			6/8
Kroh et al. [25]	*	*	*	*	*	*	*	*	8/8
Lodewick et al. [26]	*	*	*	*	*	*			6/8
Peng et al. [27]	*	*	*	*		*			5/8
Runkel et al. [9]	*		*	*		*			4/8
VanVledder et al. [28]	*	*	*	*	*	*	*	*	8/8
Wu et al. [29]	*	*	*	*	*	*			6/8
Yabusaki et al. [30]	*	*	*	*	*	*	*	*	8/8
Yang et al. [14]	*	*	*	*	*	*			6/8
Yang et al. [31]	*	*	*	*	*	*			6/8
Berardi et al. [7]	*	*	*	*	*	*			6/8
Kim et al. [32]	*	*	*	*		*			5/8
Marasco et al. [10]	*	*	*	*	*	*	*	*	8/8
Hou et al. [33]	*	*	*	*	*	*	*	*	7/8
Zhou et al. [34]	*	*	*	*	*	*			6/8
Wijk et al. [35]	*	*	*	*		*			5/8
Liu et al. (2020) [5]	*	*	*	*		*	*	*	7/8
Xiong et al. [36]	*	*	*	*		*	*	*	7/8
Pessia et al. [37]	*	*	*	*	*	*	*	*	8/8
Xu et al. [38]	*	*	*	*	*	*	*	*	8/8
Furukawa et al. [8]	*	*	*	*	*	*	*	*	8/8

2.6. Meta-Analysis

The studies that were included in the analysis were reviewed, and the data were tabulated. Due to differences in the methodology used in each study, not all of the examined data were available in every study. The data were then organized into groups and inputted into the SPSS platform, which provided the results subsequently analyzed in detail below.

Due to the large number of studies in the meta-analysis, it was necessary to sub-categorize them for better statistical management. Therefore, the studies were grouped based on the parameters analyzed to yield more significant statistical results.

The null hypothesis for Cochran's Q is that the percentage of "hits" is equal for all groups. The alternative hypothesis, on the other hand, suggests that the ratio varies at least among one group. If the calculated critical value Q is greater than a critical χ^2 value, then the null hypothesis is rejected. If the variation is only due to within-study error, then its expected value would be the degrees of freedom for this meta-analysis, where df = 25. Therefore, it follows that Q < df. By calculating I^2, it shows that $I^2 = 0$, indicating that the heterogeneity of the sample is not statistically significant for the meta-analysis (Figure 2).

Cochran Test

Frequencies

	Value	
	0	1
Sarcopenia	751	1127
Survival	694	1184

Test Statistics

N	1878
Cochran's Q	3.028[a]
Df	1
Asymp. Sig	0.082

a. 1 is treated as a success

Figure 2. Cochran's Q Test.

The research studies were divided into categories based on their focus on the complication rate in sarcopenic patients. By analyzing these groups, the odds ratio (OR) of sarcopenic patients who developed complications in the various studies was determined, and a forest plot was created for the studies included.

3. Results

In this study, a total of 6103 patients underwent hepatic resection of one or more segments or metastasectomy. The study aimed to investigate the effect of sarcopenia on the survival, mortality and complication rate of the patients.

The study analyzed patients based on their sex, age and whether they had sarcopenia. The data were also categorized based on the stage of the disease and the initial location of the tumor, as well as the presence of preoperative chemotherapy. The patients' demographics and characteristics are shown in Table 2. The patients were followed up for varying periods, and their postoperative complications, mortality and survival were studied.

Table 2. Patient demographics and characteristics.

Author	Population	Groups	Sex	Age (mean)	BMI (mg/m^2)	SMI	Primary Tumor Location	Tumor Stage	Neoadjuvant Chemotherapy
Bajric et al. [24]	315	Sarcopenic, n = 78 (24.7%); non-sarcopenic, n = 237 (75.3%)	135 M, 220 F	68 (60–74)	25.5 (23.3–28.7)	NA	Colorectal cancer	IV (100%)	NA
Harimoto et al. [2]	186	Sarcopenic, n = 75 (40.3%); non-sarcopenic, n = 111 (59.7%)	145 M, 41 F	66 (55–77)	Sarcopenic, 20.5 (18.1); non-sarcopenic, 24 (21.2–26.8); $p < 0.001$	Sarcopenic, 37.8; non-sarcopenic, 49.7; $p < 0.001$	Liver	Sarcopenic, I n = 11 (14.7%), II n = 38 (50.7%), III n = 20 (26.6%), IV n = 6 (8%); non-sarcopenic, I n = 18 (16.2%), II n = 57 (51.3%), III n = 29 (26.2%), IV n = 7 (6.3%)	NA
Harimoto et al. [11]	146	Sarcopenic, n = 146	106 M, 40 F	68 (28–89)	22.7 (14.8–31.4)	36.8	Liver	NA	NA
Hayashi al. [3]	303	Sarcopenic, n = 106 (34.9%); non-sarcopenic n = 197 (65.1%)	Sarcopenic, 96 M / 10 F; non-sarcopenic, 125 M / 72 F	Sarcopenic, 72 (38–89); non-sarcopenic, 70 (36–85)	Sarcopenic, n = 21.9 (13.4–32.5); non-sarcopenic, 23.8 (16.5–45.2); $p < 0.001$	NA	Liver	Sarcopenic, I n = 20 (18.9%), II n = 41 (38.7%), III n = 34 (32.1%), IV n = 11 (10.3%); non-sarcopenic, I n = 49 (24.9%), II n = 84 (42.6%), III n = 50 (25.4%), IV n = 14 (7.1%)	NA

Table 2. Cont.

Author	Population	Groups	Sex	Age (mean)	BMI (mg/m²)	SMI	Primary Tumor Location	Tumor Stage	Neoadjuvant Chemotherapy
Hu et al. [16]	153	Sarcopenic, n = 45 (29.4%); non-sarcopenic, n = 108 (70.6%)	133 M, 45 F	60 (51–66)	<25, n = 109; >25, n = 44	Sarcopenic: 41.84; non-sarcopenic: 49.20 ($p < 0.001$)	Liver	I n = 95 (62.1%), II–IV n = 58 (37.9%)	NA
Kobayashi et al. [4]	124	Sarcopenic, n = 24 (19.3%); non-sarcopenic, n = 100 (80.7%)	78 M, 46 F	65 (59–70)	22.7 (20.3–24.7)	NA	Colon, n = 69; Rectum, n = 55	I/II, n = 28 (24%); III/IV, n = 91 (76%)	52%
Kroh et al. [25]	70	Sarcopenic, n = 33 (47.1%); non-sarcopenic, n = 37 (52.9%)	49 M, 21 F	67 (54–80)	26.64 (22.02–31.26)	47.98	Liver	T1, n = 22 (31.5%) T2, n = 25 (35.7%) T3, n = 23 (32.8%) *	NA
Lodewick et al. [26]	80	Sarcopenic, n = 31 (38.7%); non-sarcopenic, n = 49 (61.3%)	51 M, 29 F	66 (28–82)	24.9 (18.7–46.4)	NA	Colorectal/HBC	NA	NA
Peng et al. [27]	259	Sarcopenic, n = 41 (15.8%); non-sarcopenic, n = 218 (84.2%)	155 M, 104 F	58 (46–70)	<30, n = 191; ≥30, n = 68	NA	Colon, n = 191; Rectum, n = 68	T1/T2, n = 41 (15.8%) T3/T4, n = 218 (84.2%) *	NA
Runkel et al. [9]	94	Sarcopenic, n = 94	58 M, 36 F	61 (34–83)	26 (13.8–45.6)	NA	Colorectal cancer	IV (100%)	62.8%
VanVledder et al. [28]	196	Sarcopenic, n = 38 (19.4%); non-sarcopenic, n = 158 (80.6%)	120 M, 76 F	64.5 (31–86)	Sarcopenic, 23.7 (20.7–26.7); non-sarcopenic, 26.7 (23.2–30.2)	NA	Colon, n = 116; Rectum, n = 80	T2 n = 25 (13.2%), T3 n = 148 (78.3%), T4 n = 16 (8.5%) *	Sarcopenic, 47%; non-sarcopenic, 46.2%

Table 2. Cont.

Author	Population	Groups	Sex	Age (mean)	BMI (mg/m²)	SMI	Primary Tumor Location	Tumor Stage	Neoadjuvant Chemotherapy
Wu et al. [29]	1172	Sarcopenic, n = 421 (35.9%); non-sarcopenic, n = 751 (65.1%)		Sarcopenic: <65, n = 329; ≥65, n = 92; non-sarcopenic: <65, n = 613; ≥65, n = 138	Sarcopenic, 25.47 (21.77–26.32); non-sarcopenic, 22.94 (20.76–25.63) p < 0.001	Sarcopenic, 37.84; non-sarcopenic, 46.68 p < 0.001	HCC	Sarcopenic, I n = 191 (45.3%), II n = 100 (23.7%), III n = 121 (28.8%), IV n = 9 (2.2%); non-sarcopenic, I n = 342 (45.6%), II n = 180 (23.9%), III n = 217 (28.9%), IV n = 12 (1.6%)	None
Yabusaki et al. [30]	195	Sarcopenic, n = 89 (45.6%); non-sarcopenic, n = 106 (54.4%)	157 M, 38 F	66 (22–80)	23.2 (14.3–37.3)	NA	HCC	I, n = 20 (10.3%) II, n = 112 (57.4%) III, n = 42 (21.5%) IVA, n = 19 (9.7%) IVB, n = 2 (1.1%)	NA
Yang et al. [14]	155	Sarcopenic, n = 89 (57.4%); non-sarcopenic, n = 66 (42.6%)	135 M, 20 F	60 (51–66)	23.37 (23.14–23.6)	47.05	HCC	I–II, n = 138 (89.1%) III–IV, n = 17 (10.9%)	NA
Yang et al. [31]	171	Sarcopenic, n = 86 (50.2%); non-sarcopenic, n = 85 (49.8%)	99 M, 72 F	59 (50–67)	22.86 (20.94–25.08)	42.22	HCC, n = 47 CLM, n = 44 Other HBC **, n = 80	NA	NA
Berardi et al. [7]	234	Sarcopenic, n = 143 (61.2%); non-sarcopenic, n = 91 (38.8%)	158 M, 76 F	66 (58–74)	27.12 (23.28–29.55)	46.22	HCC, n = 101; Colorectal cancer, n = 96	NA	Sarcopenic, 36.4%; non-sarcopenic, 39.5%

Table 2. Cont.

Author	Population	Groups	Sex	Age (mean)	BMI (mg/m^2)	SMI	Primary Tumor Location	Tumor Stage	Neoadjuvant Chemotherapy
Kim et al. [32]	159	Sarcopenic, n = 74 (46.5%); non-sarcopenic, n = 85 (53.5%)	133 M, 26 F	59 (49–69)	24.8 (21.1–28.42)	51.08	HCC	I–II, n = 65 (40.9%); III–IV, n = 94 (59.1%)	NA
Marasco et al. [10]	159	Sarcopenic, n = 82 (51.6%); non-sarcopenic, n = 77 (48.4%)	128 M, 31 F	68 (58–75)	Sarcopenic, 25.6 (23.8–27.8); non-sarcopenic, 27.5 (25.6–29.4)	F: 39.2; M: 48.9	HCC	NA	NA
Hou et al. [33]	153	Sarcopenic, n = 77 (50.3%); non-sarcopenic, n = 76 (49.7%)	128 M, 25 F	>55, n = 68; ≤55, n = 85	Sarcopenic, 21.64 (19.73–23.78); non-sarcopenic, 24.27 (21.93–25.62)	NA	Combined HCC–CC	HCC: Stage I n = 21 (13.7%), stage II n = 18 (11.8%), stage III n = 92 (60.1%), stage IV n = 22 (14.4%); CC: Stage I n = 22 (14.4%), stage II n = 23 (15%), stage III n = 108 (70.6%)	NA
Zhou et al. [34]	67	Sarcopenic, n = 33 (49.3%); non-sarcopenic, n = 34 (50.7%)	22 M, 45 F	61 (47–81)	22.2 (24.4–28.7)	41.2	IHCC	I–II, n = 44 (65.7%); III–IV, n = 23 (34.3%)	None
Wijk et al. [35]	128	Sarcopenic, n = 83 (64.8%); non-sarcopenic, n = 45 (35.2%)	89 M, 39 F	65.5 (57–74)	25.6 (22.5–28.7)	NA	Colorectal cancer	NA	NA

Table 2. Cont.

Author	Population	Groups	Sex	Age (mean)	BMI (mg/m²)	SMI	Primary Tumor Location	Tumor Stage	Neoadjuvant Chemotherapy
Liu et al. [5]	182	Sarcopenic, n = 48 (26.4%); non-sarcopenic, n = 134 (73.6%)	106 M, 76 F	59.5 (28–85)	24.3 (20.7–27.9)	NA	Colorectal cancer	T1 n = 3 (1.6%), T2 n = 22 (12.1%), T3 n = 73 (40.1%), T4 n = 84 (46.2%) *	Sarcopenic, 21%; non-sarcopenic, 19%
Xiong et al. [36]	114	Sarcopenic, n = 58 (50.8%); non-sarcopenic, n = 56 (49.2%)	91 M, 23 F	62.5 (57–70)	<18.5, n = 20; ≥18.5, n = 94	Sarcopenic, 34.2; non-sarcopenic, 42.7	Gastric cancer	NA	Sarcopenic, 53.5%; non-sarcopenic, 58.9%
Pessia et al. [37]	74	Sarcopenic, n = 48 (64.8%); non-sarcopenic, n = 26 (35.2%)	NA	NA	Sarcopenic, 24.2; non-sarcopenic, 27.6	Sarcopenic, 39.3; non-sarcopenic, 52.7	Colorectal cancer	NA	100%
Xu et al. [38]	1420	Sarcopenic, n = 458 (32.2%); non-sarcopenic, n = 962 (67.8%)	NA	NA	Sarcopenic, 24.2; non-sarcopenic, 27.6	Sarcopenic, 39.3; non-sarcopenic, 52.7	HCC	NA	NA
Furukawa et al. [8]	63	Sarcopenic, n = 33 (52.3%); non-sarcopenic, n = 30 (47.7%)	31 M, 37 F	67.5 (28–90)	NA	NA	Colorectal cancer	NA	Sarcopenic, 37%; non-sarcopenic, 34%

M, male; F, female; NA, not applicable; HBC, hepatobiliary carcinoma; HCC, hepatocellular carcinoma; CLM, colorectal liver metastases; CC, cholangiocarcinoma; IHCC, intrahepatic cholangiocarcinoma. * The AJCC TNM system was used for HCC, HBC, CC or IHCC staging. When information on lymph nodes (N) or metastasis (M) was not available, only the tumor extent (T) was used to present the data. ** Cholangiocarcinoma, n = 67, Gallbladder cancer, n = 7, Mixed liver cancer, n = 6.

After collecting the data, statistical analysis was conducted, and several results were extracted. Out of the 6103 patients included in the study, 2232 were diagnosed with sarcopenia, while 3841 were not. Among the total number of patients, 2167 were male, and 1126 were female, resulting in a male-to-female ratio of 2:1. The average age of all patients was 64.3 years. The average BMI for patients with sarcopenia was 22.9, whereas for non-sarcopenic patients, it was 25.8. On average, the SMI of sarcopenic individuals was 38.9, while for non-sarcopenic patients, it was 49.6.

According to the data, the average rate of complications in patients with sarcopenia is 35.4%, while in non-sarcopenic patients, it is 23.1% (35.4% vs. 23.1%; $p = 0.002$). The diagram in Figure 3 shows that the complication rate in sarcopenic patients is significantly higher than in non-sarcopenic patients. Furthermore, Figures 4 and 5 show the OR of the complication rates in the nine studies that compared the complications between sarcopenic and non-sarcopenic patients. However, it was not possible to classify the complications further based on Clavien–Dindo classification, as it was only used in very few studies. The morbidity of sarcopenic patients in comparison to non-sarcopenic patients and the specific complications and their incidence reported in each of the included studies are shown in Tables 3 and 4.

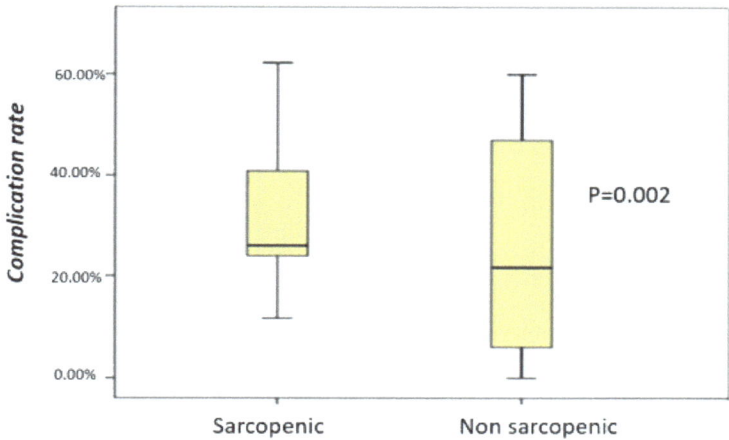

Figure 3. Complication rate of sarcopenic vs. non-sarcopenic patients.

Studies	OR	CI(-)	CI(+)
Bajric et al. (2022)	29.347	6.5752	126.7205
Harimoto et al. (2013)	0.6343	0.362	1.1113
Hayashi et al.(2023)	0.9607	0.6512	1.4175
Hu et al.(2022)	1.3176	0.7396	2.3474
Kroh et al.(2019)	0.897	0.3166	2.5414
Yabusaki et al.(2016)	0.9321	0.4731	1.8364
Yang et al. (2022)	6.6667	2.2776	19.5135
Yang et al. (2023)	3.6667	1.2084	11.1256
Marasco et al.(2022)	19.7273	1.1366	342.4008

Figure 4. Odds ratio of complication rate in sarcopenic patients. OR, odds ratio [2,3,10,14,16,24,25,30,31].

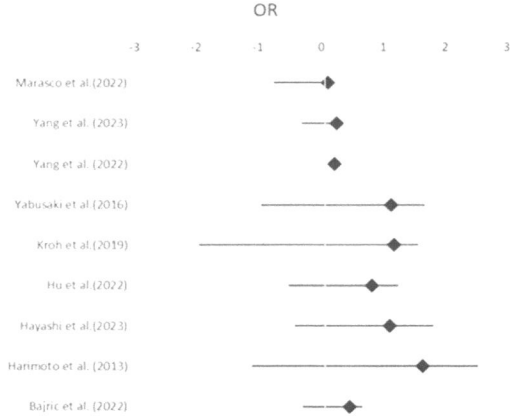

Figure 5. Forest plot. OR, odds ratio [2,3,10,14,16,24,25,30,31].

Table 3. Morbidity of sarcopenic vs. non-sarcopenic patients undergoing hepatectomy for liver cancer.

Study		Population	Complication Rate	Follow-Up (Months)
Bajric et al. [24]		315		30
	Sarcopenic	78 (24.7%)	24.9%	
	Non-sarcopenic	237 (75.3%)	9.7%	
			$p = 0.01$	
Harimoto et al. [2]		186		NA
	Sarcopenic	75 (40.3%)	32%	
	Non-sarcopenic	111 (59.7%)	50.5%	
			$p = 0.613$	
Harimoto et al. [11]		146		NA
	Sarcopenic	146	8.2%	
	Non-sarcopenic	0	-	
			-	
Hayashi et al. [3]		303		60
	Sarcopenic	106 (34.9%)	58%	
	Non-sarcopenic	197 (65.1%)	60%	
			$p = 0.812$	
Hu et al. [16]		153		12
	Sarcopenic	45 (29.4%)	62.3%	
	Non-sarcopenic	108 (70.6%)	47.2%	
			$p = 0.162$	
Kroh et al. [25]		70		60
	Sarcopenic	33 (47.1%)	24%	
	Non-sarcopenic	37 (52.9%)	27%	
			$p = 1$	

Table 3. Cont.

Study		Population	Complication Rate	Follow-Up (Months)
Peng et al. [27]		249	23%	NA
	Sarcopenic	41 (15.8%)	-	
	Non-sarcopenic	218 (84.2%)	-	
			-	
Runkel et al. [9]		94		NA
	Sarcopenic	94	62.8%	
	Non-sarcopenic	0	-	
			-	
Wu et al. [29]		1172		NA
	Sarcopenic	421 (35.9%)	Significantly higher	
	Non-sarcopenic	751 (65.1%)	-	
			$p < 0.001$	
Yabusaki et al. [30]		195		37
	Sarcopenic	89 (45.6%)	20.2%	
	Non-sarcopenic	106 (54.4%)	21.7%	
			$p = 0.8$	
Yang et al. [14]		155		NA
	Sarcopenic	89 (57%)	40.9%	
	Non-sarcopenic	66 (43%)	6.06%	
			$p < 0.001$	
Yang et al. [31]		171		NA
	Sarcopenic	86 (50.2%)	26.1%	
	Non-sarcopenic	85 (49.8%)	4.5%	
			$p = 0.032$	
Berardi et al. [7]		234	30.3%	3
	Sarcopenic	91 (38.8%)	-	
	Non-sarcopenic	143 (61.2%)	-	
Marasco et al. [10]		159		30
	Sarcopenic	82 (51.6%)	11.8%	
	Non-sarcopenic	77 (48.4%)	0	
			$p = 0.032$	
Wijk et al. [35]		128	40.6%	NA
	Sarcopenic	83 (64.8%)	-	
	Non-sarcopenic	45 (35.2%)	-	
			-	
Kim et al. [32]		159	41.5%	1
	Sarcopenic		-	
	Non-sarcopenic		-	
			-	

Table 3. Cont.

Study	Population	Complication Rate	Follow-Up (Months)
Liu et al. [5]	182	33%	32.5
Sarcopenic		38.3%	
Non-sarcopenic		27.7%	
		-	
Xiong et al. [36]	114	29.3%	60
Sarcopenic		43.7%	
Non-sarcopenic		33.6%	
		-	

Table 4. Complications reported after hepatectomy.

Complications after Hepatectomy			
Complication	Number of Cases	Complication	Number of Cases
Bile leakage	83	Liver failure	109
Ascites	8	Pleural effusion	80
Pneumonia	4	Surgical site infection	50
Intra-abdominal abscess	62	Postoperative bleeding	10
Brain infarction	1	Hepatic encephalopathy	1
Obstruction of blood dialysis shunt	1	Reintubation	1
Biloma	2	Sepsis	1
Portal vein thrombosis	1	Cardiopulmonary	3
Gastrointestinal	2	Hematological	3
Bacteremia	2	Miscellaneous infections	6

No further statistical analysis could be performed on complications experienced by patients, as they were not further analyzed in most studies. The most commonly reported complications include surgical wound infection and delayed gastric emptying. In the studies that do provide information regarding complications, they are typically classified using the Clavien–Dindo system, with the majority falling into grade I or II.

The average 5-year OS rate of the patients included in our study was 64.7%. The patients who were diagnosed with sarcopenia had an average OS rate of 43.8%, which ranged from 13.4% to 91.1%. On the other hand, the non-sarcopenic patients had an average OS rate of 63.6%, ranging from 9.7% to 99.1%. Sarcopenic patients had a statistically significantly lower 5-year OS than non-sarcopenic patients, with a p-value < 0.01. No statistical correlation was found between mortality incidence in sarcopenic and non-sarcopenic patients (p-value > 0.1) (Table 5).

A sub-categorization was created to include studies that included the rate of complications experienced by patients after hepatectomy. Additionally, data evaluation on the initial location of the tumor and the occurrence of sarcopenia led to the conclusion that patients with hepatocellular carcinoma or liver metastasis do not exhibit a statistically significant difference in the occurrence of sarcopenia (p-value > 0.01). However, a significant difference is observed in patients who underwent hepatectomy due to a tumor in the right or left colon. Patients who underwent right colectomy are more likely to experience sarcopenia as compared to those who underwent left colectomy or low anterior resection. This difference can be attributed to the removal of the cecum and terminal ileum during the right colectomy.

This was followed by the survival study of sarcopenic and non-sarcopenic patients after hepatectomy. We should take into account that the studies were conducted in different time periods, and the follow-up period of these patients was different in every study.

As is evident from the diagram in Figure 6, a lower survival rate appears in sarcopenic patients compared to non-sarcopenic patients. At 30 months of follow-up, there is an increase in the line, which is not actually the case, as there were two studies that had the same follow-up months with different results in terms of survival rates. The Log-rank test was 1.0146, with a p-value 0.3131.

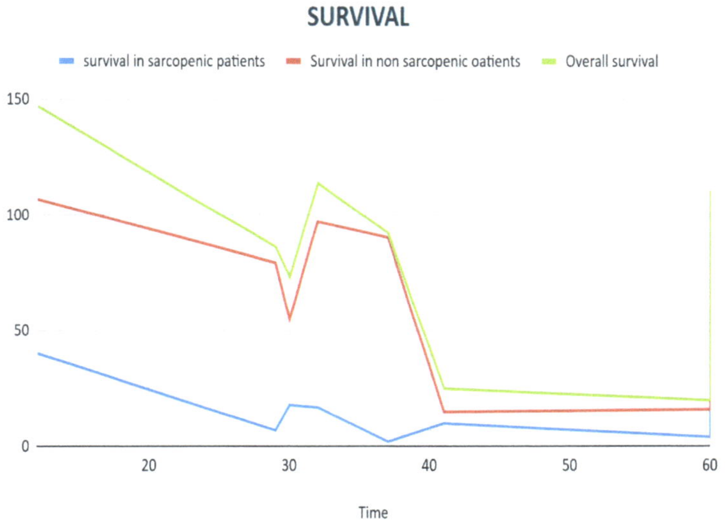

SURVIVAL

Figure 6. Kaplan–Meier curve.

The subgroup of patients who underwent hepatectomy for metastatic colorectal cancer was then created. It was studied in terms of the odds ratio (Table 6), and then, a forest plot (Figure 7) was created, wherein those studies that included this subgroup were distinguished.

Table 5. 5-year overall survival and mortality of sarcopenic vs. non-sarcopenic patients undergoing hepatectomy for liver cancer.

Study	Population	5-Year Overall Survival	Mortality (30 Days)	Follow-Up (Months)
Bajric et al. [24]	315			30
Sarcopenic	78 (25%)	20.3%	38.2%	
Non-sarcopenic	237 (75%)	23.1%	34.3%	
		$p = 0.01$	$p > 0.05$	
Harimoto et al. [2]	186			NA
Sarcopenic	75 (40.3%)	71%	-	
Non-sarcopenic	111 (59.7%)	83.7%	-	
		$p = 0.001$		

Table 5. Cont.

Study	Population	5-Year Overall Survival	Mortality (30 Days)	Follow-Up (Months)
Hayashi et al. [3]	303			60
Sarcopenic	106 (34.9%)	-	0	
Non-sarcopenic	197 (65.1%)	-	0.5%	
		$p = 0.023$	$p = 0.353$	
Hu et al. [16]	153			12
Sarcopenic	45 (29.4%)	91.1%	2.2%	
Non-sarcopenic	108 (70.6%)	99.1%	0	
		$p = 0.043$	-	
Kobayashi et al. [4]	124			NA
Sarcopenic	24 (19.3%)	-	-	
Non-sarcopenic	100 (80.7%)	-	-	
		$p = 0.343$	$p = 0.946$	
Kroh et al. [25]	70			60
Sarcopenic	33 (47.1%)	45%	3%	
Non-sarcopenic	37 (52.9%)	13.6%	8%	
		$p = 0.035$	$p = 0.616$	
Lodewick et al. [26]	80	-	-	3
Sarcopenic	31 (39%)	-	10.5%	
Non-sarcopenic	49 (61%)	-	3.5%	
		-	-	
Peng et al. [27]	259	40%	0.8%	NA
Sarcopenic	41 (16%)	-	-	
Non-sarcopenic	218 (84%)	-	-	
		-	-	
Vledder et al. [28]	196	-	-	29
Sarcopenic	38 (19%)	20%	42.9%	
Non-sarcopenic	158 (81%)	49.9%	-	
		$p < 0.001$	-	
Wu et al. [29]	1172			NA
Sarcopenic	421 (35.9%)	(Significantly worse)	-	
Non-sarcopenic	751 (65.1%)	-	-	
		$p < 0.001$	-	
Yabusaki et al. [30]	195			37
Sarcopenic	89 (45.6%)	85.3 months	2.2%	
Non-sarcopenic	106 (54.4%)	96.3 months	2.8%	
		$p = 0.72$	$p = 0.8$	
Berardi et al. [7]	234	-	-	3
Sarcopenic	91 (38.8%)	-	1.3%	
Non-sarcopenic	85 (53.5.%)	-	0	
		-	-	
Kim et al. [32]	159	70.2%	27%	1
Sarcopenic	74 (46.5%)	-	-	
Non-sarcopenic	85 (53.5%)	-	-	
		-	-	

Table 5. *Cont.*

Study	Population	5-Year Overall Survival	Mortality (30 Days)	Follow-Up (Months)
Hou et al. [33]	153	21.4%	71.2%	41.3
Sarcopenic	77 (50.3%)	-	-	
Non-sarcopenic	76 (49.7%)	-	-	
		-	-	
Zhou et al. [34]	195	-	79.1%	NA
Sarcopenic	89 (45.6%)	21 months	-	
Non-sarcopenic	106 (54.4%)	6 months	-	
		$p < 0.001$	-	
Liu et al. [5]	182	63%	-	32.5
Sarcopenic	48 (26.4%)	-	-	
Non-sarcopenic	134 (73.6%)	-	-	
		-	-	
Xiong et al. [36]	114	34.3%		60
Sarcopenic	58 (50.8%)	-	-	
Non-sarcopenic	56 (49.2%)	-	-	
		-	-	
Pessia et al. [37]	74			32
Sarcopenic	48 (64.8%)	Significantly worse	-	
Non-sarcopenic	26 (35.2%)	-	-	
		$p = 0.0297$	-	
Xu et al. [38]	1420			12
Sarcopenic	458 (32.2%)	Significantly worse	-	
Non-sarcopenic	962 (67.8%)	-	-	
		$p = 0.002$	-	
Furukawa et al. [8]	63			36
Sarcopenic	33 (52.3%)	63.9%	-	
Non-sarcopenic	30 (47.7%)	77.7%	-	
		$p = 0.02$	-	

Table 6. Odds ratio for right and left colon.

Studies	Patients	Right Colon	Left Colon	Odds Ratio	Lower 95% CI	Upper 95% CI
Bajric et al. (2022) [24]	355	180	175	4	3.2083	6.1028
Kobayashi et al. (2017) [4]	124	69	55	0.5555	0.2993	1.031
Lodewick et al. (2015) [26]	80	24		1.8452	0.9799	3.4748
Peng et al. (2011) [27]	259	191	68	0.8176	0.5317	1.2572
Runkel et al. (2021) [9]	94	60	34	1.751	0.9954	3.081
Vledder et al. (2012) [28]	196	116	80	0.8026	0.5121	1.2578
Berardi et al. (2020) [7]	234		96	1.5511	1.0884	2.2106
Wijk et al. (2021) [35]	128	58	70	2.6167	1.678	4.0806
Liu et al. (2020) [5]	182	82	100	1.0654	0.6918	1.6406
Pessia et al. (2021) [37]	74	34	40	2.6118	1.4566	4.6831
Furukawa et al. (2021) [8]	118	48	70	1.3345	0.7948	2.2407

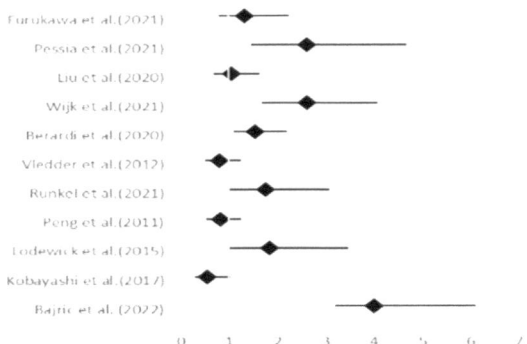

Figure 7. Forest plot for right and left colon [4,5,7–9,24,26–28,35,37].

4. Discussion

In our systematic review, we assessed the effects of preoperative sarcopenia on the survival and postoperative complications of patients undergoing hepatectomy for HCC or CRLM. The meta-analysis showed that OS was statistically significantly shorter in sarcopenic patients compared to non-sarcopenic patients and that patients with preoperative sarcopenia had a statistically significantly higher complication rate than non-sarcopenic patients. Regarding postoperative mortality, no difference was reported between the two groups of patients. Interestingly, patients who had undergone right colectomy were more likely to develop sarcopenia compared to those who had undergone left colectomy. During right colectomy, the cecum and terminal ileum are resected, which are important parts of the large intestine for absorbing water, electrolytes and nutrients. Therefore, special attention should be paid to the postoperative nutrition of these patients, which is addressed later in this section. Short OS and increased morbidity of patients undergoing hepatectomy for liver metastases were also reported by O'Connel et al. in their meta-analysis. At the same time, they noted that obesity was not associated with worse oncological outcomes [39]. Poor prognosis of patients with sarcopenia treated for HCC was also reported in a recent meta-analysis by Kong et al. [40]. Furthermore, Thormann et al. concluded that low skeletal muscle mass led to significantly more postoperative complications after surgery for hepatic metastases but not after surgery for HCC or cholangiocarcinoma [41]. Conversely, Erikson et al. did not find a correlation between muscle loss and worse OS in their study of patients treated for colorectal liver metastases [17]. The different conclusions may be explained when considering that other factors, such as muscle strength or physical performance of the patients, could also affect the perioperative risk [42]. However, sarcopenia has been associated with short OS and high rates of complications in various studies in the literature, including patients with other hepatopancreatobiliary malignancies, gastric, colorectal or small-cell lung cancer [43–47].

In order to diagnose sarcopenia, the muscle mass of the patient needs to be calculated first. A CT scan is used to measure muscle density at the level of the third lumbar vertebra, which is then normalized for the patient's height. The resulting value is known as the SMI. A patient with an SMI below a certain cut-off value is characterized as sarcopenic. Various means of determining an SMI cut-off value have been described in the literature. The most common method is using data from healthy individuals to calculate the mean SMI. Sarcopenia is defined as more than two standard deviations below the mean [48,49]. Another means commonly used both in the literature and in the studies included in our review is optimal stratification of the data, which results in the ideal cut-off value for both men and women [28,50]. Even though the methods for cut-off calculation are standard, the cut-off value itself varies greatly among the different studies. For instance, some SMI cut-offs used for patients with respiratory or gastrointestinal tract tumors were 38.5, 30.88

or 41.1 for women and 52.4, 40.33 or 43.75 for men [28,48–50]. Efforts should be made to introduce a standard and universal sarcopenia definition, so that the effects of sarcopenia on patients with cancer can be more systematically assessed.

Another confounding factor is that the administration of NAC in patients undergoing curative intent surgery for hepatic malignancies is not systematically addressed in the literature. In our review, only 10 out of 26 studies reported the administration of neoadjuvant chemotherapy, as shown in Table 2, while in 2 out of 10 studies [29,34], none of the patients received systematic therapy. Even though the administration of preoperative chemotherapy is similar among sarcopenic and non-sarcopenic patients, there are not enough data regarding the tolerance or completion of it [18]. Furthermore, loss of skeletal muscle has been reported after NAC, which may further worsen the performance status of sarcopenic individuals and lead to poor outcomes. This was shown in a study by Miyamoto et al. after NAC administration for unresectable colorectal cancer [51]. However, Eriksson et al. did not report worse OS after NAC in patients with resectable colorectal liver metastases who had lost over 5% of skeletal muscle during therapy [17]. It is evident that chemotherapy may indeed affect the patient's preoperative status, but unfortunately, insufficient data are available in the literature. Future studies should focus on reporting the effects of chemotherapy on preoperative nutritional status, so that the timing of the operation and the perioperative support can be optimized.

Sarcopenia is frequent in patients with cancer and especially in patients with liver cancer. Its impact on survival dictates the necessity for adequate prevention, which is challenging due to its multifactorial nature [52]. Body composition, such as myosteatosis, central or sarcopenic obesity and visceral fat amount seem to gain popularity as predictors of survival too, which implies the critical role of nutritional status [7,35]. Two major strategies have been described to improve body composition. The first is nutritional therapy, which includes preoperatively adding branched-chain amino acids, leucine, lipids, dextrose and L-carnitine to the patient's diet. Fan et al. divided their patients undergoing hepatectomy for HCC into two groups: one who received nutritional support and one control group. They showed that the worsening of liver function, sepsis-related complications and overall postoperative morbidity were lower in the nutrition compared to the control group (34% vs. 55%) [53]. The second is physical activity, which could inhibit the progress of sarcopenia by recruiting more myofibers, although reversing it remains unclear. Another promising method to reverse sarcopenia is the use of selective androgen receptor modulators (SARMs). Due to their anabolic effects, SARMs increase bone and muscle mass and inhibit protein degradation, decreasing sarcopenia's progression rate [54]. To conclude, multidisciplinary support should be considered in select cases of sarcopenic patients who undergo surgical and systematic therapy in order to improve or even reverse sarcopenia and optimize the outcomes.

One limitation of our systematic review is that the studies included were retrospective cohort studies, thereby prone to recall or selection bias. Another limitation is that there are no standard SMI cut-offs for diagnosing sarcopenia. Even when the same statistical method was applied to determine the cut-offs, different thresholds occurred in different populations. Furthermore, patients did not undergo the same type of hepatectomy, which may have affected survival, as larger operations tend to have more complications. Of note, operations were performed in different institutes by different teams with variable experience. In our study, we included patients with both primary and metastatic liver disease. A more advanced disease is by nature a poor prognostic factor, and patients with metastatic disease usually present with worse performance status, which in turn may affect the postoperative outcomes independently. Of note, none of the studies reported the administration of preoperative nutritional support. Finally, some patients received neoadjuvant chemotherapy, but the timing from last therapy to surgery was not available. Also, the follow-up varied greatly among the studies and was unavailable in many of them. In future, studies should focus on standardizing sarcopenia assessment and determining universal cut-off values based on data from large populations, as well as on incorporating methods for improvement of preoperative patient status in order to optimize patient care.

5. Conclusions

In conclusion, sarcopenia could lead to poor OS and high complication rates in patients undergoing hepatectomy for HCC or CRLM. We showed that sarcopenic patients had a significantly decreased OS and significantly more postoperative complications compared to non-sarcopenic patients. However, by integrating perioperative nutritional support and physical activity, the effects of sarcopenia could be reversed, with potentially improved postoperative outcomes. Future research should focus on conducting large prospective studies in high-volume centers with standardized protocols in an attempt to achieve optimal results for select patients with liver malignancy undergoing curative intent surgery.

Author Contributions: A.G. and M.P. contributed equally to the final manuscript. Conceptualization, A.G. and M.P.; methodology, A.G.; validation, P.B., P.D.L. and E.L.; data extraction, A.G. and M.P.; data curation, P.C. and A.D.G.; writing—original draft preparation, A.G and M.P.; writing—Results section, P.C.; writing—Discussion section, A.D.G.; writing—review and editing, A.M., I.M. and D.A.; project administration, D.G.; supervision, V.N.P. All authors have read and agreed to the published version of the manuscript.

Funding: This research received no external funding.

Institutional Review Board Statement: Not applicable.

Informed Consent Statement: Not applicable.

Data Availability Statement: Not applicable.

Conflicts of Interest: The authors declare no conflicts of interest.

References

1. Hamaguchi, Y.; Kaido, T.; Okumura, S.; Ito, T.; Fujimoto, Y.; Ogawa, K.; Mori, A.; Hammad, A.; Hatano, E.; Uemoto, S. Preoperative intramuscular adipose tissue content is a novel prognostic predictor after hepatectomy for hepatocellular carcinoma. *J. Hepato-Biliary-Pancreat Sci.* **2015**, *22*, 475–485. [CrossRef] [PubMed]
2. Harimoto, N.; Shirabe, K.; Yamashita, Y.-I.; Ikegami, T.; Yoshizumi, T.; Soejima, Y.; Ikeda, T.; Maehara, Y.; Nishie, A.; Yamanaka, T. Sarcopenia as a predictor of prognosis in patients following hepatectomy for hepatocellular carcinoma. *Br. J. Surg.* **2013**, *100*, 1523–1530. [CrossRef]
3. Hayashi, H.; Shimizu, A.; Kubota, K.; Notake, T.; Masuo, H.; Yoshizawa, T.; Hosoda, K.; Sakai, H.; Yasukawa, K.; Soejima, Y. Combination of sarcopenia and prognostic nutritional index to predict long-term outcomes in patients undergoing initial hepatectomy for hepatocellular carcinoma. *Asian J. Surg.* **2023**, *46*, 816–823. [CrossRef]
4. Kobayashi, A.; Kaido, T.; Hamaguchi, Y.; Okumura, S.; Shirai, H.; Kamo, N.; Yagi, S.; Taura, K.; Okajima, H.; Uemoto, S. Impact of Visceral Adiposity as Well as Sarcopenic Factors on Outcomes in Patients Undergoing Liver Resection for Colorectal Liver Metastases. *World J. Surg.* **2018**, *42*, 1180–1191. [CrossRef] [PubMed]
5. Liu, Y.-W.; Lu, C.-C.; Chang, C.-D.; Lee, K.-C.; Chen, H.H.; Yeh, W.S.; Hu, W.-H.; Tsai, K.-L.; Yeh, C.-H.; Wee, S.-Y.; et al. Prognostic value of sarcopenia in patients with colorectal liver metastases undergoing hepatic resection. *Sci. Rep.* **2020**, *10*, 6459. [CrossRef] [PubMed]
6. Hamaguchi, Y.; Kaido, T.; Okumura, S.; Kobayashi, A.; Fujimoto, Y.; Ogawa, K.; Mori, A.; Hammad, A.; Hatano, E.; Uemoto, S. Muscle Steatosis is an Independent Predictor of Postoperative Complications in Patients with Hepatocellular Carcinoma. *World J. Surg.* **2016**, *40*, 1959–1968. [CrossRef] [PubMed]
7. Berardi, G.; Antonelli, G.; Colasanti, M.; Meniconi, R.; Guglielmo, N.; Laurenzi, A.; Ferretti, S.; Sandri, G.B.L.; Spagnoli, A.; Moschetta, G.; et al. Association of Sarcopenia and Body Composition with Short-term Outcomes After Liver Resection for Malignant Tumors. *JAMA Surg.* **2020**, *155*, e203336. [CrossRef] [PubMed]
8. Furukawa, K.; Haruki, K.; Taniai, T.; Hamura, R.; Shirai, Y.; Yasuda, J.; Shiozaki, H.; Onda, S.; Gocho, T.; Ikegami, T. Osteosarcopenia is a potential predictor for the prognosis of patients who underwent hepatic resection for colorectal liver metastases. *Ann. Gastroenterol. Surg.* **2021**, *5*, 390–398. [CrossRef] [PubMed]
9. Runkel, M.; Diallo, T.D.; Lang, S.A.; Bamberg, F.; Benndorf, M.; Fichtner-Feigl, S. The Role of Visceral Obesity, Sarcopenia and Sarcopenic Obesity on Surgical Outcomes After Liver Resections for Colorectal Metastases. *World J. Surg.* **2021**, *45*, 2218–2226. [CrossRef]

10. Marasco, G.; Serenari, M.; Renzulli, M.; Alemanni, L.V.; Rossini, B.; Pettinari, I.; Dajti, E.; Ravaioli, F.; Golfieri, R.; Cescon, M.; et al. Clinical impact of sarcopenia assessment in patients with hepatocellular carcinoma undergoing treatments. *J. Gastroenterol.* **2020**, *55*, 927–943. [CrossRef]
11. Harimoto, N.; Hoshino, H.; Muranushi, R.; Hagiwara, K.; Yamanaka, T.; Ishii, N.; Tsukagoshi, M.; Igarashi, T.; Watanabe, A.; Kubo, N.; et al. Skeletal Muscle Volume and Intramuscular Adipose Tissue Are Prognostic Predictors of Postoperative Complications After Hepatic Resection. *Anticancer Res.* **2018**, *38*, 4933–4939. [CrossRef] [PubMed]
12. Yasuta, S.; Sugimoto, M.; Kudo, M.; Kobayashi, S.; Takahashi, S.; Konishi, M.; Gotohda, N. Early postoperative decrease of skeletal muscle mass predicts recurrence and poor survival after surgical resection for perihilar cholangiocarcinoma. *BMC Cancer* **2022**, *22*, 1358. [CrossRef] [PubMed]
13. Jung, H.E.; Han, D.H.; Koo, B.N.; Kim, J. Effect of sarcopenia on postoperative ICU admission and length of stay after hepatic resection for Klatskin tumor. *Front. Oncol.* **2023**, *13*, 1136376. [CrossRef]
14. Yang, J.; Chen, K.; Zheng, C.; Chen, K.; Lin, J.; Meng, Q.; Chen, Z.; Deng, L.; Yu, H.; Deng, T.; et al. Impact of sarcopenia on outcomes of patients undergoing liver resection for hepatocellular carcinoma. *J. Cachexia Sarcopenia Muscle* **2022**, *13*, 2383–2392. [CrossRef]
15. Yoon, S.B.; Choi, M.H.; Song, M.; Lee, J.H.; Lee, I.S.; Lee, M.A.; Hong, T.H.; Jung, E.S.; Choi, M.G. Impact of preoperative body compositions on survival following resection of biliary tract cancer. *J. Cachexia Sarcopenia Muscle* **2019**, *10*, 794–802. [CrossRef] [PubMed]
16. Hu, J.; Yang, J.; Yu, H.; Bo, Z.; Chen, K.; Wang, D.; Xie, Y.; Wang, Y.; Chen, G. Effect of Sarcopenia on Survival and Health-Related Quality of Life in Patients with Hepatocellular Carcinoma after Hepatectomy. *Cancers* **2022**, *14*, 6144. [CrossRef]
17. Eriksson, S.; Nilsson, J.H.; Strandberg Holka, P.; Eberhard, J.; Keussen, I.; Sturesson, C. The impact of neoadjuvant chemotherapy on skeletal muscle depletion and preoperative sarcopenia in patients with resectable colorectal liver metastases. *HPB* **2017**, *19*, 331–337. [CrossRef]
18. Bernardi, L.; Roesel, R.; Vagelli, F.; Majno-Hurst, P.; Cristaudi, A. Imaging based body composition profiling and outcomes after oncologic liver surgery. *Front. Oncol.* **2022**, *12*, 1007771. [CrossRef]
19. Page, M.J.; McKenzie, J.E.; Bossuyt, P.M.; Boutron, I.; Hoffmann, T.C.; Mulrow, C.D.; Shamseer, L.; Tetzlaff, J.M.; Akl, E.A.; Brennan, S.E.; et al. The PRISMA 2020 statement: An updated guideline for reporting systematic reviews. *BMJ* **2021**, *372*, n71. [CrossRef]
20. Fielding, R.A.; Vellas, B.; Evans, W.J.; Bhasin, S.; Morley, J.E.; Newman, A.B.; van Kan, G.A.; Andrieu, S.; Bauer, J.; Breuille, D.; et al. Sarcopenia: An Undiagnosed Condition in Older Adults. Current Consensus Definition: Prevalence, Etiology, and Consequences. International Working Group on Sarcopenia. *J. Am. Med. Dir. Assoc.* **2011**, *12*, 249–256. [CrossRef]
21. Cruz-Jentoft, A.J.; Baeyens, J.P.; Bauer, J.M.; Boirie, Y.; Cederholm, T.; Landi, F.; Martin, F.C.; Michel, J.-P.; Rolland, Y.; Schneider, S.M.; et al. Sarcopenia: European consensus on definition and diagnosis. *Age Ageing* **2010**, *39*, 412–423. [CrossRef] [PubMed]
22. Muscaritoli, M.; Anker, S.D.; Argiles, J.; Aversa, Z.; Bauer, J.M.; Biolo, G.; Boirie, Y.; Bosaeus, I.; Cederholm, T.; Costelli, P.; et al. Consensus definition of sarcopenia, cachexia and pre-cachexia: Joint document elaborated by Special Interest Groups (SIG) "cachexia-anorexia in chronic wasting diseases" and "nutrition in geriatrics". *Clin. Nutr.* **2010**, *29*, 154–159. [CrossRef] [PubMed]
23. Wells, G.A.; Shea, B.; O'Connell, D.; Pereson, J.; Welch, V.; Losos, M.; Tugwell, P. The Newcastle-Ottawa Scale (NOS) for Assessing the Quality of Nonrandomised Studies in Meta-Analyses. Published Online 2000. Available online: https://www.ohri.ca/programs/clinical_epidemiology/oxford.asp (accessed on 12 March 2024).
24. Bajrić, T.; Kornprat, P.; Faschinger, F.; Werkgartner, G.; Mischinger, H.J.; Wagner, D. Sarcopenia and primary tumor location influence patients outcome after liver resection for colorectal liver metastases. *Eur. J. Surg. Oncol.* **2022**, *48*, 615–620. [CrossRef] [PubMed]
25. Kroh, A.; Uschner, D.; Lodewick, T.; Eickhoff, R.M.; Schöning, W.; Ulmer, F.T.; Neumann, U.P.; Binnebösel, M. Impact of body composition on survival and morbidity after liver resection in hepatocellular carcinoma patients. *Hepatobil. Pancreat Dis. Int.* **2019**, *18*, 28–37. [CrossRef] [PubMed]
26. Lodewick, T.M.; van Nijnatten, T.J.; van Dam, R.M.; van Mierlo, K.; Dello, S.A.W.G.; Neumann, U.P.; Damink, S.W.M.O.; Dejong, C.H.C. Are sarcopenia, obesity and sarcopenic obesity predictive of outcome in patients with colorectal liver metastases? *HPB* **2015**, *17*, 438–446. [CrossRef] [PubMed]
27. Peng, P.D.; van Vledder, M.G.; Tsai, S.; de Jong, M.C.; Makary, M.; Ng, J.; Edil, B.H.; Wolfgang, C.L.; Schulick, R.D.; Choti, M.A.; et al. Sarcopenia negatively impacts short-term outcomes in patients undergoing hepatic resection for colorectal liver metastasis. *HPB* **2011**, *13*, 439–446. [CrossRef] [PubMed]
28. Van Vledder, M.G.; Levolger, S.; Ayez, N.; Verhoef, C.; Tran, T.C.K.; IJzermans, J.N.M. Body composition and outcome in patients undergoing resection of colorectal liver metastases19. *Br. J. Surg.* **2012**, *99*, 550–557. [CrossRef] [PubMed]
29. Wu, D.-H.; Liao, C.-Y.; Wang, D.-F.; Huang, L.; Li, G.; Chen, J.-Z.; Wang, L.; Lin, T.-S.; Lai, J.-L.; Zhou, S.-Q.; et al. Textbook outcomes of hepatocellular carcinoma patients with sarcopenia: A multicenter analysis. *Eur. J. Surg. Oncol.* **2023**, *49*, 802–810. [CrossRef]
30. Yabusaki, N.; Fujii, T.; Yamada, S.; Suzuki, K.; Sugimoto, H.; Kanda, M.; Nakayama, G.; Koike, M.; Fujiwara, M.; Kodera, Y. Adverse impact of low skeletal muscle index on the prognosis of hepatocellular carcinoma after hepatic resection. *Int. J. Surg.* **2016**, *30*, 136–142. [CrossRef]

31. Yang, J.; Wang, D.; Ma, L.; An, X.; Hu, Z.; Zhu, H.; Zhang, W.; Chen, K.; Ma, J.; Yang, Y.; et al. Sarcopenia negatively affects postoperative short-term outcomes of patients with non-cirrhosis liver cancer. *BMC Cancer* **2023**, *23*, 212. [CrossRef]
32. Kim, H.; Choi, H.Z.; Choi, J.M.; Kang, B.M.; Lee, J.W.; Hwang, J.W. Sarcopenia with systemic inflammation can predict survival in patients with hepatocellular carcinoma undergoing curative resection. *J. Gastrointest. Oncol.* **2022**, *13*, 744–753. [CrossRef] [PubMed]
33. Hou, G.; Jiang, C.; Du, J.; Yuan, K. Sarcopenia predicts an adverse prognosis in patients with combined hepatocellular carcinoma and cholangiocarcinoma after surgery. *Cancer Med.* **2022**, *11*, 317–331. [CrossRef] [PubMed]
34. Zhou, G.; Bao, H.; Zeng, Q.; Hu, W.; Zhang, Q. Sarcopenia as a prognostic factor in hepatolithiasis-associated intrahepatic cholangiocarcinoma patients following hepatectomy: A retrospective study. *Int. J. Clin. Exp. Med.* **2015**, *8*, 18245–18254. [PubMed]
35. Van Wijk, L.; Van Duinhoven, S.; Liem, M.S.L.; Bouman, D.E.; Viddeleer, A.R.; Klaase, J.M. Risk factors for surgery-related muscle quantity and muscle quality loss and their impact on outcome. *Eur. J. Med. Res.* **2021**, *26*, 36. [CrossRef] [PubMed]
36. Xiong, J.; Wu, Y.; Hu, H.; Kang, W.; Li, Y.; Jin, P.; Shao, X.; Li, W.; Tian, Y. Prognostic Significance of Preoperative Sarcopenia in Patients with Gastric Cancer Liver Metastases Receiving Hepatectomy. *Front. Nutr.* **2022**, *9*, 878791. [CrossRef] [PubMed]
37. Pessia, B.; Romano, L.; Carlei, F.; Lazzari, S.; Vicentini, V.; Giuliani, A.; Schietroma, M. Preoperative sarcopenia predicts survival after hepatectomy for colorectal metastases: A prospective observational study. *Eur. Rev. Med. Pharmacol. Sci.* **2021**, *25*, 5619–5624. [CrossRef] [PubMed]
38. Xu, L.; Jing, Y.; Zhao, C.; Zhang, Q.; Zhao, X.; Yang, J.; Wu, L.; Yang, Y. Preoperative computed tomography-assessed skeletal muscle index is a novel prognostic factor in patients with hepatocellular carcinoma following hepatectomy: A meta-analysis. *J. Gastrointest. Oncol.* **2020**, *11*, 1040–1053. [CrossRef] [PubMed]
39. O'Connell, R.M.; O'Neill, M.; Ó Ríordáin, M.G.; Ó Súilleabháin, C.B.; O'Sullivan, A.W. Sarcopaenia, obesity, sarcopaenic obesity and outcomes following hepatic resection for colorectal liver metastases: A systematic review and meta-analysis. *HPB* **2022**, *24*, 1844–1853. [CrossRef] [PubMed]
40. Kong, Q.; Gao, Q.; Li, W.; Chen, Z. The Impact of Imaging-Diagnosed Sarcopenia on Long-term Prognosis After Curative Resection for Hepatocellular Carcinoma: A Systematic Review and Meta-analysis. *Acad. Radiol.* **2024**, *31*, 1272–1283. [CrossRef]
41. Thormann, M.; Omari, J.; Pech, M.; Damm, R.; Croner, R.; Perrakis, A.; Strobel, A.; Wienke, A.; Surov, A. Low skeletal muscle mass and post-operative complications after surgery for liver malignancies: A meta-analysis. *Langenbecks Arch. Surg.* **2022**, *407*, 1369–1379. [CrossRef]
42. Martin, D.; Maeder, Y.; Kobayashi, K.; Schneider, M.; Koerfer, J.; Melloul, E.; Halkic, N.; Hübner, M.; Demartines, N.; Becce, F.; et al. Association between CT-Based Preoperative Sarcopenia and Outcomes in Patients That Underwent Liver Resections. *Cancers* **2022**, *14*, 261. [CrossRef] [PubMed]
43. Kamarajah, S.K.; Bundred, J.; Tan, B.H.L. Body composition assessment and sarcopenia in patients with gastric cancer: A systematic review and meta-analysis. *Gastric Cancer* **2019**, *22*, 10–22. [CrossRef] [PubMed]
44. Deng, H.Y.; Hou, L.; Zha, P.; Huang, K.L.; Peng, L. Sarcopenia is an independent unfavorable prognostic factor of non-small cell lung cancer after surgical resection: A comprehensive systematic review and meta-analysis. *Eur. J. Surg. Oncol.* **2019**, *45*, 728–735. [CrossRef]
45. Levolger, S.; Van Vugt, J.L.A.; De Bruin, R.W.F.; IJzermans, J.N.M. Systematic review of sarcopenia in patients operated on for gastrointestinal and hepatopancreatobiliary malignancies. *Br. J. Surg.* **2015**, *102*, 1448–1458. [CrossRef]
46. Trejo-Avila, M.; Bozada-Gutiérrez, K.; Valenzuela-Salazar, C.; Herrera-Esquivel, J.; Moreno-Portillo, M. Sarcopenia predicts worse postoperative outcomes and decreased survival rates in patients with colorectal cancer: A systematic review and meta-analysis. *Int. J. Colorectal Dis.* **2021**, *36*, 1077–1096. [CrossRef] [PubMed]
47. Simonsen, C.; de Heer, P.; Bjerre, E.D.; Suetta, C.; Hojman, P.; Pedersen, B.K.; Svendsen, L.B.; Christensen, J.F. Sarcopenia and Postoperative Complication Risk in Gastrointestinal Surgical Oncology: A Meta-analysis. *Ann. Surg.* **2018**, *268*, 58–69. [CrossRef] [PubMed]
48. Hamaguchi, Y.; Kaido, T.; Okumura, S.; Kobayashi, A.; Shirai, H.; Yagi, S.; Kamo, N.; Okajima, H.; Uemoto, S. Impact of Skeletal Muscle Mass Index, Intramuscular Adipose Tissue Content, and Visceral to Subcutaneous Adipose Tissue Area Ratio on Early Mortality of Living Donor Liver Transplantation. *Transplantation* **2017**, *101*, 565–574. [CrossRef] [PubMed]
49. Martin, L.; Birdsell, L.; MacDonald, N.; Reiman, T.; Clandinin, M.T.; McCargar, L.J.; Murphy, R.; Ghosh, S.; Sawyer, M.B.; Baracos, V.E. Cancer Cachexia in the Age of Obesity: Skeletal Muscle Depletion Is a Powerful Prognostic Factor, Independent of Body Mass Index. *J. Clin. Oncol.* **2013**, *31*, 1539–1547. [CrossRef]
50. Prado, C.M.; Lieffers, J.R.; McCargar, L.J.; Reiman, T.; Sawyer, M.B.; Martin, L.; Baracos, V.E. Prevalence and clinical implications of sarcopenic obesity in patients with solid tumours of the respiratory and gastrointestinal tracts: A population-based study. *Lancet Oncol.* **2008**, *9*, 629–635. [CrossRef]
51. Miyamoto, Y.; Baba, Y.; Sakamoto, Y.; Ohuchi, M.; Tokunaga, R.; Kurashige, J.; Hiyoshi, Y.; Iwagami, S.; Yoshida, N.; Watanabe, M.; et al. Negative Impact of Skeletal Muscle Loss after Systemic Chemotherapy in Patients with Unresectable Colorectal Cancer. *PLoS ONE* **2015**, *10*, e0129742. [CrossRef]
52. March, C.; Omari, J.; Thormann, M.; Pech, M.; Wienke, A.; Surov, A. Prevalence and role of low skeletal muscle mass (LSMM) in hepatocellular carcinoma. A systematic review and meta-analysis. *Clin. Nutr. ESPEN* **2022**, *49*, 103–113. [CrossRef] [PubMed]

53. Fan, S.T.; Lo, C.M.; Lai, E.; Chu, K.M.; Liu, C.L.; Wong, J. Perioperative Nutritional Support in Patients Undergoing Hepatectomy for Hepatocellular Carcinoma. *N. Engl. J. Med.* **1994**, *331*, 1547–1552. [CrossRef] [PubMed]
54. Perisetti, A.; Goyal, H.; Yendala, R.; Chandan, S.; Tharian, B.; Thandassery, R.B. Sarcopenia in hepatocellular carcinoma: Current knowledge and future directions. *World J. Gastroenterol.* **2022**, *28*, 432–448. [CrossRef] [PubMed]

Disclaimer/Publisher's Note: The statements, opinions and data contained in all publications are solely those of the individual author(s) and contributor(s) and not of MDPI and/or the editor(s). MDPI and/or the editor(s) disclaim responsibility for any injury to people or property resulting from any ideas, methods, instructions or products referred to in the content.

MDPI AG
Grosspeteranlage 5
4052 Basel
Switzerland
Tel.: +41 61 683 77 34

Journal of Clinical Medicine Editorial Office
E-mail: jcm@mdpi.com
www.mdpi.com/journal/jcm

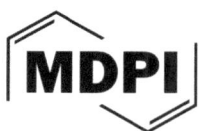

Disclaimer/Publisher's Note: The statements, opinions and data contained in all publications are solely those of the individual author(s) and contributor(s) and not of MDPI and/or the editor(s). MDPI and/or the editor(s) disclaim responsibility for any injury to people or property resulting from any ideas, methods, instructions or products referred to in the content.

www.ingramcontent.com/pod-product-compliance
Lightning Source LLC
LaVergne TN
LVHW072342090526
838202LV00019B/2461